Fundamental Anatomy

Walter C. Hartwig, Ph.D.
Touro University College of Osteopathic Medicine

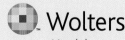 Wolters Kluwer | Lippincott Williams & Wilkins
Health

Philadelphia · Baltimore · New York · London
Buenos Aires · Hong Kong · Sydney · Tokyo

Acquisitions Editor: Crystal Taylor
Managing Editor: Kelly Horvath
Marketing Manager: Valerie Sanders
Production Editor: Paula C. Williams
Designer: Risa M. Clow
Compositor: Nesbitt Graphics, Inc.
Printer: R.R. Donnelley (Asia) Trading Limited

351 West Camden Street
Baltimore, MD 21201

530 Walnut Street
Philadelphia, PA 19106

The publisher is not responsible (as a matter of product liability, negligence, or otherwise) for any injury resulting from any material contained herein. This publication contains information relating to general principles of medical care that should not be construed as specific instructions for individual patients. Manufacturers' product information and package inserts should be reviewed for current information, including contraindications, dosages, and precautions.

Printed in China

Library of Congress Cataloging-in-Publication Data

Hartwig, Walter Carl, 1964-
  Fundamental anatomy / Walter C. Hartwig.
      p. ; cm.
  Includes index.
  ISBN-13: 978-0-7817-6888-7 (alk. paper)
  ISBN-10: 0-7817-6888-8 (alk. paper)
  1. Human anatomy. 2. Embryology, Human. I. Title.
  [DNLM: 1. Anatomy. QS 4 H337f 2008]
  QM23.2.H372 2008
  611—dc22
                              2006100519

The publishers have made every effort to trace the copyright holders for borrowed material. If they have inadvertently overlooked any, they will be pleased to make the necessary arrangements at the first opportunity.

To purchase additional copies of this book, call our customer service department at **(800) 638-3030** or fax orders to **(301) 223-2320**. International customers should call **(301) 223-2300**.

Visit Lippincott Williams & Wilkins on the Internet: *http://www.LWW.com.* Lippincott Williams & Wilkins customer service representatives are available from 8:30 am to 6:00 pm, EST.

07 08 09 10
1 2 3 4 5 6 7 8 9 10

*To Mitchell B. Day, with gratitude,
for setting the example*

Preface

The anatomy of the human body has been well-documented and thoroughly explicated in print for at least 100 years. Education pioneers, such as J.C.B. Grant, W.H. Hollinshead, and D.J. Cunningham (to name just a few), inspired the teaching of gross anatomy with enlightening but very different emphases and perspectives. The material results were profound, multiedition texts with successive titles like *Grant's Method of Anatomy*, *Hollinshead's Textbook of Anatomy*, and *Cunningham's Textbook of Anatomy*. These books expressed the personal cognitive framework of their creators for understanding how the body is constructed. Grant's approach was strikingly visual and emphasized a region-by-region study of the body. Hollinshead wrote brilliantly of function and reviewed anatomy in a combined systemic and regional approach. Cunningham's text, along with the more familiar *Gray's Anatomy*, is one of the few purely systemic approaches to the subject.

The era of extensive anatomy courses is over, however, largely because the curricular demands of medical school limit the time that can be devoted to anatomy and compel students to think about clinical applications of structure from the beginning of their training. As a result, the dominant texts of today tend to emphasize the regional approach of Grant, supplemented with clinical correlations and case studies. The days of eponymous book titles are now historical, with such titles being replaced by *Clinically Oriented Anatomy* or *Clinical Anatomy*, which also have matured through numerous revisions to become comprehensive references of gross anatomy.

I believe that students need "perspective" books in addition to comprehensive reference books. People acquire subject knowledge through two basic pathways, which sometimes are described as "bottom-up" and "top-down." The bottom-up pathway is the method of assembling facts and mastering their relationships to arrive at some understanding of the subject in general. The top-down pathway, naturally, is the reverse—a method of learning the organization of a subject before exercising its factual basis. In theory, these pathways enable the student to both understand and command a subject. I believe that a concise dose of the top-down approach can greatly improve the effectiveness of the bottom-up approach. That is the essential purpose of this book.

The present text expands two aspects of anatomic education that blend well together: **embryology,** and **systemic anatomy**. In many medical schools, embryology is taught either as a low-unit course to supplement anatomy or as a few lectures within the anatomy course. In this book, I attempt to explain the development of the body in a style that makes it clinically relevant. I also attempt this because I believe that a sense of embryology resolves a vast amount of anatomic detail into a manageable whole, as expressed by Rosse, C. & Gaddum-Rosse, P. Hollinshead's Textbook of Anatomy, 5th Edition. Baltimore: Lippincott-Raven, 1997:6:

> [T]he study of anatomy need not consist of the memorization of long lists of names; rather, it should rely on the visualization of parts and regions of the body in three dimensions based on an understanding of how these relationships have come about and why they exist. Such an understanding may be gained through the study of embryology.

The other design emphasis of this book is an expansion of systemic information. Many degree programs in the health professions now teach the body "system-by-system," which is an effective way of integrating the normal structure and function of a tissue complex with disease processes and medical management. Body systems are unified by function. The sequence of systems as presented in this book tries to balance the logic of body design with a minimum redundancy of coverage. A body-wide system, circulation, leads off as a guide to all body regions. The other organ systems follow, given their tightly related embryologies, functions, and relatively simple (anatomically, at least) innervation schemes. There is no separate chapter on the endocrine organs; rather, they are discussed in the appropriate embryologic passages. The peripheral nervous system and the musculoskeletal system are interrelated both spatially and functionally. Although the nature of how they function is similar from one region to the next, the number of named nerves, muscles, bones, and joints is quite large, so these chapters are relatively long. To maintain the pace of embryologic discourse, they are placed after the organ chapters.

Lastly, a brief chapter on skin and superficial fascia concludes the book. This is an awkward topic for a systemic book of gross anatomy, because a structure of great clinical relevance, the mammary gland, grows within a body-wide system of integument that otherwise is more microscopic (histologic) than macroscopic. The breast must be covered in an anatomy book, but as a modified sweat gland it is appropriately placed in a chapter, albeit confined, on the integument.

For students to begin to understand how anatomy relates to patient examination, diagnosis, and treatment, I have incorporated *Clinical Anatomy* boxes throughout the text. These are not meant to be comprehensive but, rather, to highlight conditions that are primarily developmental and anatomic.

Acknowledgments

I would not be an anatomy teacher today if not for the investment of the following people in my education. For prompting me to study anatomy 20 years ago, I thank Mitchell B. Day, Roderick V. Moore, F. Clark Howell, and Sylvia Hixson. I first learned anatomy in the laboratory from the late Dr. Herbert Srebnik, David Lewis, Professor Marian Diamond, and Joe Reyes at UC–Berkeley. Another graduate advisor of mine, Professor Tim White, has helped me through the years to realize how much anatomy I still do not know.

After UC–Berkeley, I went to Chicago, where Alfred L. Rosenberger, Larry Cochard, and Sandra Inouye fostered my respect for anatomy. A fortuitous postdoctoral opportunity took me to SUNY Stony Brook, where Jack T. Stern, William L. Jungers, Susan Larson, John Fleagle, Pierre Lemelin, Brian Richmond, and especially, David Eliot trained me and tolerated my weaknesses.

At Touro University College of Osteopathic Medicine, my sense of anatomy has deepened under the influence of Barbara M. Kriz and, especially, the phenomenal anatomy teacher Bruce Richardson. Other colleagues at the California College of Podiatric Medicine and at Touro University College of Osteopathic Medicine, namely Reed A. Rowan, David Eliot (again), Bruce Silverman, James Binkerd, Ghulam Noorani, Nripendra Dhillon, and Jeffrey Kwok, inspire me to keep working at the unusual craft of teaching and dissecting the human body.

At Lippincott Williams & Wilkins, I thank Betty Sun for first endorsing this project. Crystal Taylor, Kelly Horvath, and Jen Clements developed this project from beginning to end and spent countless hours attending to my inability to follow directions. Kelly Horvath in particular nurtured my concept into an actual book with patience and good humor. Janis Acampora produced the original artwork.

For more than a decade leading to this project, I have received unconditional support and encouragement from my wife, Yeun, and from the Lee and Hartwig families. Yeun's support is a vital part of this work without which I would never have envisioned nor finished it.

TABLE OF CONTENTS

Essentials of Early Development

INTRODUCTION

The narrow goal of this chapter is to understand how the three germ layers of ectoderm, mesoderm, and endoderm come to be and what becomes of them. The broader goal is to understand how the tissue and organ systems function in the body by incorporating the germ layers. To serve the narrow goal, you will learn the names of structures that exist only transiently (literally a matter of hours) in the body but are key to the successful transition of one cellular block into another, appropriate one. You will certainly be able to treat a patient in the future without having this information for immediate recall, but as a medical student you will struggle if you lack a developmental perspective of the body.

BASIC ANATOMIC TERMS AND ORIENTATION

Anatomy is a map of the body with a language and directions all its own. Some people orient by landmarks ("turn left at the gas station") and others by universal standards ("go 2.1 km, then turn north"). Health care professionals must learn the map of the body, and everyone treating the patient must speak the same language. For this reason, universal terms of location and movement apply to a standard orientation of the human body. Language is powerful, but it must be precise. This text introduces proper terminology within a relatively relaxed narrative to facilitate understanding. Once understood, the language of professional discourse should be proper and specific. (See Clinical Anatomy Box 1.1.)

THE SIMPLE FORM OF ANIMATE LIFE

This book depicts anatomy in terms of the basic needs of an animate life form. All animals have the same simple body plan—humans are modified only slightly. The simple plan is described here in a "top-down" approach to give students a basis for mastering the details.

The animate life form survives through three basic activities: sensing the outside world, absorbing energy from the outside world, and moving about in response to the demands of those same needs. In the history of life on earth, these imperatives manifest as tissue layers: an outer layer of detection and protection, an inner layer of absorption, and a middle layer of contractility between them (Fig. 1.1). These layers first develop as cell colonies that are capable of differentiating into special shapes and sizes, and these cell colonies, or **tissues**, have specific names: **ectoderm** for the outer layer, **endoderm** for the inner layer, and **mesoderm** for the layer in between. The diversity of animal life on earth is not the result of different kinds of tissue layers in different animals but, rather, of the degree to which these three basic layers develop.

Simple life forms in biology are hardly more than these three layers set out in a tube-like body shape (Fig. 1.2). The outer layer may have basic means of detecting the environment but no specialized senses, such as smell, vision, or hearing. The inner layer absorbs what it can from particulate matter that is either ingested or carried into the animal by water. What does not get absorbed simply passes out the other end of the tube, with no separation of liquid waste and solid waste. The layer derived from mesoderm may be nothing more than basic contractile cells that give the animal an ability to pulse its way through the environment.

Contrast this with a complex life form, such as a tiger (Fig. 1.3), which has elaborations at all three levels. The outer layer develops tactile hairs and whiskers and a nervous system that can detect changes in light waves, sound waves, and "smell" waves in the atmosphere. The inner layer expands into a big sac (the stomach) for digesting protein and then elongates to maximize energy absorption. Water is retrieved from the matter that is not digested, and the tube ends as a portal for solid waste only. Most complex is the middle layer, which includes four outgrowths called limbs, for powerful and precise, conscious movement. Most dramatic and recognizable is the elaborate head,

CLINICAL ANATOMY

Box 1.1

BASIC ANATOMIC TERMS AND ORIENTATION

Reference terms for standard anatomic position, orientation, and relative direction in the human body.

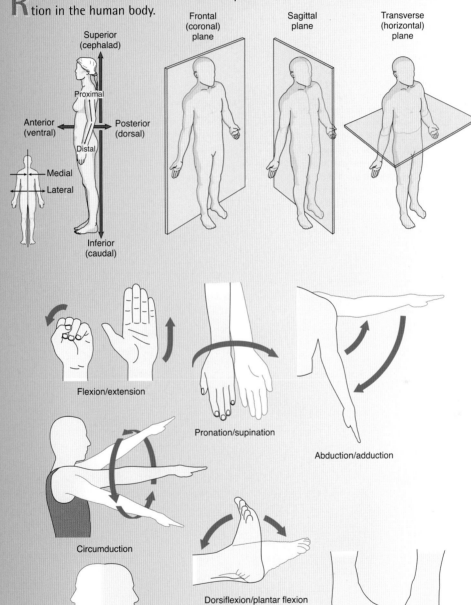

Basic anatomic terms and orientation. (From Cohen BJ, Taylor JJ. Memmler's The Human Body in Health and Disease, 10th Edition. Baltimore: Lippincott Williams & Wilkins, 2005.)

FIGURE 1.1   The basic tissue design of animate organisms.

One tissue (ectoderm) senses the outside world and protects the organism from it. Another tissue (endoderm) also is in contact with the outside world, but through a guarded entrance ("mouth") and a guarded exit ("anus"). This layer absorbs, with little power to resist, whatever contacts it. A third layer (mesoderm) fills the space between the inner and outer tissues. Mesoderm can develop into structures that are very loose (fat) or very rigid (bone). It can develop into structures that contract when stimulated (muscle), including both voluntary (skeletal muscle) and involuntary (smooth or cardiac muscle) contraction. It also can squeeze the endodermal tube (peristalsis) and move one bone against another (locomotion). Mesoderm is what makes the animate organism animated.

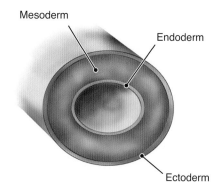

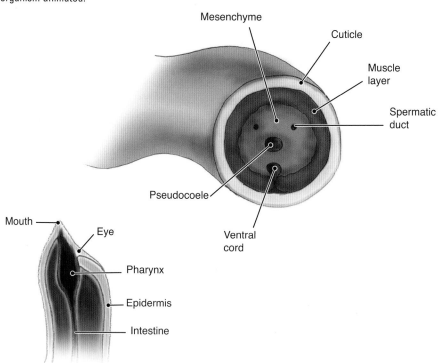

FIGURE 1.2   A simple animate life form, in this case a nematomorph worm.

The basic three tissue layers are barely changed in this adult state, which presents a protective but unspecialized outer layer, an absorbent but unmodified inner layer, and an intermediate lining of musculature with no limb buds. The "head" and "tail" ends are barely modified for "intake" and "outflow" of energy.

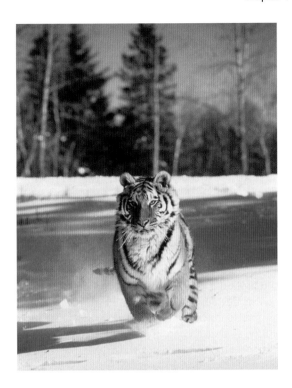

FIGURE 1.3   **An example of a complex life form, in which the three basic tissue layers have been modified greatly.**

Of the three layers, mesoderm is the most dynamic, which is why animate organisms display so many varieties of size, posture, and locomotion. (Reprinted with permission from Tom Brakefield/Photodisc Green/Getty Images.)

which houses the expanded and specialized "top" end of all three layers. Even with this complexity, however, the tiger is just a collection of ectoderm, endoderm, and mesoderm cell purposes.

Some of the most primitive forms of animate life are barely animate. Their simplistic body surfaces provide only binary signals of the world around them, and they have wide, open portals at the "front" and "back" end for the input and output, respectively, of particulate matter. They lack appendages, and they cannot control the effect of gravity on their position or movement. Humans are highly developed by comparison, but we are still just a highly developed set of neural tissues, digestive tissues, and support tissues. Much of what you have to remember in anatomy is how these connective tissues are governed by the nervous system and how they relate to one another. Deriving them from the simple **trilaminar** ("three-layered") **germ disc** of ectoderm, endoderm, and mesoderm is the best way to begin learning anatomy, and this is the subject of embryology.

Three Basic Tissue Families: Sensing, Moving, Absorbing

The **ectoderm** layer detects the environment. From the ectoderm, the skin and the entire nervous system, including the central nervous system (brain and spinal cord) and peripheral nervous system (the fibers that lead from the central system and make contact with the environment through endings near the skin), are derived. Even the "special" senses of smell, sight, hearing, and taste represent nothing more than neural (ectodermal) tissues that are directly exposed to specialized skin (e.g., the cornea or the tympanic membrane). Even pigment cells, which are directly altered by exposure to the environment, represent ectoderm that has migrated, like a special agent, from the centralized tube that becomes the thinking center.

Now consider the **endoderm**, which remains relatively unchanged during development and is represented in the adult body only by thin layers of cells that line most of the "wet" internal surfaces. In keeping with our animal design heritage, this endodermal tube remains open at the top end (the mouth) and at the bottom end (the anus). Between these two points, the entire tube of cells responsible for absorbing nutrient energy for the body remains exposed to the outside world. Thanks to the third (germ) layer, however, we can close ectoderm over these holes so that things do not just fly, drop, or blow in there.

Except for two places, the **mesoderm** layer occupies every available point between the ectodermal plate and the endodermal plate. One unoccupied point is at the cranial end of the embryo, and the other is at the caudal end. At these spots, the mesoderm cannot break the seal of ectoderm on endoderm; this is the case both during development and in the adult body. Think about where the dry skin bends inward and becomes wet and absorbent. These are the direct transitions from ectoderm to endoderm, end-to-end. Everywhere else, you have mesoderm under the skin.

Mesoderm develops into all the muscle and connective tissue (e.g., bone, ligament, tendon, and fascia) and into specialized tissues as well (e.g., blood vessels). Mesoderm enables you to maintain a certain position or to mobilize that position as conditions warrant. Mesoderm develops into some rigid connective tissue, such as bone, and some very compliant connective tissue, such as fascia. It remains closely affixed to the endodermal tube so that it can provide rhythmic contraction to the gut tube and move food particles in a process called **peristalsis**. Mesoderm is why you have posture and the ability to change it.

Some forms of animate life, including most vertebrates, have developed complex mesodermal buds on their bodies—the limbs— that enable them to move along or within their environments. The body's **axial skeleton** supports cavities (the trunk), and its **appendicular skeleton** enables coordinated movement. No endoderm is found in the limbs; their anatomy is a study in the potential of connective tissue.

As the text covers the systems of the body, we will return to the story of development. We must account for how the embryonic layers fold to become a trunk and how the endoderm manages to stay so thin but become so very, very long. We also must account for how the brain develops from the top end of the ectodermal tube and, in so doing, allude to why our faces are relatively flat and forward-looking compared to those of our mammalian cousins. The full stories of development are engaging, but most medical curricula do not allow another course of the same size as anatomy to be concerned solely with them.

Body Growth Through Cell Division: Differentiation Versus Proliferation

You are the result of what once was a single cell. Through cell division, a wide variety of very different types of cells are produced—a process known as **differentiation**. The capacity of some cells to divide into cells of other types is known as **pluripotency**. In the earliest stages of growth, the first few generations of cells are **totipotent**, because each of them has the capacity to produce all the various cell types in a living person. The qualities of totipotency and pluripotency, however, are transient—a condition at the heart of debates about stem cell research. At some point during embryonic growth, all the different types of cells have appeared, and from that point forward, growth is a matter of the **proliferation** of existing cell types.

The 9-month prenatal period begins as a few weeks of aggressive cellular differentiation, followed by an extended period (several months) of minor cellular differentiation and major multiplication, or proliferation. The severity of a "birth defect" (or, more appropriately, a **congenital anomaly**) is the result, in part, of the point during prenatal growth when the problem arose. An unbearable burden to the embryo at a time when its cells are still pluripotent will result in descendant cells of different types carrying the effects of the insult. Thus, problems that occur during these early stages of growth can be incompatible with life, and the embryo does not survive. By contrast, if the burden is introduced later, at a time when cells are no longer differentiating, the result tends to be less severe, because only a single type or line of cells is affected. Knowledge of embryologic anatomy will enable you to communicate to worried parents as a professional in terms that make them aware and assured, not uncertain and bewildered.

EARLY HUMAN DEVELOPMENT

Try to think of the human body in comparison to other animate life forms. These life forms must survive to reproduce, and they must reproduce to survive. Part of survival involves detecting what is around you (e.g., food or danger), and part of it involves getting energy from the environment. Part of it also involves moving from place to place to avoid danger and to encounter food. In a very real sense, humans are no more animate than worms. We develop from the same basic cell clusters: one for sensing the environment, one for processing the materials of the environment, and one for moving from place to place. The difference lies in the degree to which we develop. It is fair to say that all of anatomy is contained within the embryonic period of development.

The First 3 Weeks of Growth

The fertilized human egg, or zygote, must first protect itself, feed, and then grow. As the zygote gravitates to a receptive surface of the maternal uterus, the inexorable process of cell division transforms it from one cell to two, and each of those cells to two descendants, and so forth, until it becomes a critical mass of 16 cells (Fig. 1.4). This is called the **morula** stage, from the Latin word for mulberry, because in mammals, the cells adhere in the clustered or beaded form of a mulberry. The division to this point takes approximately 96 hours, or 4 days, after which the developing embryo tries to dig into the wall of the uterus (**implantation**) using cells that it produced but that remain outside of the embryo itself (or **extraembryonic**). Also at this time, cells inside the

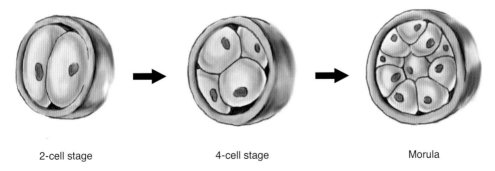

2-cell stage   4-cell stage   Morula

FIGURE 1.4   **Maturation of the zygote into a 16-cell morula.**

embryo yield their totipotency as they divide into descendants with a purposeful and asymmetric position. The simple plan is begun.

The morula cells cluster into two distinct layers, one inside of the other. The outside layer of cells is called, logically, the **outer cell mass**, and its purpose is to handle the extraembryonic goals of the embryo. The inside layer is called the **inner cell mass** (or **embryoblast**), and its purpose is to divide into every cell that becomes part of you. In concept, the genetic code is commissioning some of its cells to establish a perimeter, or a support structure, that is ultimately expendable. It commissions the rest of the cells to develop into actual body tissues within the relatively safe confines of the protective outer mass. The successor of the morula is called the **blastocyst**, which means, loosely, a cell-producing cavity (Fig. 1.5).

The story of implantation is not central to embryonic development, but it does illustrate a governing principle of how the embryo survives and flourishes. Think of the embryo as a parasite, an organism that draws its livelihood from the energy of a host. Human embryos must do this, because mammals give birth to live offspring instead of to a covered "egg." For animals that develop within a shelled egg, nutrition comes from the egg itself, and basically, the animal hatches after it has exhausted the food supply "donated" by its mother. Mammalian embryos, however, develop in connection with the mother, and this relationship involves some amount of siphoning resources from her.

The outer cell mass is the parasitic half of the organism. It forms a ring (**cytotrophoblast**) around the inner cell mass to protect it from the natural instinct of the host (the mother), which is to dissolve, reject, or expel it. Some of the cells of the cytotrophoblast divide into a productive colony of cells that infiltrate the uterine tissue and neutralize its antagonism. These cells are often found as conglomerations of nuclei without defined cell walls, a design called a **syncytiotrophoblast** (Fig. 1.6). This basic configuration expands significantly and, ultimately, will connect to blood islands of the uterus for diffusion of nutrients back to the embryo. The interfacing layers of the trophoblast are dynamic, but the basic original ring of cells around the embryo is not. The parasite must maintain a tough barrier against continued efforts by the host to cut it loose.

FIGURE 1.5   The morula becomes a blastocyst.

The morula differentiates into an outer layer of cells and an inner, two-layered sandwich. The outer layer will manage the relationship between the embryo and the mother. The inner layer is the strict ancestor of all the cells that become you.

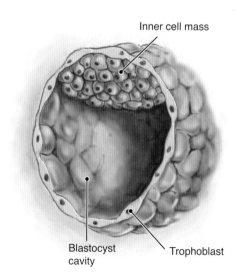

Inner cell mass

Blastocyst cavity

Trophoblast

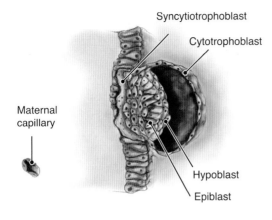

Syncytiotrophoblast

Cytotrophoblast

Maternal capillary

Hypoblast

Epiblast

FIGURE 1.6   Implantation begins.

The cytotrophoblast remains a barrier between the embryo proper (shown here as an epiblast layer and a hypoblast layer) and the uterus. As the cytotrophoblast invades the uterus, it produces a loose network of cells that lack rigid cell walls (syncytiotrophoblast). These cells incorporate further into the uterine wall and seek out blood pools to bring maternal nutrients into the embryo. In the meantime, the embryo is about to store its own yolk in the cavity between the hypoblast and the cytotrophoblast.

While implantation is completing on days 7, 8, and 9, the inner cell mass continues to grow. The layer of cells that faces the cavity formed by the outer cell mass produces a new layer of cells that coat it from side to side. This layer of new cells is called the **hypoblast,** because it is formed "underneath" the original inner cell mass cluster, which now is called the **epiblast**. Both of these cell layers will expand to form shells that line the inside of the cytotrophoblast ring as a means to isolate further the cells that will form the body (the "true" embryo). This process of cell proliferation is called the formation of the **bilaminar germ disc** (Fig. 1.7).

The bilaminar germ disc would like to be still more removed from the host mother, however, so it extrudes a new layer of buffer cells between it and its own protective cytotrophoblast. This layer of **extraembryonic mesoderm** will encircle the entire bilaminar germ disc (along with its amniotic and primary yolk sac membranes), then pinch against it in two important ways. One way is along the margin of the just-created **primary yolk sac,** where it pinches the primary sac into a smaller, **secondary yolk sac** (Fig. 1.8). Another way is along the boundary between the epiblast and hypoblast, where the extraembryonic mesoderm pries the germ disc away from the cytotrophoblast and suspends it by a **connecting stalk** (Fig. 1.9). The future umbilical cord derives, in part, from this connecting stalk. As the extraembryonic mesoderm is maturing, it self-cavitates so that the embryo is effectively dangling from a connecting stalk within its own cocoon-like sac in a fluid-filled **chorionic cavity** that is, itself, lined by a shell of extraembryonic mesoderm against the cytotrophoblast.

Gastrulation

The embryo has reached a point of balance in its efforts to draw nourishment from the mother, to be protected against cellular assault, and to harbor enough of its own food supply in the secondary yolk sac. Now is the time for the dynamic inner cell mass to differentiate into the three functional cell layers of animate life: a protective and sensitive outer layer, an energy-absorbing inner layer, and a connective layer between them that is capable of contractile movement. These three layers will be called the **ectoderm, endoderm,** and **mesoderm**, respectively, and how the basic **trilaminar**

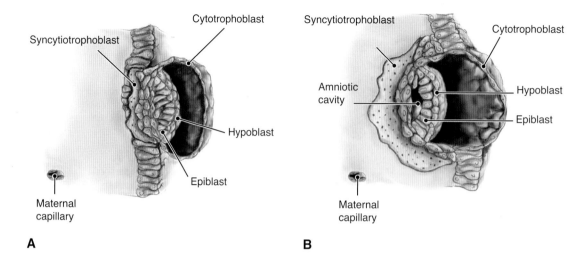

Cytotrophoblast

Syncytiotrophoblast

Hypoblast

Epiblast

Maternal
capillary

A

Syncytiotrophoblast

Cytotrophoblast

Amniotic
cavity

Hypoblast

Epiblast

Maternal
capillary

B

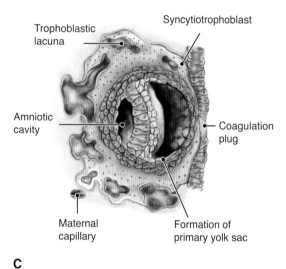

Trophoblastic
lacuna

Syncytiotrophoblast

Amniotic
cavity

Coagulation
plug

Maternal
capillary

Formation of
primary yolk sac

C

FIGURE 1.7   **The embryo forms two cavities within the protective shell of the cytotrophoblast.**

The epiblast forms an amniotic cavity above itself, and the hypoblast produces cells below itself in anticipation of storing food (**A–C**). The amniotic cavity eventually will envelop the embryo and fetus and provide it with a "homegrown" fluid environment.

germ disc is formed is called the process of **gastrulation**. From this point, the embryo's own food supply will dwindle, and its cell layers will morph into precursors of the three tissue layers.

One of the first indications that the embryo is differentiating is the appearance of an orientation, or an axis, that suggests two ends (a head end and a tail end, presumably) and a long side to the embryonic disc. A dimpling appears in the surface of the epiblast cells near one of the ends. Its position in the "midline" of the disk indicates an axial position that, eventually, will define the area of the vertebral column and the spinal cord. For the moment, however, it defines the place where cells produced by the epiblast will be funneled down to replace the hypoblast and create the definitive endoderm and mesoderm cells. It is the **primitive streak** (Fig. 1.10).

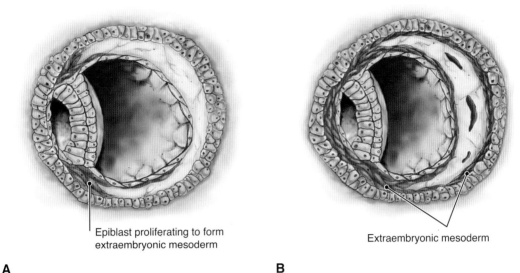

Epiblast proliferating to form
extraembryonic mesoderm

Extraembryonic mesoderm

A

B

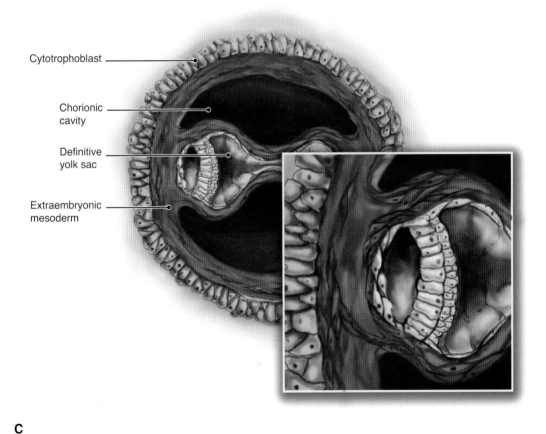

Cytotrophoblast

Chorionic
cavity

Definitive
yolk sac

Extraembryonic
mesoderm

C

FIGURE 1.8   **Note how a new layer of cells proliferates between the embryo and the cytotrophoblast.**

This aggressive cell layer insulates the embryo (**A, B**) and suspends it from the inner lining of the
cytotrophoblast. The embryo is now bobbing in the chorionic cavity (**C**). The connecting stalk that
links it to the cytotrophoblast is the future site of the umbilical cord. The extraembryonic mesoderm
develops to further buffer and isolate the embryo. Note how it pinches off some of the embryo's own
food supply by reducing the primary yolk sac to a smaller, secondary yolk sac.

FIGURE 1.9   **The embryo suspends in a chorionic cavity.**

This figure shows the basic configuration of the embryo in a longitudinal view, with the connecting stalk located almost at the "back end" of the embryo. Note how a little slip of the yolk sac got trapped in the connecting stalk. This blind pouch is called the allantois, which is Greek for "sausage-shaped."

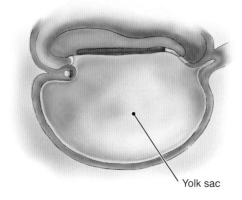

Yolk sac

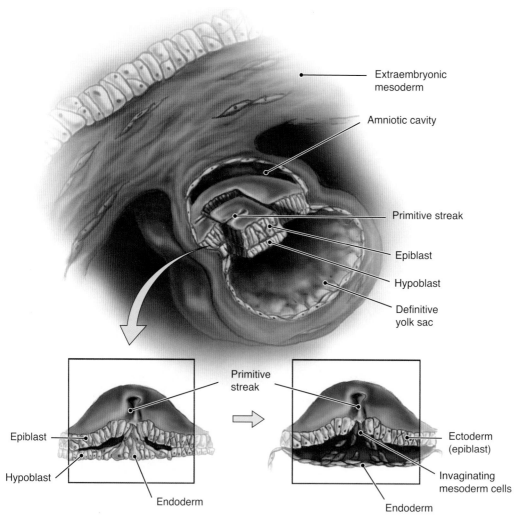

Extraembryonic mesoderm

Amniotic cavity

Primitive streak

Epiblast

Hypoblast

Definitive yolk sac

Primitive streak

Epiblast

Hypoblast

Endoderm

Ectoderm (epiblast)

Invaginating mesoderm cells

Endoderm

FIGURE 1.10   **A primitive streak dimples the epiblast and pours out endoderm cells that replace the original hypoblast cells.**

With endoderm in place, the primitive streak pours out mesoderm cells that migrate between ectoderm (blue) and endoderm (yellow) all throughout the embryonic disk. The primitive streak also produces cells that form a primitive axis to the body in the form of a notochord.

During this process, the cells that are becoming mesoderm are pouring into the space between the epiblast (now the ectoderm layer) and the endoderm (the space formerly occupied by hypoblast cells). If left unchecked, this deposit of mesoderm cells would completely separate the endoderm from ectoderm, like the inner layer of a sandwich separates the two slices of bread. Think, however, about the adult body. At the mouth end of the body, you have a transition from the protective outer layer of skin to the absorbing inner layer that is continuous with the esophagus. Likewise, the anal region presents the same transition of ectoderm to endoderm. Thus, there are two points in the developing embryo where mesoderm should not intervene between ectoderm and endoderm. In fact, along the axis defined by the primitive streak are two "plates" of fusion between ectoderm and endoderm. The one at the presumptive head end of the embryo is called the **oropharyngeal membrane,** and the one at the tail end is called the **cloacal membrane** (Fig. 1.11).

As the mesoderm pours into position, it forms three distinct clumps, or columns, of cells. These clumps are best appreciated in a cross-sectional diagram of the embryo. The innermost clump forms beside the central axis of the embryo and is called **paraxial mesoderm.** The next layer of cells toward the sides of the embryo is called **intermediate mesoderm,** and the outermost cell group is called **lateral plate mesoderm.** Eventually, the lateral plate mesoderm makes contact with the extraembryonic mesoderm when it reaches the margin of ectoderm and endoderm. This is an important interface, because it represents where intrinsic cells of the embryo contact extrinsic cells of its immediate environment (Fig. 1.12).

As the mesoderm is forming in every available space between the ectoderm and endoderm, the primitive streak busily extrudes a rod-like cell group from the node of cells at its tip. This cell group is called the **notochord,** and it assumes a midline position in the cranial half of the disc as the primitive streak regresses behind it (Fig. 1.13). As we will see, the notochord has the unique ability to compel the ectoderm above it to warp into a new shape. Before this happens, however, the primitive streak should fully regress. If the primitive streak does not fully resorb, the result is a **congenital anomaly** called **sacrococcygeal teratoma.** (See Clinical Anatomy Box 1.2.)

At this point, human development is believed to mimic that seen in birds, reptiles, and other mammals, in which the three definitive germ layers of the body appear first in a sandwich-like, pancake-layer pattern. This **trilaminar germ disc** is perched on the balloon-like, secondary yolk sac, but soon, the relative sizes of the two will reverse as the embryo grows and the yolk sac diminishes. The developing human now has the precursors to all necessary adult tissues, but these precursors do not conform in shape

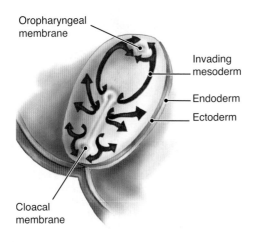

Oropharyngeal membrane

Invading mesoderm

Endoderm

Ectoderm

Cloacal membrane

FIGURE 1.11   Mesoderm cells migrate everywhere they can between the ectoderm and endoderm layers.

They cannot penetrate the adhesion at the head end of the embryo called the oropharyngeal membrane, and they cannot penetrate the adhesion at the tail end called the cloacal membrane. The mesoderm also cannot displace the notochord cells that have streamed out of the primitive streak and remained in the midline between the streak and the head end.

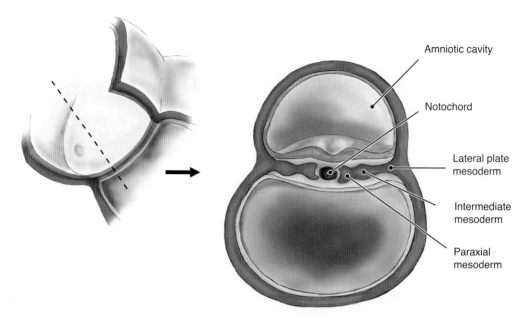

FIGURE 1.12   **Cross-sectional view of the embryo at the time of mesoderm migration.**

The mesoderm cells coalesce into three distinct clumps, or colonies. The paraxial mesoderm tracks the path of the notochord. The intermediate mesoderm hovers just beside it for a short stretch of the embryo's length. The lateral plate mesoderm fills the rest of the space and forms an important contact with the ectoderm above (dorsally), the endoderm below (ventrally), and the extraembryonic shell to the outside.

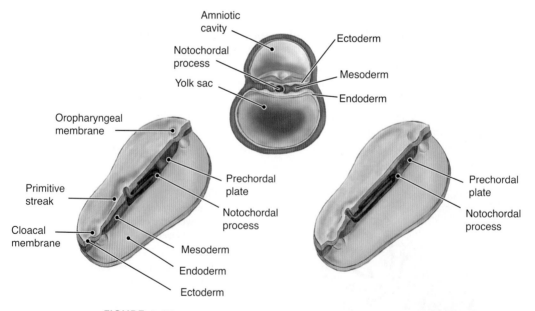

FIGURE 1.13   **The primitive streak produces a rod of cells in the midline of the embryonic disc.**

This is the notochord, and you can see from the cross-section that it forms a kind of axis for the embryo. As it gets bigger, the primitive streak itself regresses toward the tail end of the embryo. If it does not regress completely, the ectoderm over this part of the body will be abnormal. In the adult, this part of the body is the bottom of the spinal column, and the condition of a primitive streak that does not regress completely is called a sacrococcygeal teratoma.

CLINICAL ANATOMY

Box 1.2

SACROCOCCYGEAL TERATOMA

Remnants of the primitive streak may persist near the sacral end of the developing vertebral column. These remnants develop into a tumor mass called sacrococcygeal teratoma, which is the most common tumor in newborns. This tumor often arises from the tip of the coccyx. Because cells that emerge from the primitive streak can produce many different types of adult cells (a condition called pluripotency), the tumor may contain examples of those cells. For unknown reasons, approximately 75% of sacrococcygeal tumors occur in females. The prognosis is good if the tumor is excised shortly after birth; if the tumor is not diagnosed soon after birth, it can become malignant. This type of congenital anomaly may represent one of the few circumstances in which an error that occurs very early in development (day 21, approximately) is survivable.

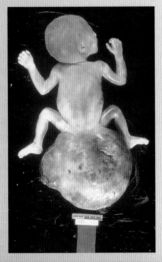
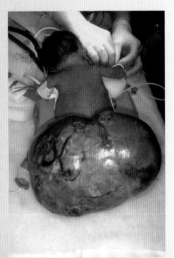
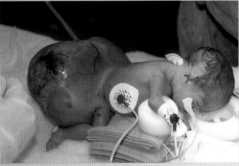
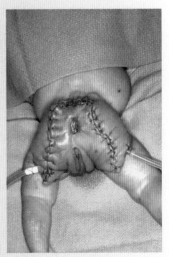

Sacrococcygeal teratoma. (Reprinted with permission from www.virtualpediatrichospital.org.)

to the animate condition. The ectoderm must envelop the organism to form a sensitive and protective surrounding. The endoderm must convert from a plate surface to a tube so that matter may enter the body at one end and exit the other, passing "through" the body as it is being absorbed. The mesoderm must differentiate into the three-dimensional support and contractile structures that give the organism independent movement. These complex conversions take place fairly rapidly, during the critical events of **neurulation** and **embryonic folding** in the third and fourth week after conception.

Neurulation

Neurulation forms nervous tissue from the layer of ectoderm cells. Imagine that the cells destined to sense the outside world, and to protect you from it, partially retreat into the shell of the body, with "feelers" (some special and some regular) remaining in contact with the outside world. The rapid cell migration that occurs internally along the midline of the forming body is called **neurulation,** and it results in a spinal cord from the neck down and an elaborate swelling called the brain from the neck up. "Nerves" are what connect the brain and spinal cord to the ectoderm that maintains a "skin" or envelope around the other embryo tissues.

The notochord induces the ectoderm cells immediately above it to expand and sag downward, thus giving the ectodermal surface of the embryo a **plated** and then a **grooved** appearance (Fig. 1.14). The idea is to convert some ectoderm cells into specialized processors and to sink these cells into a protected area by first grooving the ectodermal surface, then folding the groove inward on itself, and finally closing the **fold** completely to form a **tube**, which then is "pinched off" by the surface ectoderm. When the tube is pinched off, it is then trapped just below the surface in a midline position.

As neurulation proceeds through days 21 to 26, the fold does not close into a tube all at once. Closure begins in the middle of the length of the neural fold, and from there it proceeds both toward the head and toward the tail (Fig. 1.15). The effect is one of "zippering," with an opening at the tail end (caudal neuropore) and an opening at the head end (cranial neuropore). For the future spinal cord and brain to form and work properly, these pores must resolve completely.

As you study this part of development, think about the larger lesson of how the neural tube gets to be where it is. In the body, this tube is encircled by 29 or so vertebral bones that grow as bodies in front of the tube and arches around the tube toward the back. You are studying development both to learn why things look the way they do in the adult body and to anticipate the nature of **congenital anomalies**. You should study neurulation as a means of understanding the position of the nervous system along the axis of the body and to anticipate that many congenital anomalies of the nervous system are the result of incomplete closure of the mesoderm around it. Broadly speaking, these conditions are variations of **spina bifida**. (See Clinical Anatomy Box 1.3.)

The completion of the head end of the embryo is such a fascinating process that it deserves a later chapter of its own. For now, however, try to appreciate that by having an undetermined boundary at the cranial end, the neural tube can swell in size if the other growth vectors around it comply. Differences in brain size are obvious distinctions among animal groups, such as amphibians, reptiles, and mammals, and particularly among different groups of mammals. Everything about growth involves a trade-off, however, so keep this in mind as you study how the rest of the head grows.

Some ectoderm cells get liberated when the neural fold pinches itself into a tube (see Fig. 1.14). These **neural crest** cells are not part of the "healed" ectoderm, and they are not part of the self-enclosed tube. Rather, they are adrift in the mesoderm between the two. **Neural crest cells give rise to all neurons outside of the brain and spinal**

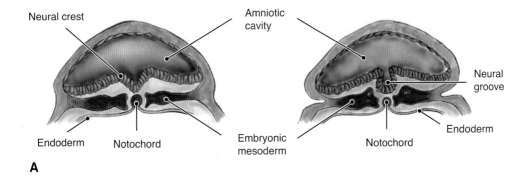

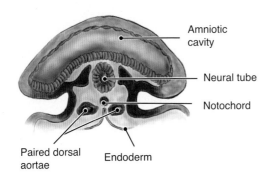

FIGURE 1.14   **Cross-sectional views of neurulation in the three-layered embryonic disk.**

Follow the blue ectoderm layer as it first folds, then grooves, just above the notochord (**A**). The groove then folds in on itself to become a tube, and the tube pulls away from the ectoderm above it to become embedded underneath the ectoderm (**B**). This process is called neurulation, and it results in a tube just under the skin of your future back. The tube will become the spinal cord and brain. (Adapted from Sadler T. Langman's Medical Embryology, 9th Edition Image Bank. Baltimore: Lippincott Williams & Wilkins, 2003.)

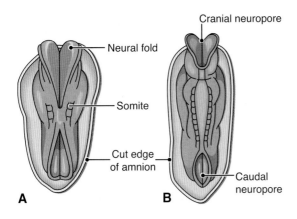

FIGURE 1.15   Top-down view of the ectoderm layer as it "zippers" closed the neural groove into a neural tube.

This process starts in the middle of the embryonic disc and continues from there both toward the head and toward the tail (**A**). The head part of the tube eventually balloons into a big brain; the tail part of the tube should close up on itself. You can see how the paraxial mesoderm follows the grooving in the form of somites (**B**), which are the precursors to the vertebral column. (LifeART image copyright (c) 2006 Lippincott Williams & Wilkins. All rights reserved.)

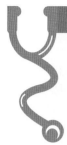

CLINICAL ANATOMY

Box 1.3

NEURAL TUBE DEFECTS

Failure of the neural tube to close properly results in a broad spectrum of problems that range from cosmetic to fatal. Mesoderm around the neural tube is intimately involved in its closure, because it forms the protective neural arches of the vertebrae. **Spina bifida** refers to a failure of the spinous processes and/or neural arches to form, which results in exposure of the spinal cord and/or its meninges. The terms describing the types of spina bifida refer to how much of the central nervous system is implicated in the defect. **Spina bifida occulta** is failure of the mesoderm to ossify fully and is the mildest of the conditions. In **spina bifida cystica,** a swelling of cerebrospinal fluid and the surrounding meninges balloons into the defect (a **meningocele**). Displacement of the spinal cord into a meningocele is a **meningomyelocele.** The final type of exposure is absolute failure of the ectoderm to close, resulting is frank exposure of the spinal cord to the outside world.

These conditions also apply to neural tube closure at the head end of the embryo. In this area, however, cranial bones rather than vertebral arches surround the large brain, and they form from direct induction by the growing brain itself. The range of neural tube defects at the cranial end includes meningoceles, which can look much more severe than they are; encephaloceles, which include portions of the brain; and **anencephaly** and **raschisis,** which involve absolute failure of the neural tube to complete.

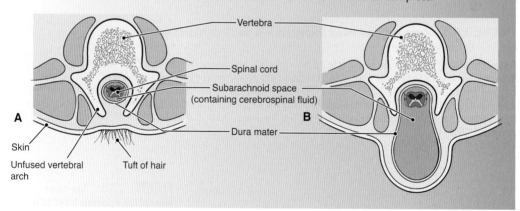

cord. They also derive ganglia, the medulla of the suprarenal gland, and melanocytes—the cells that produce pigment. Melanocytes exemplify the role of neural crest, because they represent cells that detect the outside world (as is the function of their ectodermal origin) and respond to it in a protective manner (the other domain of ectoderm) by coloring the dermis of the body to block the penetration of harmful light waves. Neural crest cells interact with mesoderm to develop into a wide variety of adult structures, including parts of some bones in the head as well as cartilages of other bones in the head. Neural crest cells confirm the essential purpose of the ectoderm layer and the creative manner in which its daughter cells play out all the possibilities.

Neurulation is a classic story of proliferation and differentiation. The end result is that a connected core of cells sinks under the ectoderm in the form of a long cord and a (soon-to-be) swollen brain. These cells are capable of detecting the outside world through connections to the overlying ectoderm layer (called nerves) and through a few

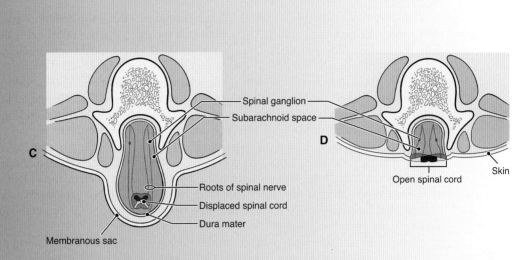

Spinal ganglion
Subarachnoid space
C
D
Roots of spinal nerve
Displaced spinal cord
Dura mater
Membranous sac
Open spinal cord
Skin

Neural tube defects. If neurulation fails to complete at the top (cranial neuropore) or the bottom (caudal neuropore) of the neural tube, the mesoderm fails to enclose the tube completely in a bony ring. This is called **spina bifida**, and it can take forms ranging from **occulta (A)**, in which the only apparent sign is a strange tuft of hair over the lower lumbar region of the back, to **cystica (B)**, in which the overlying ectoderm is "bubbled up" by an expanded cyst of fluid bathing the spinal cord. Cystic forms of spina bifida can range from exposure of the neural meninges (**meningocele; B**) to exposure of the meninges and the neural tissue (**meningomyelocele; C**) to radical exposure of neural tissue to the amniotic fluid (**raschisis; D**). At the cranial end of the neural tube, the same dynamics are in play. As long as the neural tissue is mature and bathed in cerebrospinal fluid, surgery can reduce the effect of the failed mesodermal growth. As a health care professional, it is essential that you understand how these conditions arise so that you can inform parents about their options and console the shock factor that the anatomy alone creates. (Modified from Stedman's Concise Medical Dictionary for the Health Professions, 4th Edition. Baltimore: Lippincott Williams & Wilkins, 2001.)

highly specialized sensory cell clusters in the head (the "organs" that see light waves, hear sound waves, smell molecules, and taste chemical compounds). More importantly, however, the cells respond to the sensations with chemical and electrical signals that cause the mesoderm cells, which are always in contact with them, to contract. How we can direct this activity consciously is a field of study all unto itself called neuroscience; the purpose of the next section is to show how the anatomy of it all arises logically during folding of the embryonic disc into a true body form.

Lateral and Longitudinal Folding of the Embryo

Three tube-like structures run along the axis of the adult body. One is the spinal cord, which, of course, is not a tube but is developed from a tube of cells. Another is the vertebral column, which again is not a literal tube but is a cylindrical column completely parallel to the spinal cord behind it and to the esophagus in front of it. The esophagus is the third tube, and it literally is a tube. The esophagus represents the beginning of the gut tube, which continues as the stomach, intestines, and rectum. These axial columns arise from ectoderm, mesoderm, and endoderm tissues, respectively, in keeping the with basic embryonic disc design described so far.

The skin that covers the vertebral column continues around the body in a complete wrap, making for a "volume" to the body that exceeds the space taken up by the three basic tubes. This requires that, at some point, the three germinal layers must have expanded from a simple "sandwich" design into a more three dimensional configuration. This critical step in animate development happens just after neurulation, during the fourth week after conception. The process involves changes at both the sides of the embryonic disc (**lateral folding**) and at the ends of the embryo (**longitudinal folding**). The result is a basic, fish-like body plan that characterizes all vertebrate life.

The ectoderm layer derives the outer layer of the skin (the epidermis), but before folding, it exists only as the upper, or dorsal, layer of the germ disc. This layer must assume an encompassing position during the folding episode, which means that it must wrap down around the mesoderm layer beneath it and the endoderm layer beneath that. It cannot move too fast, however, or it will interrupt the simultaneous change in the endoderm layer.

Before folding, the endoderm exists only as the lower, or ventral, layer of the germ disk. It must eventually become an enclosed tube, which in the body extends from the throat down to the anal canal in one continuous, open sleeve. At the same time (recall Fig. 1.12), the endoderm layer is exposed to the yolk sac, a nutrient pouch that hangs down from it much like a bubblegum bubble that you blow out of your mouth. If the endoderm layer folds in on itself to create a tube, then something must happen to this yolk sac.

Indeed, as the endoderm commences lateral folding, it sheds its connection to the yolk sac in almost all locations except near the very middle of the disc. This is logical, because by this time of growth the embryo has exhausted its own food supply, is fully connected to the mother, and so is ready to take most of its energy needs from her. The yolk sac is expendable, and lateral folding of the embryo expends most of it. The endoderm must accomplish this lateral folding before the closure of the ectodermal fold, and the real engineer of this coordinated tissue migration is the mesoderm.

Remember that as the mesoderm fills in the space between ectoderm and endoderm, it assembles three tissue clusters called the **paraxial mesoderm**, **intermediate mesoderm**, and **lateral plate mesoderm** (see Fig. 1.15). We now follow the destiny of the lateral plate region, which has the unique property of being in contact with extraembryonic cells along the margin of the embryonic disc. During folding of the disc, these extraembryonic cells need to be kept outside of the embryo. For this to occur, the mesoderm must "grab" the final group of ectoderm cells and the final group of endoderm cells along the sides of the disc and then tightly "tuck" inward. Because it is in a sandwich-like contact with both ectoderm and endoderm, the lateral plate mesoderm can do this, but the endoderm has already started to curl inward and to slough off the yolk sac membrane. The lateral plate mesoderm accommodates by splitting itself into two sheets, one just for the undercoating of the ectoderm and one just for the overcoating of the endoderm.

Just before the commencement of lateral folding, the lateral plate mesoderm cell group cavitates through the fascinating process of programmed cell death (Fig. 1.16). This leaves one layer of the lateral plate mesoderm in contact with the ectoderm and a separate layer of the lateral plate mesoderm in contact with the endoderm, with a cavity between them that is open to the chorionic fluid cavity, in which the entire

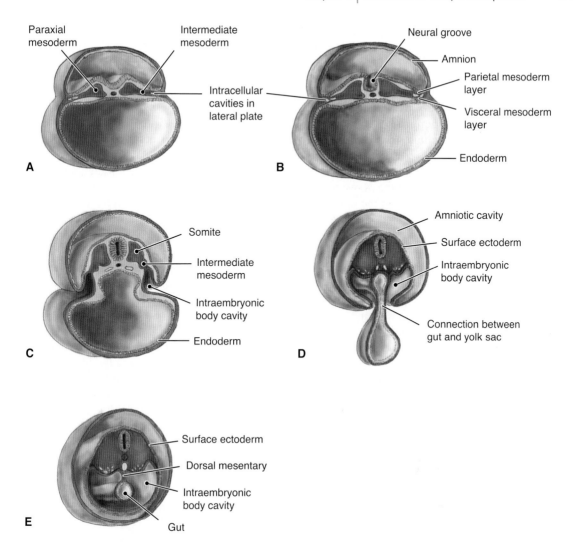

FIGURE 1.16   **The lateral plate mesoderm splits into two "tails" at the side of the embryonic disc.**

One tail grabs onto the overlying ectoderm, and one tail grabs onto the underlying endoderm (**A, B**). Both tails will then tuck downward, taking the ectoderm and endoderm with them (**C**). The endoderm transforms from a flat plate of cells with a big yolk sac cavity into a narrow tube of cells with the cavity pinched away and disintegrating (**D**). The ectoderm transforms from a flat plate into a complete wrap around the embryo, which now looks more like a cylinder than a sandwich. Because the outside of the cylinder is the ectoderm layer, the cavity above it (amniotic cavity) now completely surrounds the embryo, and while it is folding, the ectoderm expands along the midline into a neural tube that embedded just below the surface. Because the lateral plate split before folding, the area between the two "tails" is carried with the fold and becomes part of the embryo as the cavity in which the endo-dermal tube is suspended (**E**). The mesoderm that surrounds the endodermal tube hangs down from the "core" of the embryo body in the form of an important structure called a mesentery. (Adapted from Sadler T. Langman's Medical Embryology, 9th Edition Image Bank. Baltimore: Lippincott Williams & Wilkins, 2003.)

embryonic bulb is suspended by the connecting stalk. This cavity extends everywhere that the lateral plate mesoderm is formed, which means around the cranial end of the disc in front of the oropharyngeal membrane (see Fig. 1.11). The resulting cavity is in the shape of a horseshoe when seen from above (Fig. 1.17).

The subtlety of this transition is worth some patient study. The mesoderm layer that stays in an undercoating contact with the ectoderm is called **somatic or parietal mesoderm**. The layer that stays in an overcoating contact with the endoderm is called **splanchnic or visceral mesoderm**. Somatic mesoderm is destined to become many connective tissues in the body, but splanchnic mesoderm stays in intimate contact with the endoderm and becomes a thin, strong coat of smooth muscle that helps to squeeze the tube as needed.

The splanchnic mesoderm helps the endoderm layer to fold in on itself and form a tube (in much the same manner as the neural tube). In a zipper-like fashion from the cranial to the caudal end of the embryonic disc, the splanchnic mesoderm tucks inward from the sides of the embryo and meets itself in the midline. This collision pinches off the yolk sac lining and enables the endoderm cells from one sideline of the embryonic disk to merge with the endoderm cells from the other sideline as an intact tube. The splanchnic mesoderm cells likewise survive the collision and merge to form a sling around the new endodermal tube.

You should now think about two important features of the new endodermal tube. First, the tube does not completely form in the very middle of the embryo. A remnant of the yolk sac remains, dangling downward (ventrally) from the tube like a deflated balloon. (We will see what happens to this pouch when we look at longitudinal folding.) Second, the new endodermal tube is no longer adjacent to the neural tube along the midline of the embryo. As the disk has been folding laterally, the paraxial mesoderm has surrounded the neural tube, forming a vertebral body between the neural tube and the gut tube. For this and other reasons, the new endodermal tube rests in a kind of "sling" formed by the splanchnic mesoderm and by suspensions of mesoderm from the "wall" of the embryonic body (see Fig. 1.16).

Embryologists refer to the three sections of the gut tube that result as the **foregut**, **midgut**, and **hindgut**. Think of them as the fully closed tube before the yolk sac rem-

FIGURE 1.17   **Splitting of the lateral plate mesoderm (green arrow) creates an internal cavity in the embryo.**

The split stretches around the edge of the embryonic disc in a horseshoe shape (see added green arrows). This is important because as the two "sheaths" of the lateral plate mesoderm tuck downward, they bring along the cavity between them. This cavity becomes the abdominal cavity, chest cavity, and pericardial cavity as the embryo develops, but the part of it that arches around the top end of the embryonic disc cannot stay there. It must fold downward as well.

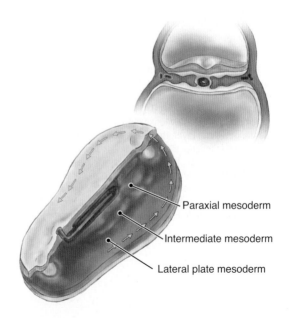

Paraxial mesoderm

Intermediate mesoderm

Lateral plate mesoderm

nant (foregut), the incompletely closed tube from which the remnant yolk sac dangles (midgut), and the fully closed tube after the yolk sac remnant (hindgut). Of these, the foregut is notable because all the accessory organs of digestion (e.g., liver and pancreas) arise from it.

As this is happening, the somatic mesoderm adheres to the final layer of ectoderm cells at the sides of the embryonic disc and tucks itself inward, just as occurs with the splanchnic mesoderm. In this case, however, rather than pinching off the lining of cells that formed the bubble around it, the somatic mesoderm drags the bubble lining behind it. In this process, the ectoderm expands to a complete circumference, as the somatic mesoderm from one side merges into the somatic mesoderm from the other side in the ventral midline (ventral to the now-folded endodermal tube; see Fig. 1.16). Just as with the splanchnic mesoderm layer, this collision in the ventral midline results in a merger of ectoderm from both sides with somatic mesoderm from both sides in a seamless heal.

Because the somatic mesoderm drags the amniotic membrane of cells behind it, the amniotic membrane from one side of the disc merges with the amniotic membrane from the other side to form an intact **amniotic cavity** that encloses the entire embryo. The amniotic fluid in this cavity is endogenous to the embryo and serves as an intermediary body of molecular exchange between the embryo and mother. Despite greatly expanding during lateral folding of the embryo, the amniotic cavity remains in its original cellular position—lined by extraembryonic cells that form a chorionic cavity in which the whole embryo package is suspended from the uterine wall by the connecting stalk.

It is self-evident that a protective layer surrounds the entire body, but note that everywhere in the body, this coating of ectoderm is lined inside, or underneath, by mesoderm. For this reason, skin is actually composed of ectodermal **epidermis** and mesodermal **dermis**. More importantly, this layer of somatic mesoderm has the capacity to become other types of connective tissue, such as muscle, bone, and deep fascia. Thus, the body is everywhere equipped for the formation of structures that will enable movement. Moreover, when the somatic mesoderm folded in around the inner tube created by the splanchnic mesoderm, a cavity was created that now lies within the body. This cavity has the awkward name of the **intraembryonic coelom**.

Both the somatic and splanchnic mesoderm layers end up inside of the embryo, and they are continuous with one another as a lining of the coelomic space. The adult body still has a coelom, but it has been partitioned into a cavity of the abdominal region called the **peritoneal sac** and a cavity of the chest region called the **pleural sac**. The coelom is an empty sac (just a little residual fluid inside) completely lined by mesoderm. **Things will push against the lining of the sac, but nothing will pierce it.** It gives the trunk of the body a "barrier space" between the organs and the wall of muscle and bone that encloses them.

If lateral folding were the end of the story, we would all look like tubes with open holes at both ends, very much like living worms. Instead, both ends are covered by specialized ingrowths and outgrowths that must have come from somewhere. Coincident with the process of lateral folding is a slight bending at the head and tail ends called **longitudinal folding**. To understand this, we need to revisit how the embryo looks just before the folding starts (Fig. 1.18).

The most notable feature at the head end during early development is the fixed adhesion of endoderm and ectoderm cells called the **oropharyngeal membrane** (see Fig. 1.11). Here, the mesoderm was unable to penetrate between the endoderm and ectoderm, but it did manage to spread above, or anterior, or forward, to this point. This region of mesoderm that bridges the two sides of the embryo is called the **septum**

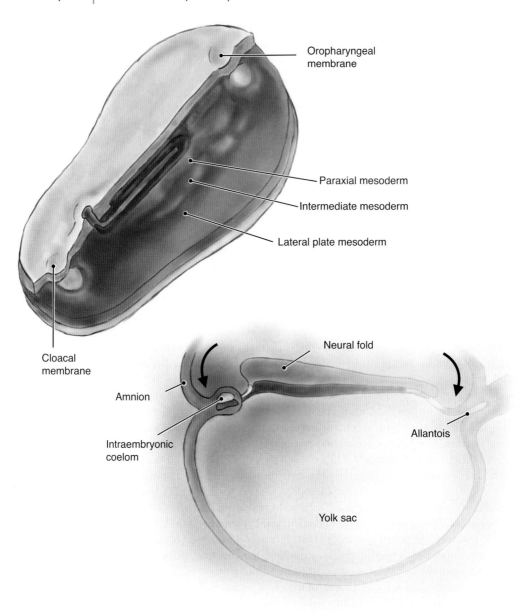

Oropharyngeal membrane

Paraxial mesoderm

Intermediate mesoderm

Lateral plate mesoderm

Cloacal membrane

Amnion

Intraembryonic coelom

Neural fold

Allantois

Yolk sac

FIGURE 1.18   **The embryonic disc as seen from above (left) and from the side before longitudinal folding.**

The side view is cut through the midline of the embryo, which is why you see the notochord (purple) but no mesoderm. Focus on the two places where the ectoderm and endoderm are fused together. These will curl under the embryonic disc during longitudinal folding. Whatever lies in front of or behind these two membranes will go along for the ride. At the head end, this means the "bend in the horseshoe" that includes the intraembryonic coelom and the transverse septum of mesoderm. At the bottom end, this means the connecting stalk and the slip of yolk sac (allantois) that got trapped within it. (Adapted from Sadler T. Langman's Medical Embryology, 9th Edition Image Bank. Baltimore: Lippincott Williams & Wilkins, 2003.)

transversum, or transverse septum (see Fig. 1.18). Behind the transverse septum in the midline between the ectoderm and endoderm are the **oropharyngeal membrane,** the **notochord,** and the **cloacal membrane.**

Growing within the mesoderm forward to the oropharyngeal membrane and just inferior to the coelom is a condensation of cells that will become the **heart.** The full story of how the circulatory system develops will come soon, so for now, please just bear with this advance preview. It is important to realize that the original position of the heart muscle is forward, or cranial, to the mouth area and just behind, or caudal, to the transverse septum of mesoderm at the apex of the head end of the disk (Fig. 1.19).

Remember that the cranial end of the neural tube is not bounded by the paraxial mesoderm clusters that will become the future vertebral column. They end near the location of the oropharyngeal membrane. The folding of the embryo in this longitudinal plane is "caused" mostly by unrestricted ballooning growth of the cranial end of the neural tube—as if the swelling brain forces the mouth membrane, the future heart, and the transverse septum to curl downward, or ventrally, to make room. The important thing to remember in this complicated process is that the order of structures toward the cranial end (mouth, heart, and transverse septum) acts like the minute-hand of a clock as you look at longitudinal folding in a side view (see Fig. 1.19). As the brain expands and the head end of the embryo folds downward, the mouth membrane rotates almost 180° so that the endodermal surface that once faced upward, toward the ectoderm plate, now faces downward, toward the diminishing yolk sac. The heart condensation that once was cranial to the mouth now curls below, or caudal, to it, taking the top of the coelom horseshoe with it. Finally, the transverse septum, which was once the most cranial structure in the embryo, now lies caudal to the heart. It is as if the minute-hand rotated from 45 minutes after the hour back to 15 minutes after the hour. The axis of the rotation was the base of the oropharyngeal membrane, which now represents the most cranial limit of mesoderm in the developing embryo.

After longitudinal folding the head end of the embryo is now a curl of ectoderm that covers a large, expanded neural tube (the future brain); the oropharyngeal membrane inferior to that; and the lateral plate mesoderm around the heart, coelom, and transverse septum that is still more inferior. The transverse septum is one of the few areas of the embryo in which a continuous layer of mesoderm crosses the midline. What is the only muscle in the adult body that really crosses from one side to the other? The thoracic **diaphragm,** which is derived from the transverse septum. The diaphragm is not at the top end of the body, however, so one outcome of longitudinal folding is to move the transverse septum from its origin at the very cranial end of the embryonic disc to a spot between the future chest and the future abdomen. Getting the diaphragm to form completely is a complicated affair, and mistakes that occur along the way lead to some relatively common developmental anomalies.

Muscles tend to have origins and insertions, and which is which depends on what happens when a muscle contracts. The diaphragm originates along a perimeter of the inside of the rib cage, but it has no proper insertion. The diaphragm inserts on itself in the center of itself, an area called the **central tendon** (Fig. 1.20). Think of the formation of the diaphragm as the arrival of a central structure that needs help from the sidelines to form a good seal between the chest cavity and the abdominal cavity. Much of this seal comes from tissue folds that migrate inward from the body wall to pinch off the coelom into a thoracic half and an abdominal half. The thoracic half is then called the **pleural coelom,** or pleural sac; the abdominal half the **peritoneal coelom,** or peritoneal sac; and the migrating tissue fold the **pleuroperitoneal fold** (Fig. 1.21).

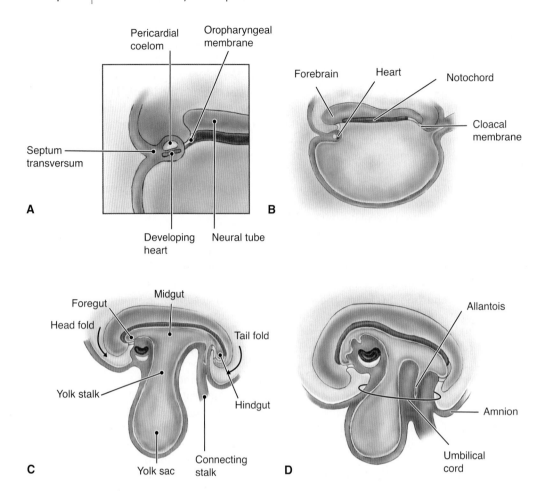

FIGURE 1.19   **The sequence of longitudinal folding.**

The top end of the neural tube expands, forcing the mesoderm layer to curl under (**A, B**). This sweeps the oropharyngeal membrane around by 180º. The transverse septum ends up below the coelom and the developing heart (**C**). The top end of the embryo becomes dominated by the expanded neural tube (**D**). Whatever was once in front of the neural tube and against the edge of the amniotic membrane gets folded down and tucked in below the developing brain. If the oropharyngeal membrane is the site of the future mouth, you can see how the endodermal lining just behind it gets folded into the beginnings of a tube that will become the esophagus (**E**). (Adapted from Sadler T. Langman's Medical Embryology, 9th Edition Image Bank. Baltimore: Lippincott Williams & Wilkins, 2003.)

Two other tissues complete the making of the diaphragm. A small amount of the **dorsal mesentery** (recall Fig. 1.16) of the esophagus contributes to the median reach of the diaphragm. The final contributor is a small region of lateral plate mesoderm that seals the perimeter of the diaphragm to the rib cage. Because of this last element, the sensory innervation of this part of the diaphragm is the same as that of the body wall at this point. The motor innervation was dragged down by the transverse septum, which was once near the very top of the embryo. Thus, portions of the ventral rami of cervical spinal nerves 3, 4, and 5 merge together as the **phrenic nerve** to form the

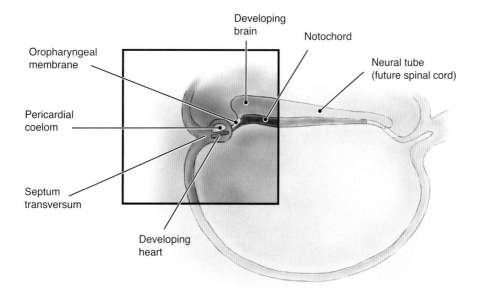

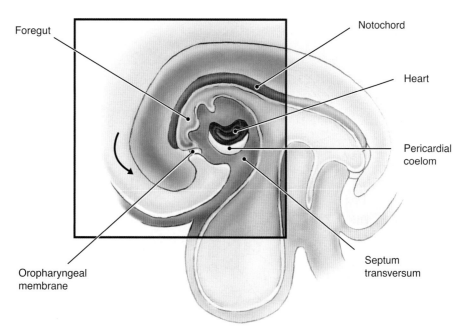

E

FIGURE 1.19 (*Continued*).

complete motor and partial sensory supply to the diaphragm. Knowing that the bulk of the diaphragm originally came from the top end of the embryo will help you to remember why a muscle at the bottom of the thorax is innervated by nerves from the top of the neck.

Given the complex sequence of events leading up to division of the thoracic and peritoneal cavities, developmental defects in the diaphragm are not uncommon. If the pleuroperitoneal folds fail to migrate completely, a gap remains between the thoracic and abdominal cavities. Because abdominal contents are under greater pressure than

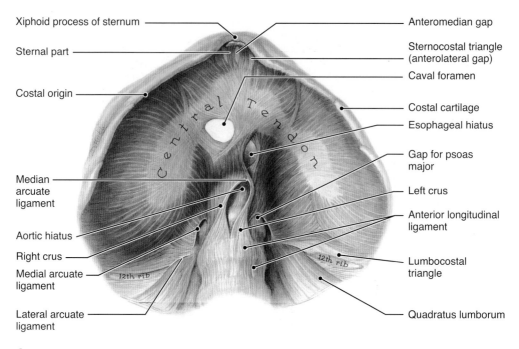

Xiphoid process of sternum ————————————— Anteromedian gap

Sternal part ——————————————— Sternocostal triangle
(anterolateral gap)

Caval foramen

Costal origin ——————————— Costal cartilage

Esophageal hiatus

Gap for psoas
major

Median
arcuate
ligament ——————————— Left crus

Anterior longitudinal
ligament

Aortic hiatus —————

Right crus ————— Lumbocostal
triangle

Medial arcuate ————— 12th rib   12th rib
ligament

Lateral arcuate ——————————— Quadratus lumborum
ligament

A

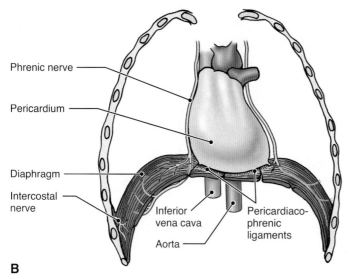

Phrenic nerve ————

Pericardium ————

Diaphragm ————

Intercostal ————
nerve
            Inferior ———   ——— Pericardiaco-
            vena cava   phrenic
                                    ligaments
            Aorta ———

B

FIGURE 1.20   The adult diaphragm.

The muscle attaches to the entire perimeter of your trunk—the inner lining of the rib cage and the vertebral column. It inserts on itself in the form of a central tendon (**A**). When it contracts against this central region, it changes from a dome-shaped, loose muscular coat into a flatter band of tissue that spans the space between the abdomen and the thorax (**B**). (Adapted from Moore KL, Dalley AF. Clinically Oriented Anatomy, 4th Edition. Baltimore, Lippincott Williams & Wilkins, 1999.)

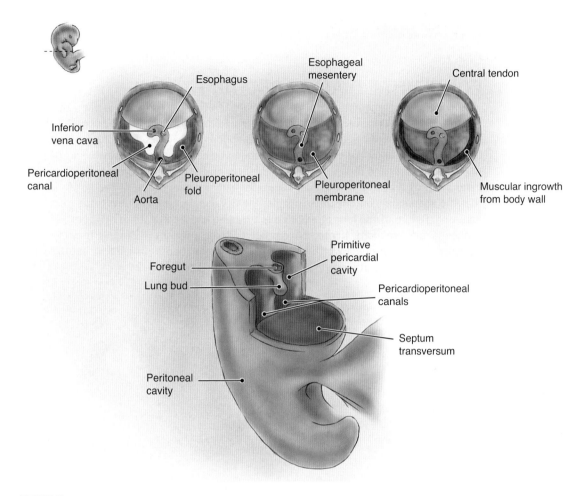

FIGURE 1.21   **Formation of the diaphragm.**

The diaphragm forms from the transverse septum, ingrowth of the pleuroperitoneal membrane from the lining of the cavity, a bit of dorsal mesentery of the foregut, and lastly, ingrowth of mesoderm from the body wall. The diaphragm is not a circular disc, of course. It is a sheet of muscle that lies across the body over the liver and the stomach. It is shaped like a dome, mostly because the extra contributors migrate in from the perimeter to give the central part more room to form a dome. Because it is formed from different sources, its sensory and motor supplies also come from separate sources. Motor fibers follow the transverse septum down from the head region (via the phrenic nerve of the cervical region), and sensory fibers come from both the phrenic and the same nerves that serve the body wall in this area (via intercostal nerves). (From Sadler T. Langman's Medical Embryology, 9th Edition Image Bank. Baltimore: Lippincott Williams & Wilkins, 2003.)

the thoracic contents, they may get pushed up through this foramen and come to lie in the thoracic cavity. This condition is called **congenital diaphragmatic hernia**, and it usually occurs on the left side, where closure is normally later than on the right. (See Clinical Anatomy Box 1.4.)

Somewhere in the near future, a neck must take shape between the oropharyngeal membrane and the heart. Do not worry if you are unable to visualize the folding process from these words and diagrams. The important concept to draw from embryonic folding is that even in complex anatomic arrangements, such as the head and

CLINICAL ANATOMY

Box 1.4

CONGENITAL DIAPHRAGMATIC HERNIA

Congenital diaphragmatic hernias are thought to occur as frequently as 1 in 2,000 to 2,500 newborns. They typically result from failure of the pleuroperitoneal fold to complete closure between the thoracic and abdominal cavities. The folds exist on both sides of the body, but congenital diaphragmatic hernias almost always occur on the left side. Early and prolific growth of the liver on the right side probably secures maturation of that side of the diaphragm. The major complication of the hernia is that the abdominal contents press against the developing lung and prevent it from maturing. Failure of the lungs to mature is a leading cause of death in newborns, so congenital diaphragmatic hernias are considered to be a serious risk to life. They can be detected by ultrasound, which has opened the possibility of fetal surgery, but this procedure introduces other serious risks to both fetus and mother.

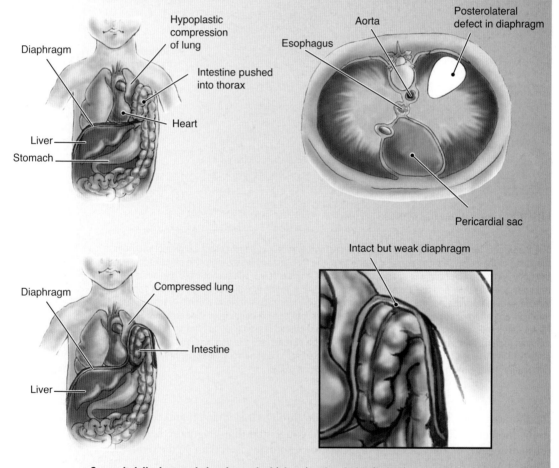

Congenital diaphragmatic hernia, typical (above) and variation (below).

face, you are still composed of nothing more than a protective outer layer, an absorbing inner layer, and connecting tissue in between.

The longitudinal folding of the tail end is less complicated. Recall what the tail end of the embryo looks like before folding (see Fig. 1.18). The primitive streak is almost completely regressed. The ectoderm and endoderm are fused together as a cloacal membrane, and the only significant structure more caudal to this is the connecting stalk. The connecting stalk was formed as the embryonic disc extruded protective cell layers and achieved a state of suspension in a pocket of fluid. It represents the vital connection between parent and offspring, and before folding it is located at virtually the tail end of the three-layered disc.

You should appreciate the fold of endoderm that was trapped in the connecting stalk at this stage. This fold is called the **allantois,** and it began as a simple artifact of the embryo pulling away from its own implantation. As the tail fold proceeds, however, this simple artifact will take on a new significance. The pivot point for the downward, or ventral, tail fold is the terminal part of the primitive streak (Fig. 1.22). Just as the oropharyngeal membrane swung around in the head fold, the cloacal membrane rotates ventrally in the tail fold. The allantois, which was once caudal to the cloacal membrane, pivots almost 180° and ends up cranial to the cloacal membrane.

These changes seem almost minor compared to the reorientation of the connecting stalk. In the tail fold, the connecting stalk follows the pivot and curls under, or ven-

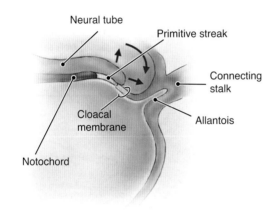

A

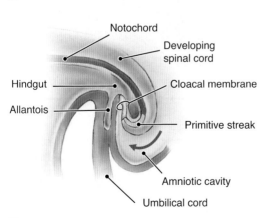

B

FIGURE 1.22   **A sagittal view of longitudinal folding of the caudal end of the embryo.**

The connecting stalk is being swept under the embryonic disc toward the very middle, or "belly," of the ventral surface (**A**). It takes the allantois with it, which changes the relative position of the allantois from behind to in front of the cloacal membrane (**B**). The cloaca is the primitive exit port for anything in the endodermal tube. Simple animal forms eliminate both solid and liquid waste from the same hole, called the cloaca. More complex animals, particularly those that give birth to live offspring, separate the reproductive pathways from the waste pathways and further separate liquid from solid waste. This implies more complex development of the cloacal membrane shown here.

tral, to the folding embryo until it collides with the remains of the yolk sac in the center of the embryo's new "belly" region (Fig. 1.23). This collision results in the connecting stalk incorporating the yolk sac remnant and still retaining the allantois pouch, or diverticulum. The new bundle is the official **umbilical cord**, and it is positioned midway along the newly folded endodermal tube. This is the one remaining portion of the developing embryo that is not fully covered by ectoderm, which, given the need of the embryo to be ported into the mother's circulatory system, is logical.

The goal here is not to master the transformations of one cartoonish drawing into another as the embryo changes but, rather, to understand how three plates of tissue migrate into staging positions for the rest of growth. The external plate, or the ectoderm, has invaginated its own control center, the neural tube, and then spread out to enclose the other two plates. The internal plate, or the endoderm, has radically withdrawn into a narrow tube that runs the length of the embryo in midline. It holds on to a remnant of its original food supply, and it contacts the outside world through only two patches of exposure: the oropharyngeal membrane, and the cloacal membrane. The middle plate, or the mesoderm, engineers the changes in the ectoderm and endoderm and assumes four distinct positions within the folded embryo: a paraxial position

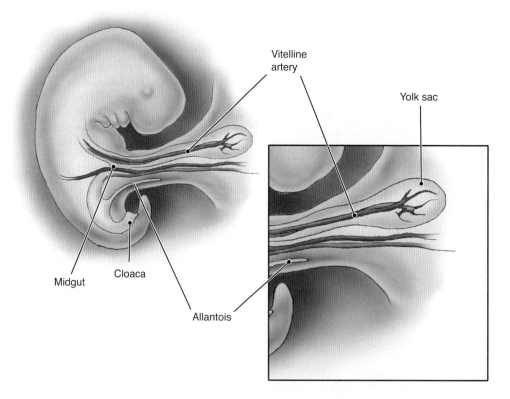

FIGURE 1.23   **Formation of the umbilical cord.**

Remember that the original yolk sac gets pinched off by lateral and longitudinal folding except for a dwindling pouch in the very center of the embryo. This is now called the vitelline duct, and it is a blind pouch that simply dangles there until the connecting stalk crashes into it during longitudinal folding, after which the vitelline duct and the blind pouch called the allantois are incorporated with the connecting stalk as the umbilical cord. (Adapted from Sadler T. Langman's Medical Embryology, 9th Edition Image Bank. Baltimore: Lippincott Williams & Wilkins, 2003.)

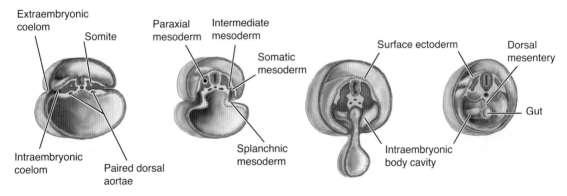

FIGURE 1.24   **Mesoderm differentiates and migrates.**

Review how the mesoderm engineers an inward fold of the ectoderm and endoderm. The end result is that mesoderm completely coats the undersurface of the ectoderm and completely "overcoats" the outer surface of the endoderm. (Adapted from Sadler T. Langman's Medical Embryology, 9th Edition Image Bank. Baltimore: Lippincott Williams & Wilkins, 2003.)

for building structure to the axis of the body; an intermediate position, which eventually will become the urogenital structures; a somatic lining position underneath the ectoderm everywhere in the body; and a splanchnic lining against the endodermal tube from top to bottom (Fig. 1.24). Given the extent of mesoderm proliferation by the end of the fourth week, now is a good time to explore its activity.

Mesodermal Growth

Although we think of our bodies in terms of four limbs, a trunk, and a big head, the trunk is really the major entity. The limbs will be little more than unusual growths of the body wall, and the head and neck will elaborate from the upper end of the trunk tubes. The trunk, however, provides the axial symmetry of the body, the chambers for its energy-absorbing structures, and the ultimate position of the self-regulated pump that keeps it alive—the **heart**. Before we have a recognizable head and limbs, we are a primitive trunk, and the defining structure of the trunk is the vertebral column, which derives from paraxial mesoderm.

The paraxial region of mesoderm condenses into segments called **somites**. The number of somites that are apparent in an embryo is one measure of how mature that embryo is; eventually, the body will have from 42 to 44 total pairs, most of which contribute to the vertebrae. The somite, however, is a study in the complete package of connective tissue that the mesoderm provides. It begins as a block of tissue on the side of the neural tube, separated from its partner on the other side by the notochord. First and foremost, it must provide support to the neural tube, so many of the cell lines are destined to become the hardest of the connective tissues—**bone**—and remain in their original position (Fig. 1.25). Somite cells from each side fuse to form vertebral bodies, and in doing so, they cannibalize the notochord cells between them. From the vertebral body will grow the arch of bone that wraps around the neural tube dorsally. Other cell clusters in the somite, however, extend to the ectodermal blanket covering the neural tube and have a different fate.

Embryologists consider the somite to be a parent cell cluster for two daughter clusters: a **sclerotome** group, and a **dermomyotome** group. These words aptly define a

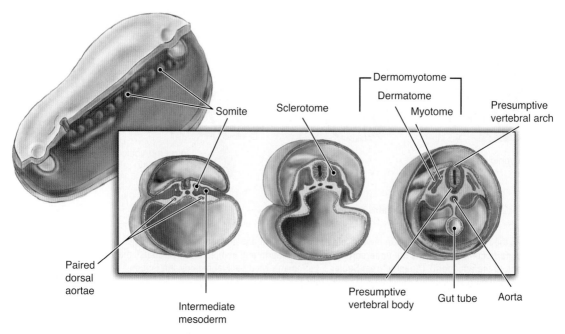

A

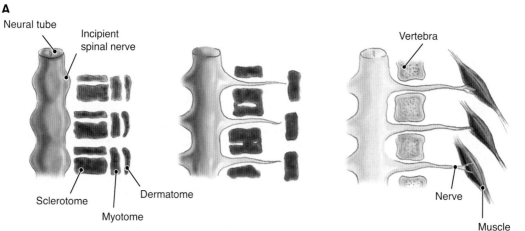

B

FIGURE 1.25   Transformation of the paraxial mesoderm.

Paraxial mesoderm develops vertebrae around the neural tube muscles that move the vertebrae, and dermis for the body. The muscle and dermis cell colonies are called dermomyotomes (**A**). Each somite of mesoderm contributes to two vertebrae by cleaving of the sclerotomes (**B**). In this way, each muscle cluster derived from a somite can span a vertebral space. As the sclerotomes from each side merge in the midline to form vertebral bodies, they cannibalize the notochord (**C**). The notochord persists in the spaces between adjacent vertebral bodies, where it becomes subsumed in an articular disc.

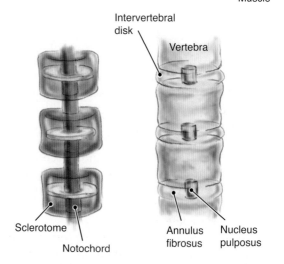

C

source of bony material (sclerotome) and a source of dermis and muscle material (dermomyotome). Thus, whereas most of the somite is dedicated to laying down a hard connective tissue to support the neural tube (a sclerotome), some of it is dedicated to more pliant tissue that bridges the space between the ectoderm and the tube. The dermomyotome begins in the back of the body, but with its ability to lay down muscle and dermis, it rapidly migrates around the wall of the trunk in two distinct cell clusters. This may seem abstract at this stage, while the embryo is little more than a bean-shaped tube, but it will help you to understand later the design of a **spinal nerve**.

In the trunk of the body, you have a group of muscles that connect one vertebra to another. These sometimes are called the intrinsic muscles of the back, or deep back muscles, and they are the muscles that feel stiff and sore in the absence of regular stretching exercises. Another group of muscles spans the circumference of the trunk, both between the ribs and around the abdominal wall (the infamous "sit-up" muscles). These two zones of muscles give the trunk of the body support and the capacity to move. They grow as distinct sets, however, because one group is dedicated just to the vertebral column and the other group to everything *but* the vertebral column. Both develop from a myotome, but from different ends of the myotome.

As the myotome grows, it splits into a cluster called an **epimere** and a cluster called a **hypomere**, which refer to whether the cluster lies above or below, respectively, a kind of imaginary line from the transverse process of the vertebra to the skin (Fig. 1.26). The muscles that arise from epimeric cells will serve the vertebral column, and the muscles that arise from hypomeric cells will serve the circumference of the trunk from the transverse process around to the front. The significance of this is that as the neural tube reaches out to access the ectoderm, it will provide dedicated and separated spinal nerve fibers to the epimeric versus the hypomeric muscles. Because the limbs grow from the trunk wall, the muscles that dominate their movement are all hypomeric muscles. The nerve fibers that serve them are substantial in size, making the design of a typical spinal nerve very asymmetric. In general, the epimeric region of the body is limited to the vertebral column and the narrow strip of deep muscles that run along either side of the vertebral spines. (Clinicians sometimes lump all the separate muscles together and call them the **paraspinous muscles**.) The dominance of the hypomeric tissues is the story of how animate life transformed from simple, segmented,

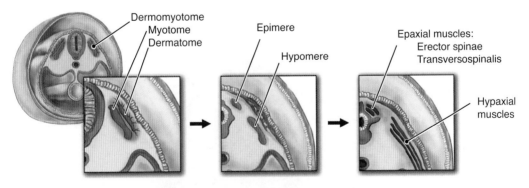

Dermomyotome
Myotome
Dermatome

Epimere

Hypomere

Epaxial muscles:
Erector spinae
Transversospinalis

Hypaxial
muscles

FIGURE 1.26   **Dermomyotomes cleave into dorsal and ventral components.**

Each dermomyotome cleaves into cell clusters that are dedicated to either the dorsal zone of the body axis (epimeric region of the body) or the much larger ventral zone (hypomeric region of the body). Muscles that develop strictly to move the vertebrae are epaxial muscles; all other muscles of the trunk (and future limbs) are hypaxial muscles.

tubular forms to complex, limbed, quadrupedal, bipedal, or even flight-capable forms—and it all begins at the time the body first develops a type of axis.

Because paraxial mesoderm is the source of almost all skeletal, or voluntary, muscle tissue in the body, the role of the somatic layer of lateral plate mesoderm is more limited. This somatic layer joins with the dermatome of the paraxial region to form the dermis of the skin. The splanchnic layer of lateral plate mesoderm, however, does form muscle, specifically the smooth muscle that surrounds the gut tube. Arterial walls also have smooth muscle, but this forms from local mesoderm cells, as you will see when you study the circulatory system.

Early Development of the Heart and Circulatory System

To this point, we have seen how the three basic tissue layers arise and migrate as the embryo assumes a three-dimensional form. To complete our sense of a functioning animal, however, we must connect a nutrient supply and an impulse wiring to these tissues. The nutrient supply is administered by the circulatory system, and the impulse network is trafficked by nerve fibers. We begin with the circulatory system.

For the first several days of development, the embryonic disc receives nutrition from its own yolk sac and from diffusion of maternal blood into the cytotrophoblast cell network (see Fig. 1.6). This is enough to sustain the embryonic disc until it develops its own system of vessels that can connect directly to maternal arteries through the connecting stalk. Because the embryo quickly exhausts its own food supply and outpaces the yield from diffusion, it must develop its own nutrient inflow and waste outflow system as soon as possible. The cardiovascular system begins to function during the fourth week of embryonic development and, thus, is the first "operating system" of the embryo. Logically, it is the mesoderm that differentiates into the anatomic structures that form the cardiovascular system.

The mesoderm that migrated cranially to the oropharyngeal membrane during gastrulation is destined to become the future heart and so is called the **cardiogenic area** (Fig. 1.27). This area congeals into parallel endocardial tubes on either side of the midline, and as you move backward toward the tail, each tube splits into a lateral endocardial tube and a dorsal aorta.

FIGURE 1.27 **Superior view of the embryonic disc showing the cardiogenic area.**

Mesoderm that migrates cranially in the embryonic disc differentiates into the primordial cells of the heart. The initial cardiogenic area pulses fluid through a primitive tubing design that, ultimately, will form distinct inflow (endocardial tube) and outflow (aorta) paths from the contractile cells of the cardiogenic area.

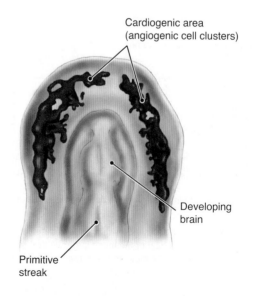

Cardiogenic area (angiogenic cell clusters)

Developing brain

Primitive streak

How the mesoderm cells in this area transform into cooperative tubular units is fascinating but beyond the scope of this introduction to gross anatomy. We pick up the story late in the third week of embryonic development, at the point just before lateral folding. As the **lateral endocardial tubes** and the **dorsal aortae** approach the cranial end of the embryo, they merge into one another. Soon, this "divining rod" configuration will merge into the one from the other side when the embryo folds laterally. The result is a single-chamber tube with four ports (Fig. 1.28).

At the same time that the cardiogenic area is forming, mesoderm cells throughout the embryonic disc coalesce into blood islands and, eventually, into canalized tubes around the blood molecules. They are like loose cords looking for a wall socket, and the folding of the embryo provides just that. The lateral fold brings both the endocardial tubes into contact with one another and the dorsal aortae into contact with one another. The contact fuses the like tubes into single tubes, one of which remains throughout the life as the **aorta** and the other of which becomes the muscular pump that is the **heart** (see Fig. 1.28). Toward the bottom of where the endocardial tubes merge is the region of the primitive heart called the **sinus venosus** that is receptive to blood vessels carrying molecules that are depleted of oxygen. In other words, the fused endocardial tubes develop a port for the future veins of the body (Fig. 1.29).

Longitudinal folding of the embryo ensures that the merged endocardial tubes end up in the future thorax. Because the transverse septum was cranial to the heart tube (recall Fig. 1.19) and also bent inward during the fold, it now lies inferior to the heart, just as the diaphragm does in the body. The longitudinal fold also creates an interesting loop in the dorsal aorta. Before the fold, the dorsal aorta plugged into the heart tube from below, or from the caudal end of the embryo. As the heart tube follows the longitudinal fold, the dorsal aorta gets arched above and cranial to it, resulting in the adult orientation of an aorta that appears to rise out of the heart and arch toward the head.

Development of the heart is a complicated process to visualize, but it is a very basic process conceptually. If you can understand how the mesoderm responds to the circulatory needs of an air-breathing animal, you can anticipate the types of congenital heart defects that you will see in clinical practice (some of which are illustrated below).

The heart begins not as a four-chambered cardiac muscle but, rather, as a central point in the inflow–outflow tubular network of blood vessels. The chambers arise later (see below), in response to the need to inspire oxygen as a source of energy. For now, however, the heart is just a section of pipe, with one end formed by the convergence

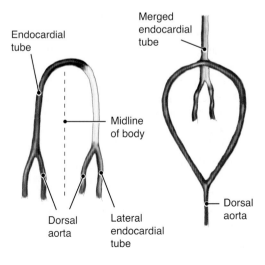

Endocardial tube

Merged endocardial tube

Midline of body

Dorsal aorta

Lateral endocardial tube

Dorsal aorta

FIGURE 1.28 **The effect of lateral folding on the cardiogenic area.**

The lateral folding of the embryo occurs along the dotted line in this figure. The beginnings of the heart and the aorta will come together, but they do not merge completely. When the embryo folds inward, these "divining rods" will merge so that the endocardial tubes become a single endocardial tube (heart), the dorsal aortae merge toward the tail but stay separate near to the heart, and the lateral endocardial tubes remain apart and become input channels to the heart.

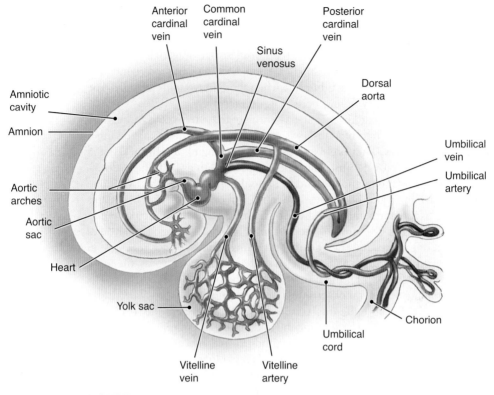

FIGURE 1.29   **Circulation in the embryo.**

Three regions are served with primary inflow and outflow tubes. The body of the embryo itself is served by the aorta pathway on each side and returns blood back to the heart through cardinal veins. The diminishing yolk sac is served by vitelline arteries and returns blood via vitelline veins. The connecting stalk delivers the vital umbilical veins to the embryo and receives embryonic outflow through the umbilical arteries. (Adapted from Sadler T. Langman's Medical Embryology, 9th Edition Image Bank. Baltimore: Lippincott Williams & Wilkins, 2003.)

of vessel tubes attracted to the merger of the endocardial tubes and the other formed by the enduring outflow pipe of the dorsal aortae (which eventually fuse into the singular aorta). Some of the cardiogenic cells cluster into nodes that transmit nerve impulses into rhythmic contractions, which is the unique property of heart muscle.

Two other aspects of cardiovascular development deserve mention at this time. One, the incipient veins that port into the new heart tube represent the logical sources of where blood must be drained in the embryo. On each side of the body is a **cardinal vein** for draining the body tissue, a **vitelline vein** for draining what is left of the yolk sac, and an **umbilical vein** for bringing in blood from the mother. These six veins transform into just two major veins (superior and inferior vena cavae) and one minor vein (coronary sinus)in the neonatal body (see below). The arterial system is much simpler, in one sense, because it all derives from a singular aorta. The second important aspect to consider is that all of this transformation is happening next to the intact coelom cavity that paralleled the cardiogenic area around the cranial end of the embryo. The cavity folds with the heart tube. This means that the heart, much like the formation of the gut tube, grows against a fluid-lined space defined by a layer of splanchnic, or visceral, mesoderm cells. We will see the tremendous clinical significance of this relationship when we revisit heart formation later in this book.

Development of the Peripheral Nerves

So far, we have seen how the **central** part of the system, the future brain and spinal cord, arise as an invagination of the ectoderm layer. This command center of ectoderm cells must maintain a physical connection to the outside world, however, and must connect to the mesoderm layer that is capable of contraction. These connections are the nerves. Anatomists refer to this part of the system as the **peripheral nervous system**, which includes everything that is not the brain and spinal cord.

The peripheral nervous system grows via an unusual type of cell called a **neuron**. This type of cell is unusual because it produces an arm-like growth called an **axon** that can achieve remarkable lengths. Many of the named nerves in gross anatomy actually are just collections of very long, single cells wrapped in supporting membranes. Neurons descend from **neural crest** cells (see above), which also contribute a great deal of the **ganglia**, or collections of nerve cell bodies, and supporting cells, such as **glial cells** and **Schwann cells**, to the system.

One way to understand how these structures develop is to consider what the peripheral nervous system must accomplish. It must sense the environment, so some nerves should reach the skin and transmit basic sensory information—pain, pressure, touch, and temperature—back to the neural tube. It must respond to the environment, so some nerves should reach the muscles that develop from mesoderm and cause them to contract. Some of the responses are under conscious control, and some are not. For example, the heart muscle contracts with no real conscious effort. Therefore, it is logical to expect that the nerves reaching the involuntary muscles of the body will be different than the nerves reaching the voluntary muscles. The nerves of involuntary contraction constitute the **autonomic nervous system**.

Other things that seem to be "actions" actually do not require the nervous system. Digestion, for example, can be thought of as the process of absorbing what you put into contact with the gut tube, or the endodermal membrane. The movement of the food matter through the tube is a result of involuntary contraction of the smooth muscles that overcoat the gut tube, but the actual absorption of molecules and compounds across the endoderm layer is a chemical process.

The animate body plan is a segmented body plan. As the mesoderm proliferates during gastrulation, it collects into those three familiar cell clusters: paraxial mesoderm, intermediate mesoderm, and lateral plate mesoderm. Recall that the paraxial mesoderm condenses as a series of blocks called somites, ultimately with some 42 to 44 pairs (Fig. 1.30). They even give the embryo a segmented appearance when viewed from the outside, and they contribute to the most obvious reflection of segmentation in the adult body—the vertebral column.

This segmentation affects the formation of the nerves that fulfill the obligations of the central nervous system tube. They emerge from it as a series of parallel, or segmented, **spinal nerves**. Because it proliferates from the top of the tube, the top of the spinal cord, the brain, is much less segmented, and the nerves that emanate from it, which are called **cranial nerves**, likewise are less uniform (Fig. 1.31). You will study the cranial nerves in great detail both in gross anatomy and other medical courses; the goal for the moment is to understand how a basic spinal nerve develops.

Because the embryo is shaped more like a general vertebrate than like an upright human, we refer to the back side as dorsal rather than posterior. Likewise, the front side is ventral rather than anterior. These traditional terms are important to grasp here, because they stay with the nomenclature of the nervous system through adulthood. Different signal pathways reside in the dorsal half of the cord compared to the ventral half of the cord. At the end of the fourth week of embryonic development, columns of

FIGURE 1.30   **Lateral view of a 5-week-old embryo.**

The column of somites emphasizes the segmented nature of the embryo at this stage. Note the already large cranial end and the undifferentiated limb buds. The peripheral nervous system abides by this segmented body plan and contacts the body surface and inner tissues through a parallel series of nerves called spinal nerves. (Reprinted with permission from Blechshmidt E. The Stages of Human Development Before Birth. Philadelphia: WB Saunders, 1961.)

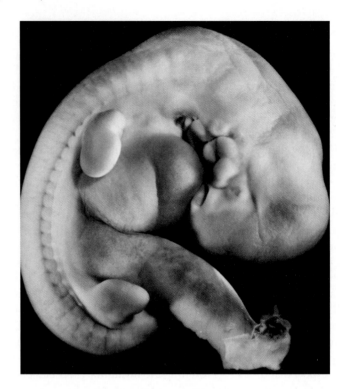

cells in these regions begin to specialize as sensory, motor, or association neurons. Begin to memorize now that the dorsal column of the spinal cord develops **association neurons** and the ventral column **motor neurons**.

The neurons of the dorsal column link the motor neurons of the ventral column to true sensory neurons that grow into the spinal cord from ganglia that arose from neural crest cells (Fig. 1.32). Technically, a **ganglion** is a collection of cell bodies outside the central nervous system. What is important to remember is that the **ganglia** (plural) of the spinal nerves arise from **neural crest cells,** which explains why the ganglia are external to the spinal cord, which was the neural tube. Sensory neurons collect at each segment of the cord in the neighborhood of the dorsal column and plug into the cord with a root called the **dorsal root. The dorsal root conducts only sensory information into the spinal cord,** where it gets routed, at least in part, through association neurons into the motor column. Anatomically, the structure that results is a root sticking out of the dorsal part of the cord and leading to a swelling of cell bodies called the **dorsal root ganglion.** Because the sensory neurons are bipolar in shape, they also have a projection that leads from the ganglion away from the spinal cord. This is also part of what is called the dorsal root.

Just as the sensory information must get into the cord, the motor response must get out of the cord. From the ventral column of cells, a root projects out of the cord in parallel to the dorsal root (see Fig. 1.32). This is logically called the **ventral root,** and it carries fibers of both the conscious motor system and the autonomic, or subconscious, motor system. As detailed later in this book, the autonomic nervous system forms **sympathetic fiber bundles** and **parasympathetic fiber bundles,** which direct the very different subconscious reactions of excitation or equilibrization, respectively. For now,

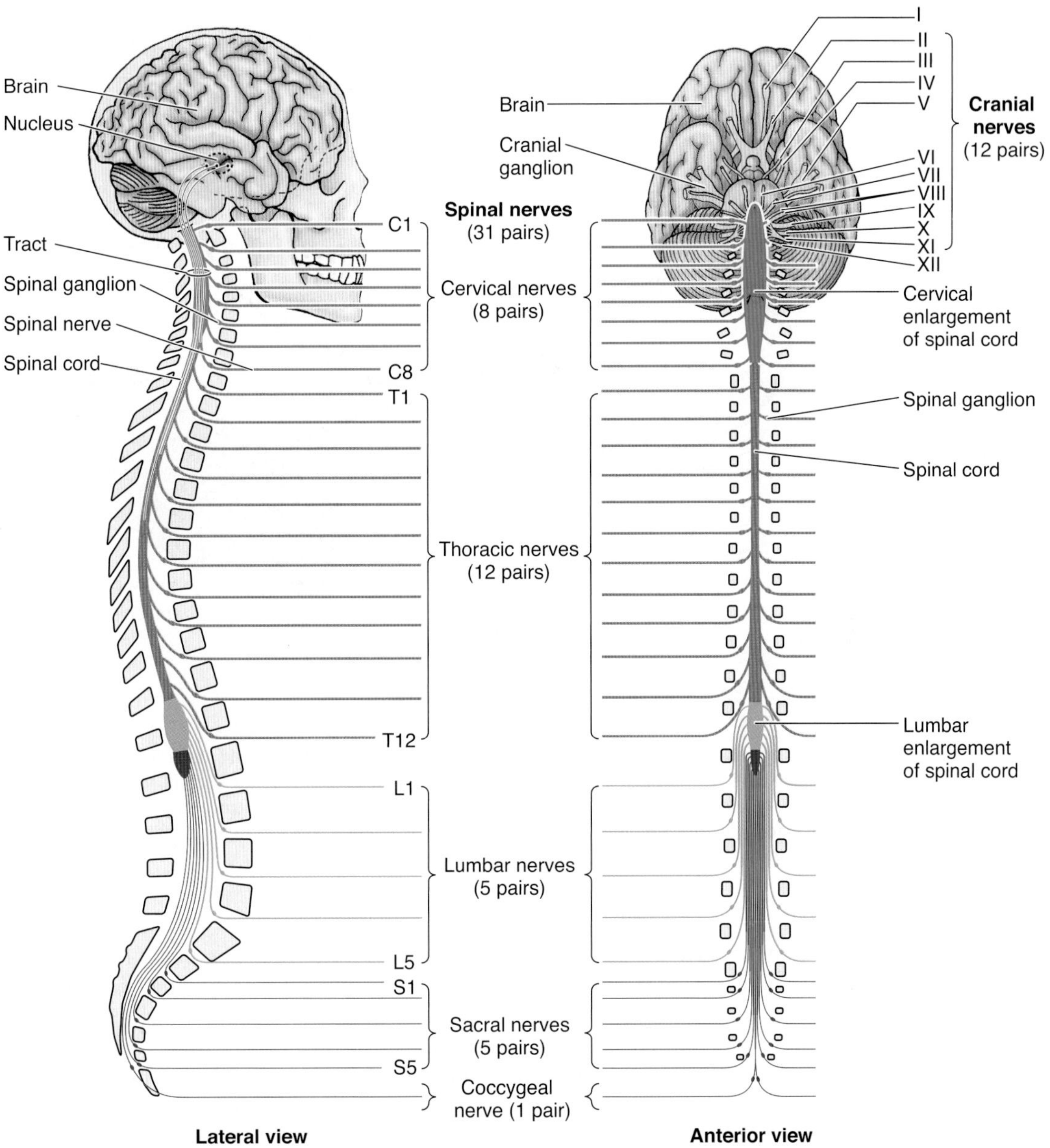

Brain
Nucleus
Tract
Spinal ganglion
Spinal nerve
Spinal cord
C1
C8
T1
T12
L1
L5
S1
S5
Spinal nerves
(31 pairs)
Cervical nerves
(8 pairs)
Thoracic nerves
(12 pairs)
Lumbar nerves
(5 pairs)
Sacral nerves
(5 pairs)
Coccygeal
nerve (1 pair)
Brain
Cranial
ganglion
I
II
III
IV
V
VI
VII
VIII
IX
X
XI
XII
Cranial
nerves
(12 pairs)
Cervical
enlargement
of spinal cord
Spinal ganglion
Spinal cord
Lumbar
enlargement
of spinal cord
Lateral view
Anterior view

FIGURE 1.31 **Spinal nerves form in parallel to the body's connective tissue segmentation.**

Twelve pairs of cranial nerves serve the motor and sensory needs of the head and neck. (From Moore KL, Dalley AF. Clinically Oriented Anatomy. 4th Edition. Baltimore, Lippincott Williams & Wilkins, 1999.)

simply realize that the cell bodies of the **sympathetic** part of this system are found in a column of cells somewhat between the dorsal and the ventral columns called the **intermediolateral cell column**. This column does not extend the entire length of the cord but, rather, is limited to the region between the first thoracic spinal nerve and the second or third lumbar spinal nerve ("**T1-L2**," a heuristic phrase worth repeating over and over again).

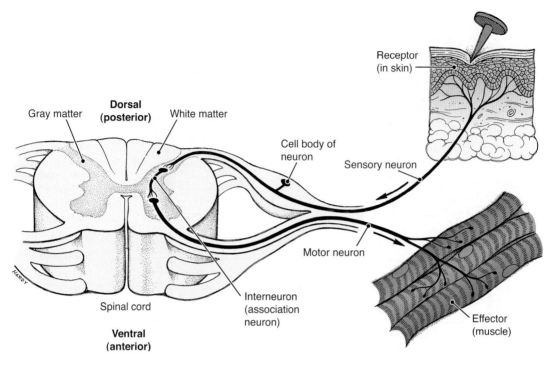

FIGURE 1.32   **Formation of a typical spinal nerve.**

Sensory information enters the spinal cord only through the dorsal root, and motor information leaves the spinal cord only through the ventral root. The roots come together into a single, wrapped bundle very near the spinal cord. From there, both motor and sensory fibers can travel together in the dorsal ramus and the ventral ramus. In gross anatomy, some of these rami are so large that they have their own individual name. (From Neil O. Hardy. Westport, CT.)

Cell bodies of the **parasympathetic** part are located in the brain (and follow some cranial nerves) or in the sacral segments of the spinal cord. Because these locations are on either side of the sympathetic cells (technically above and below them in the neural tube), the system is logically called parasympathetic. The axons of the sympathetic system and the sacral part of the parasympathetic system project out of the cord just as the voluntary motor axons do and, thus, also are found in the ventral root (see Fig. 1.32).

It makes perfect sense that nerve cells with different capacities (sensory versus motor) are separate from one another as they integrate with the central nervous system, but it would be impractical for them to keep separate routes throughout the body. Indeed, the two roots actually merge into a single bundle almost immediately. Anatomically, this takes place where the arches of the vertebral column pass by the side of the spinal cord (Fig. 1.33). This union of the dorsal root and the ventral root is sometimes called the **spinal nerve** proper. It is the first position in which both sensory and motor fibers can be found in a single bundle.

Two important things happen as the fiber bundles move from the spinal nerve proper toward the rest of the body. First, they divide into two cables, one headed dorsally and the other headed ventrally. These cables are now called the **dorsal ramus** and the **ventral ramus**, respectively. Second, the sympathetic fibers that left the cord through the ventral root now leave the spinal nerve bundle to enter their own inde-

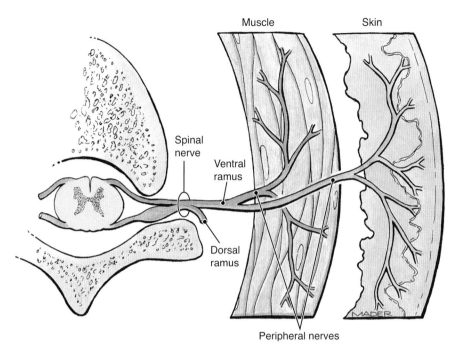

Muscle   Skin

Spinal
nerve

Ventral
ramus

Dorsal
ramus

Peripheral nerves

FIGURE 1.33   **Schematic cross-section of a spinal nerve.**

Topographically, the spinal nerve "comes together" at the intervertebral foramen, where the sensory-bearing dorsal root and the motor-bearing ventral root merge into a combined fiber bundle. (From Agur AMR, Dalley AF. Grant's Atlas of Anatomy, 11th Edition. Baltimore: Lippincott Williams & Wilkins, 2005.

pendent nerve channel structure. This is called the **sympathetic trunk**, and in the adult body it drapes like a chain or a necklace along the sides of the vertebral bodies. This is why the ganglia of the sympathetic trunk sometimes are called **paravertebral ganglia**.

Remember that neural crest cells form many of the nerve cell ganglia in the body. They also congregate to form the ganglia of the sympathetic fiber network. The ganglia, however, must connect to the spinal nerve for the sympathetic fibers to reach them and synapse. The extension of nerve fibers out of the spinal nerve and into the sympathetic ganglia is called a **white ramus communicans**, or a **white ramus**. The color term refers to the fact that this sheath of nerve cells is still coated by a myelin sheath, but in practice, you will not be able to detect the color as you dissect this region of the body.

As described below, the sympathetic nerve fibers must reach all the smooth muscle in the body, which includes the smooth muscle that lines the arteries of the body and the smooth muscle in the sweat glands of the skin. This means that some of the sympathetic fibers are better off traveling with the spinal nerve fibers, so a second communicating ramus called a **gray ramus** runs from the sympathetic ganglion back to the spinal nerve (Fig. 1.34). From here, the sympathetic fibers track along with all the nerves of the body until they can exit onto a blood vessel or sweat gland.

To reach the full extent of mesoderm, the spinal nerve develops very economically. Rather than move out in an infinite number of independent fibers toward the dermis and muscle cells, the spinal nerve fibers link to the precursor mesoderm cell clusters before those adult structures form. Spinal nerves link into somites while they

FIGURE 1.34   **Distribution of a typical spinal nerve.**

Each ramus carries motor and sensory fibers, but the ventral rami canvas a much larger part of the body. Fibers that carry sympathetic impulse from the spinal cord gather outside the spinal nerve in a chain of ganglia, from which they route to their targets either directly or back through the course of a spinal nerve ramus. (From Stedman's Medical Dictionary, 27th edition. Baltimore: Lippincott Williams & Wilkins, 2000.)

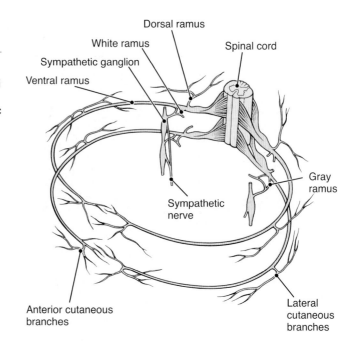

are still somites. As the somite differentiates into a sclerotome and a dermomyotome, the spinal nerve dedicates itself to the future of the dermomyotome. It has not traveled a long distance, and it links into the cell cluster in time to be carried with it throughout the body. For this reason, the pattern of somatic (or body) motor and sensory innervation is segmental. Mastering the basic segmental plan of skin innervation is essential for proper physical diagnosis and effective clinical evaluation of the patient.

Recall that the dermomyotome of each segmental somite divides into two unequal halves (revisit Fig. 1.26). One half is becoming the dermis and musculature that serves the vertebral column exclusively; this is the **epimere**. The other larger half is becoming the dermis and musculature that serve the body wall from the transverse process of the vertebra all the way around to the front of the body; this is the **hypomere**. The spinal nerve links into the dermomyotome at this moment; therefore, it has a separate link into the growing epimere and into the growing hypomere (see Fig. 1.34). The connections between the spinal nerve proper and the epimeric and hypomeric mesoderm cell clusters are thus called the **dorsal ramus** and **ventral ramus**, respectively.

Be careful to distinguish between root and ramus as you study. The dorsal and ventral roots carry fibers of a particular function, or modality. The **dorsal root** is **sensory**, and the **ventral root** is **motor**. The dorsal ramus and ventral ramus, however, are mixed bundles—they each carry sensory and motor fibers. This naming scheme is easy to confuse. You will want to master it, however, because of its relevance to victims of spinal nerve injury. An injury to a ramus will have different signs and symptoms than an injury to the corresponding root, even though they are only millimeters from one another in the anatomy of the vertebral column/spinal cord.

In the adult, the dorsal ramus is considerably smaller than the ventral ramus, because the amount of the body that grows from the hypomeric cell cluster is much greater than the amount that grows from the epimeric cell cluster. This directly reflects the animate body plan. Basic animate life forms are segmental, in keeping with the somite plan. For many of them, movement is limited to a basic contraction or expansion of the linear segments, much like a worm or anemone. The advent of limbs in

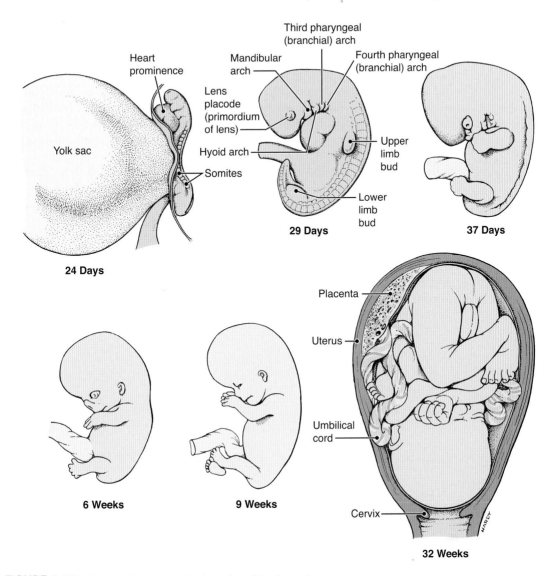

FIGURE 1.35   **Progressive stages of embryonic and fetal maturity.**

Lateral views. (Reprinted with permission from Blechshmidt E. The Stages of Human Development Before Birth. Philadelphia: WB Saunders, 1961; from Sadler T. Langman's Medical Embryology, 9th Edition Image Bank. Baltimore: Lippincott Williams & Wilkins, 2003.)

more complex animals enables a much greater range of possible motions. These limbs, as described below, emerge from the hypomeric part of the body wall, so given the amount of cells that have to be served, the ventral ramus going to the hypomere will carry most of the nerve fibers that are bundled together in the spinal nerve proper. Very few dorsal rami are given individual names in gross anatomy. Ventral rami, however, achieve a large caliber, travel great distances, and render major symptoms when injured, so they usually receive specific names (e.g., radial nerve or sciatic nerve).

This book gives some parts of the developing body more attention than others. This should convey to you how important it is to know those parts very well conceptually. The anatomic design of the nervous system is one of those areas about which everything you learn will be useful at one time or another.

From this basic body plan, we must develop the interacting systems of the body. As mammals, we must develop some means of drawing air into our bodies and absorbing oxygen from it. More generally, we must develop a digestive system for absorbing energy from the environment. We must develop structures that enable us to eliminate the waste products that are left over from consuming the environment. We must elaborate some structures for reproducing ourselves. We must develop projections of our body that help us move about in the world, and as humans, these projections will be slightly different in the upper half (arms) compared to the lower half (legs). Last but not least, we must elaborate the part of our body that holds the top of the neural tube and the inlet for the absorbing pathway—the head and neck. The anatomies that result are best understood in terms of the processes of their growth (Fig. 1.35).

To keep the study of gross anatomy as efficient as possible, this text now moves from a description of ectoderm, endoderm, and mesoderm to a systemic, or system-by-system, approach. Within each system, you will study how the components complete development, and you will study the logic of how the components are arranged and named. Remember that the goal here is to master the organization of the body so that you can put the specific regional details into a logical and stimulating context.

2

Cardiovascular System

INTRODUCTION

The body must somehow deliver expendable energy to its living tissues. One surface of the embryo—the endoderm—grows into a surface for absorbing oxygen and a surface for absorbing particulate matter (food). These useful materials are routed to the body tissues by a **circulatory system**. The circulatory system is driven by a very hardworking muscular pump—the **heart**—and reaches the tissues through ever-narrowing channels called **arteries** and **capillaries**. Blood that is depleted of its oxygen and other nutrients returns to the heart through a passive system of collecting **veins**. Tissues and the spaces between them contain other fluids, principally water. A specialized network of ducts and nodes called the **lymphatic system** attends to these fluids and to infections and foreign bodies that invade the bloodstream. Lymphatic channels are similar in design to the venous system and track them closely throughout the body; ultimately, all lymphatic drainage in the body empties into the large veins near the heart. Early formation of the heart and blood tubes was described earlier. We now resume the story of how the heart and great vessels form.

HEART FORMATION

The heart tube that formed during the embryonic fold now lies atop the migrated septum transversum and between the two developing lung buds. Like the lung buds and the gut tube, it pushes against a closed sac of fluid—in this case, the **pericardial sac**. The pericardial sac is the product of the division of the intraembryonic coelom by the pleuropericardial folds. Remember that the "top" of the "horseshoe" of the embryonic cavity bends "downward" during longitudinal folding. The pleuropericardial folds isolate the part of the cavity that is adjacent to the heart, and this becomes the pericardial sac.

The pleuropericardial folds never go away, of course. They persist as a "curtain" of tissue between the heart (and its sac) and the lungs (and their sacs) (Fig. 2.1). In the adult, this curtain virtually fuses with the outer layer of the pericardial sac, which makes the heart look like it is pressed against a single sac. The **fibrous pericardium** is the part that is derived from the pleuropericardial folds and is the "outer" layer of the sac. The **serous pericardium** is the original pericardial sac. The fibrous pericardium is generally sensitive, which is relevant to how people experience chest pain related to heart ailments. It also is somewhat fixed in space, given its fusion to the diaphragm, sternum, and great vessels. Its inelasticity aggravates pressures that might build up in the pericardial sac, such as a **cardiac tamponade**. (See Clinical Anatomy Box 2.1).

The heart tube must dedicate some of its effort to getting blood out of the regular lines (think **systemic circulation** here) and into the refueling tubes (think **pulmonary circulation** here). That is, blood must be siphoned out of the body circulation and exposed to the oxygen that is inspired into the lungs, and blood must then be returned to the heart for pumping out through the outflow tube (**aorta**). The heart tube accomplishes this anatomic detouring by first dilating and constricting parts of its walls to

FIGURE 2.1   **Division of the coelom in the thoracic cavity.**

The pleuropericardial fold that migrates inward from the body wall to divide the pleural sac from the pericardial sac stays intact during growth and becomes a "curtain" between the two sacs. For better or worse, it is called the fibrous pericardium, and as the heart matures, the outer layer of its own pericardial sac virtually fuses with the adjacent fibrous pericardium.

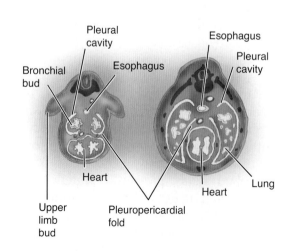

Pleural cavity

Esophagus

Pleural cavity

Bronchial bud

Esophagus

Heart

Upper limb bud

Pleuropericardial fold

Heart

Lung

CLINICAL ANATOMY

Box 2.1

CARDIAC TAMPONADE

The heart grows against a fluid-lined pericardial sac, and together they press against the remnant of the pleuropericardial membrane, the fibrous pericardium. The fibrous pericardium is anchored to surrounding connective tissue, such as the sternum, diaphragm, great vessels, and vertebrae. It is not very elastic. If fluid accumulates in the pericardial sac, the building pressure is more likely to compress the heart muscle than to distort the fibrous pericardium. This leads to a life-threatening condition called cardiac tamponade. If the pressure is not relieved, it ultimately "suffocates" the ability of the heart to contract.

Cardiac Tamponade

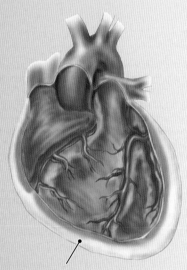

Fluid buildup within pericardial sac puts pressure on the heart, which may prevent it from pumping effectively

form initial "front-to-back" chambers. The chamber closer to the aorta becomes a **ventricle**, and the one closer to the inflow end becomes an **atrium**. So, the first step is simply to bulge out the two basic chambers, with no rerouting of blood. To make room for all this growth, the tube folds on itself, which brings the outflow end closer to the bottom of the pericardial space and the inflow end closer to the top. This requires that the inflow end somehow punctures or slips by the developing **septum transversum**. This is why the **inferior vena cava** appears to poke through the **diaphragm**.

The heart tube then "buds off" some of itself to serve the lungs by self-dividing into right and left halves, with the left halves representing the essential continuation of the original tube (Fig. 2.2). The right halves adopt the new responsibility of gathering

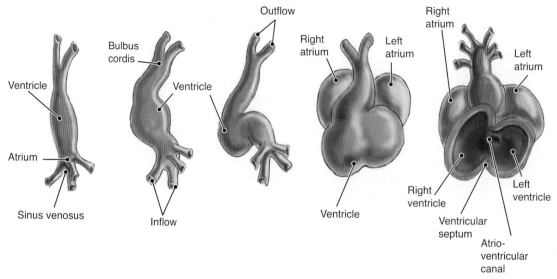

FIGURE 2.2   **The heart tube.**

During its early stages, the heart is a tube with an input end and an output end. The tube expands and curls up on itself to stay contained in the mediastinum. Expansion of the heart tube takes the form of a small atrium and a large ventricle, with a constricted area between them. These early chambers play the obvious role of receiving blood (atrium), then pumping it vigorously onward through a contraction of the expanded ventricular muscle. Because we are air-breathing creatures, the heart tube will soon divide itself into parallel right and left chambers to divert the incoming blood to the lungs before receiving it back again and pumping it through to the aorta. (Adapted from Snell RS. Clinical Anatomy, 7th Edition. Baltimore: Lippincott Williams & Wilkins, 2003.)

blood for distribution to the lungs. This is why the **right atrium** receives deoxygenated blood from the body and the **right ventricle** pumps it out to the lungs. The **left atrium** still receives oxygenated blood, just as it did from the mother when it was the inflow end of the heart tube, but this time from its own body. The **left ventricle** pumps oxygenated blood out through the aorta, just as the original ventricle did.

The heart tube dilated and constricted to form the original atrium and ventricle. The constriction that separated the two persists as the tube pinches off a set of "side" (right) chambers. Proliferation of cells adjacent to the constriction puffs the heart wall into an endocardial cushion (Fig. 2.3). Through this simple "massing" or "crowding" process, the narrow opening between the original atrium and ventricle (and, subsequently, between the right and left atria and ventricles) is maintained. In the maturing heart, the area where the cushions swell is called the **intermediate septum**. Because it is located "dead center" in the heart tube, it also must help to separate the two atria from one another and the two ventricles from one another. In principle, this seems no more complicated than keeping the "upper half" (the atria) separate from the "lower half" (the ventricles), but it is this effort that most frequently results in failure and congenital heart defects. For this reason, pay close attention to how the atria close off the wall between them and how the ventricles keep themselves separate. This helps to explain the relatively common heart defects known as **patent foramen ovale** and **ventricular septal defect** (VSD). (See Clinical Anatomy Box 2.2.)

The lungs mature, and the heart conforms to them, long before the fetus needs to breathe in its own oxygen. The fetal lung lacks the pressure gradient necessary to drive blood back to the heart through the **pulmonary veins**, so the fetal heart keeps a

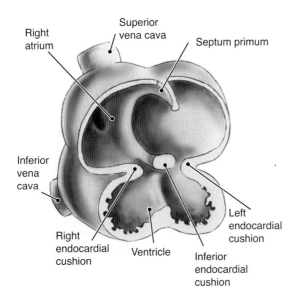

Right
atrium

Superior
vena cava

Septum primum

Inferior
vena
cava

Right
endocardial
cushion

Ventricle

Inferior
endocardial
cushion

Left
endocardial
cushion

**FIGURE 2.3   The heart
septates into chambers.**

The heart's own wall grows inward
to form a center-point boundary
pillar between the atrium and the
ventricle. This ingrowth is the
endocardial cushion. It still allows
a narrow communication between
the atrium and ventricle, and it
becomes an attachment point for
later growths that separate the
atrium and ventricle into right and
left halves.

channel open between the right and left atria until birth. In this way, blood that enters the fetal right atrium from the body can shunt straight across to the left atrium without going down through the right ventricle and to the lungs. This blood contains a large amount of oxygen anyway, because it began as richly oxygenated blood entering the fetus from the maternal circulation and routing straight to the heart. This blood then shunts from the right atrium to the left atrium, where the derivatives of the original heart tube pump it out to the rest of the fetal body through the aorta. The shunt from the right to left atria is provided by the way that the separating wall forms.

The wall separating the two atria begins to form as a flap of heart wall from the top of the atrial chamber down to the intermediate septum (Fig. 2.4). This flap is not a solid flap, however. It has a gaping hole just off-center. Soon, a second flap begins to form just to the right of the first flap, but it too has a gaping hole—in this case, just off-center in the opposite direction. The result is a "wall" between the two atria that is formed by two flaps, each of which has a hole in it. The holes do not directly overlap, but blood pressure that builds when the right atrium fills up forces blood through the hole in the right flap. This blood pushes against the left flap, finds its way through the hole in the left flap, and from there, pours into the chamber of the left atrium (Fig. 2.5). Interestingly, little reflux of blood back into the right atrium occurs, because the pressure gradient in the left atrium is relieved as soon as the collected blood drops from there into the left ventricle.

The hole in the atrial flap is called the **foramen ovale**. In normal development, the two flaps fuse together at birth, and the hole in one flap is "sealed" by the solid tissue of the other flap. This leaves a depression in the fused atrial septum called a **fossa ovalis**. In abnormal development, the atrial septum does not fuse, and the two holes permit blood to travel from the right atrium to the left atrium. This persistence of a foramen ovale is called **patent foramen ovale**, and it debilitates the newborn's ability to oxygenate its own blood sufficiently.

The story in the ventricles is similar in the sense that a wall grows from the perimeter of the chamber (the lower wall of the ventricle) toward the intermediate septum. In this case, however, it is a single wall, not two flaps. The single wall is called the **interventricular septum**, and it starts out as a very muscular and substantial barrier between the two ventricles (Fig. 2.6). As it nears its completion, however, it grows thinner, and

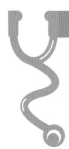

CLINICAL ANATOMY

Box 2.2

COMMON CONGENITAL HEART DEFECTS

Atrial Septal Defects

Failure of the foramen ovale to close into a fossa ovalis occurs in approximately 0.64 per 1,000 births. Oxygenated blood shunts from the left atrium to the right atrium after birth because of higher pressure on the left side. This enlarges the right atrium and ventricle and dilates the pulmonary trunk. Depending on the severity of the patency, this condition can go undetected or be largely asymptomatic in the absence of vigorous physical exertion.

Ventricular Septal Defects

Full closure of the interventricular septum is also a complex process. Failure of the septum to close occurs in 1.2 per 1,000 births, making it the most common congenital cardiac defect. This results in blood shunting from the higher-pressure left ventricle to the lower-pressure right ventricle. A large defect can lead to an overworked right ventricle, pulmonary disease (e.g., hypertension from backed-up flow), and ultimately, cardiac failure. Ventricular septal defect can be repaired surgically.

Tetralogy of Fallot

Congenital anomalies often occur in clusters and not in isolation. Four interrelated anomalies of heart development occur together in approximately 1 per 1,000 births: pulmonary stenosis, ventricular septal defect, overriding aorta, and right ventricular hypertrophy (tetralogy of Fallot). This cluster makes it very difficult for the heart to pump blood effectively, but if detected early enough, it can be corrected surgically. The primary presentation in the baby is peripheral cyanosis on exertion—a "Tet spell"—such as after an episode of aggressive crying.

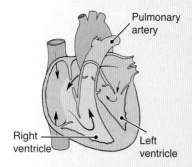

Atrial septal defect

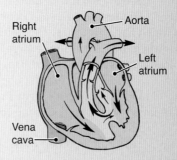

Ventricular septal defect

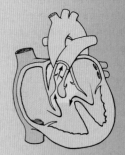

Tetralogy of Fallot

(From Neil O. Hardy. Westport, CT.)

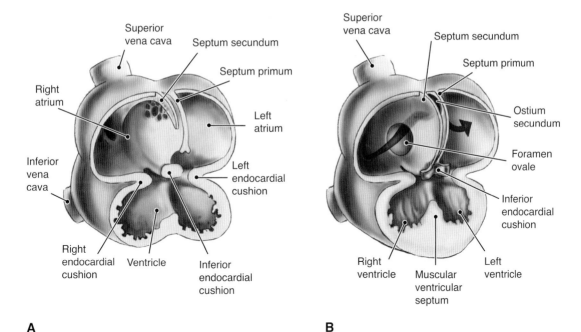

A   **B**

FIGURE 2.4   **Atrial formation.**

A septum grows down the middle of the atrium to separate it into right and left atria. This is an interesting and complicated process (**A**), because the first septum is incomplete, and the second septum is also incomplete (but in a different place). This results in a "two-flap" design that allows some blood to move from the right atrium to the left atrium (**B,** red arrow). Because the fetal heart is not transpiring oxygen into the pulmonary circulation, this is tolerated until birth. With the change in pulmonary pressure at birth (as the lungs first fill with air), these two flaps usually fuse together, and the slight opening from the right to the left side is obliterated. The slight gap in the septa is called a foramen ovale; the correctly fused septum after birth converts the foramen to a fossa.

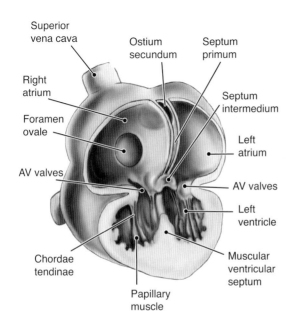

FIGURE 2.5   **Completion of the interatrial septum.**

At first, the septum between the atria forms loosely, to permit shunting of blood from right to left, and after birth, it permanently fuses. Note the simultaneous changes in the ventricle area. AV = atrioventricular.

FIGURE 2.6   **Formation of the ventricles.**

A process similar to atrial septa-tion takes place in the ventricle. The heart wall migrates up toward the endocardial cushion. The bottom half of the septum is thicker than the top half.

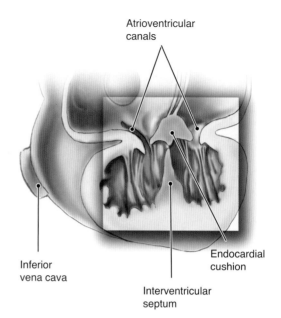

Atrioventricular canals

Endocardial cushion

Inferior vena cava

Interventricular septum

in some cases, it fails to reach the intermediate septum. This leaves at the least a very weak barrier between the two ventricles and typically a fully patent gap between them. This condition is called a **ventricular septal defect** (VSD), and it is the **most common cardiac defect at birth**.

The transformation of the heart tube extends beyond the heart into both the inflow and outflow portions of the tube. The inflow part of the heart tube burrows into part of the new right atrium. As it burrows, it becomes part of the wall of the right atrium. This explains why the inner lining of the right atrium contains a muscular part and a "smooth" part. The smooth part represents where the inflow tube invaded the atrium, and it will lead to the two big veins that empty into the right atrium: the **superior vena cava**, and the **inferior vena cava**. The left atrium also contains a large, smooth-walled surface and a small "ear-flap" of muscular tissue. In this atrium, the smooth surface is the result of **pulmonary veins** growing into the atrial wall and "pushing" the incidental mus-cular tissue aside (Fig. 2.7).

The superior vena cava and inferior vena cava drain all parts of the body **except the heart muscle itself**. The heart has a dedicated vein called the **coronary sinus** that forms at the same time as the great body veins. As the original inflow part of the tube is migrating against the atrium, a portion of it drapes around the heart tube and "degenerates," or transforms, into a vein of service to the heart muscle. In the adult heart, the coronary sinus cinches the "waist" of the heart along the posterior border between the atria and the ventricles.

The outflow portion of the heart tube undergoes an even more extensive transfor-mation as the embryo folds and the mesoderm around the top end of the neural tube and the endodermal tube proliferates to form a head and neck. In concept, this out-flow tube must get blood that is leaving the heart to go to the lungs for "refueling," then retrieve it from the heart for distribution to the entire body. It is safe to assume that the body distribution will need dedicated arteries on the right and left sides of the body for distribution to the head, the trunk, and the extremities. Because the trunk forms first, the original outflow continuation of the heart tube, the **aorta**, primarily serves the trunk. Detours from the aorta will serve the body regions that mature later (the head and extremities). For now, let us try to appreciate how the arteries get to this point.

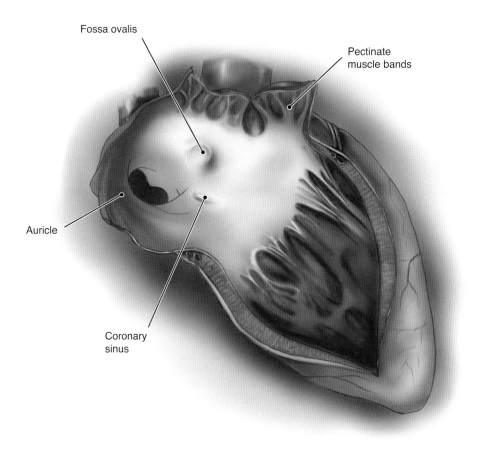

Fossa ovalis

Pectinate
muscle bands

Auricle

Coronary
sinus

FIGURE 2.7   **Internal topology of the heart chambers.**

Because the veins leading to the heart grow into the wall of the original atria, the lining on the inside
is smooth rather than muscular. Most of the actual atrial chamber is the end of the veins that dump
into it. The original muscular structure is pushed to the side as the auricle. The muscular ribbons on
the inside surface of the atrium are referred to as pectinate muscles. Note also the shallow depression in the back wall of the atrium; this is the fossa ovalis, the obliterated foramen ovale between the
right and left atrium. (Adapted from Smeltzer SCO, Bare BG. Brunner and Suddarth's Textbook of
Medical-Surgical Nursing, 9th Edition. Philadelphia: Lippincott Williams & Wilkins, 2002.)

Start with the very base of the outflow tube, where the original ventricle becomes
the aorta. In the embryo, this region is called the **truncus arteriosus**. As the ventricle
dilates and divides into two ventricles, the truncus arteriosus likewise grows in on
itself—a septum that begins as an ingrowth of the wall, much like the original division
of the foregut tube and the respiratory diverticulum. Indeed, the similarity is more than
coincidental. As the foregut pinches off a bud that becomes the lung, the blood supply that originally served this part of the foregut must go with it. Because of embryonic
folding, that blood supply is very close to the heart, which migrated in the longitudinal
fold to be right next to the developing lungs. So, as the foregut parents a respiratory
sac, the heart chambers parent a right-side atrium and ventricle, and above the ventricles, the once-single outflow tube parents a **pulmonary trunk** to stay with the right
ventricle and serve the lung buds (Fig. 2.8).

One interesting "twist" to this story is that the truncus arteriosus does just that—
it twists—as it is dividing. The result is that the mature pulmonary trunk outflow of

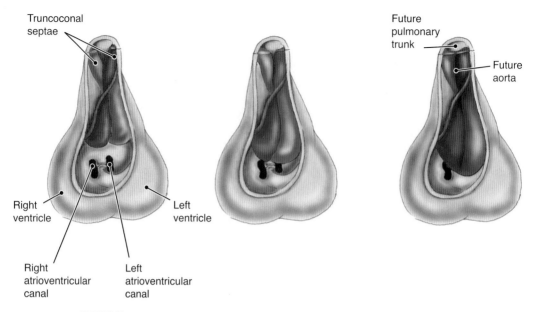

Truncoconal septae

Future pulmonary trunk

Future aorta

Right ventricle

Left ventricle

Right atrioventricular canal

Left atrioventricular canal

FIGURE 2.8   **The outflow path from the heart also septates.**

Unlike the other cardiac septa, the septum that continues into the outflow tube spirals, which explains why the adult aorta appears to arise behind the pulmonary trunk but then arch forward, over it, and then behind it again. (From Sadler T. Langman's Medical Embryology, 9th Edition Image Bank. Baltimore: Lippincott Williams & Wilkins, 2003.)

the right ventricle appears to twist around and underneath the ascending aorta outflow of the left ventricle. Once again, development explains the gross anatomy. Another interesting parallel in arterial development is the persistent communication between the pulmonary trunk and the aorta during fetal growth. Remember that the two atria stay in communication with one another until birth, because the fetal blood is not oxygenated in the fetal lung. Although a pulmonary trunk forms to route blood from the right ventricle to the lungs, this route also is unnecessary until the fetus is birthed and begins to breathe. In the meantime, blood in the pulmonary trunk can escape through a persistent duct that links it to the ascending aorta, the **ductus arteriosus** (Fig. 2.9). Like the foramen ovale, this duct usually closes over at birth, resulting in a remnant ligament, the **ligamentum arteriosum**. When this duct fails to close over (a **patent ductus arteriosus**), the newborn heart will back up with oxygenated blood and work much harder to get the volume through the pulmonary circuit. (See Clinical Anatomy Box 2.3.)

The respiratory system of vertebrates is a modification of the absorbing layer of the embryo—the endoderm. Indeed, air-breathing vertebrates derived from "water-breathing" ancestors that obtained oxygen from the aqueous medium in which they lived. They accomplished this through a system of gill slits in their neck region. In these animals, the embryonic outflow portion of the heart tube splits into dedicated arteries for each slit—the **branchial arch** or the **pharyngeal arch**. These arteries coalesce into a dorsal aorta above and behind the gills (Fig. 2.10). In air-breathing vertebrates, a similar network of arches develops along the aorta, but obviously we do not develop gills. This network must transform into the asymmetric configuration of the major arteries.

In its original state, the aorta does divide into five pharyngeal arches just beyond the heart before coalescing back into a single "descending," or thoracic and abdomi-

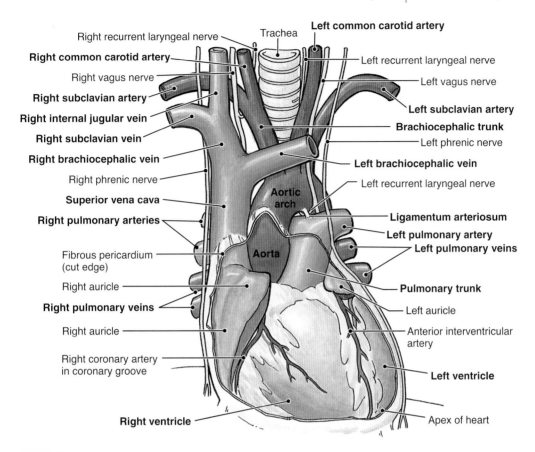

Right recurrent laryngeal nerve
Trachea
Left common carotid artery

Right common carotid artery
Left recurrent laryngeal nerve

Right vagus nerve
Left vagus nerve

Right subclavian artery
Left subclavian artery

Right internal jugular vein
Brachiocephalic trunk

Right subclavian vein
Left phrenic nerve

Right brachiocephalic vein
Left brachiocephalic vein

Right phrenic nerve
Left recurrent laryngeal nerve

Superior vena cava
Aortic arch

Right pulmonary arteries
Ligamentum arteriosum

Left pulmonary artery

Fibrous pericardium (cut edge)
Aorta
Left pulmonary veins

Right auricle
Pulmonary trunk

Right pulmonary veins
Left auricle

Right auricle
Anterior interventricular artery

Right coronary artery in coronary groove
Left ventricle

Right ventricle
Apex of heart

FIGURE 2.9   **The adult configuration of the great vessels.**

Note the band of tissue that connects the pulmonary trunk and the arch of the aorta. This is the liga-mentum arteriosum, a withered remnant of a formerly open connection between the two tubes. Note how the ligament appears to trap a nerve that curls around the arch of the aorta. (From Moore KL, Agur AM. Essential Clinical Anatomy, 3rd Edition. Baltimore: Lippincott Williams & Wilkins, 2007.)

nal, aorta (Fig. 2.11). Instead of persisting as gill slit arteries, the aortic arches become incorporated into the fates of the arch mesoderm. Because the portion of the aorta that forms the arch in the first place is the portion that precedes the "descent" into the tho-rax and abdomen along the vertebral column, these incorporations must somehow involve getting blood to the head, neck, and upper limbs. This is a complicated process—and one of the few in the development of the body that is not perfectly sym-metric. Some arch arteries disintegrate entirely, some merge with each other, and some elongate as they mature. You can appreciate this asymmetry by realizing that as the aorta arches and descends, it also drifts from right to left. In fact, it drifts so much that a single big branch is needed just to get blood from the aorta over to the right so that it can be divided into the dedicated arteries of the head and the upper limb. This extending branch is called the **brachiocephalic trunk**. On the left side of the body, the artery of the head and neck (the **carotid**) and the artery of the upper limb (the **subclavian**) each come directly off the aorta. This asymmetry is one product of aortic arch transformation. Connection of the pulmonary trunk to the pulmonary arteries is another logical product, because the ancestral aortic arches served the oxygenating

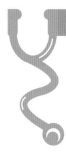

CLINICAL ANATOMY

Box 2.3
PATENT DUCTUS ARTERIOSUS

The maternal–fetal relationship alleviates the fetal circulatory system from oxygenating its own blood. At birth, the pressure gradient shifts abruptly, and this shock transition induces a remnant shunt between the pulmonary and systemic vessels to shrivel into a withered cord (the ligamentum arteriosum). When this remnant shunt fails to wither, the high pressure in the systemic tube forces blood back into the lower-pressure pulmonary tube, which ultimately causes the heart to work harder to achieve good circulation.

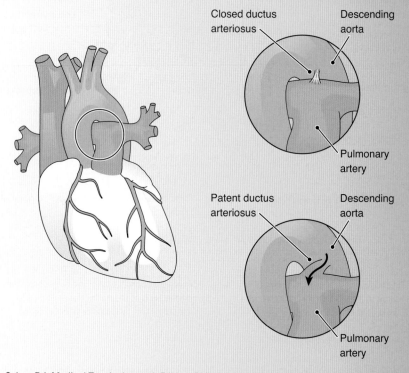

(From Cohen BJ. Medical Terminology, 4th Edition. Philadelphia: Lippincott Williams & Wilkins, 2003.)

mechanism of the original gills. As the aortic arches transform, pieces of some of them stay connected to the respiratory service.

Changes in Circulation at Birth

Consider the needs of the embryo and fetus. During the early stages, a system must get nutrients from its own feed bag (the yolk sac) into its tissues. This system consists of the **vitelline veins** (one on each side of the connecting stalk). Another system must get oxygenated blood from the mother into the fetal tissues, because the fetus is not breathing oxygen for itself. This system consists of the **umbilical veins** (again, one on each

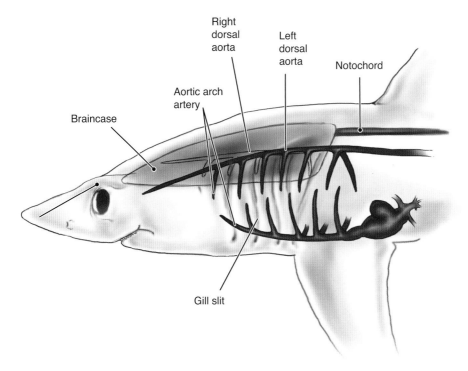

FIGURE 2.10   **Primitive design of the aortic arches.**

The human pattern of circulation beyond the heart derives from a basic water-breathing vertebrate plan in which the aorta branches into arches around the neck region to exchange gases with the water medium that flowed over gill slits in the endodermal tube. Mammals, including humans, modify this system of arches during fetal development. This explains, in part, why the pulmonary trunk exists, why the aorta arches toward the back left side, and why the aorta has three main branches directed toward the head and upper limbs.

side of the connecting stalk, or umbilical cord). And another system must route this nutrient and oxygenated blood throughout the fetal tissues and, in the process, exchange it for depleted carrier cells. This system consists of the **aortic outflow** and **cardinal vein inflow** plugged into the muscular heart tube on opposite ends. What happens to them all at birth? (See Fig. 2.12.)

You should expect that the cardinal veins and aortic circulation persist, because they developed from, by, and for the fetal body. You should expect that the umbilical veins will disappear or find another use, because they had a more limited function that, at birth, is assumed by a different part of the body (the lungs). And you should expect that the vitelline veins wither and disintegrate, because the embryo quickly exhausts its own yolk sac. Indeed, this is very close to what actually happens.

Before birth, the right umbilical vein routed directly to the heart. During gestation it degenerates, leaving the task of placental circulation delivery to the left umbilical vein alone. The left umbilical vein reaches the fetal heart by navigating from the **umbilicus** through the other large organ of development, the **liver**. In part, it skips past the liver by emptying into the **ductus venosus**, which shunts directly into the part of the **cardinal vein** system that is becoming the **inferior vena cava**. The point to remember is that maternal blood passes into and between the lobes of the liver. At birth, what remains of the left umbilical vein withers, along with the ductus venosus, into a soft ligament that binds the abdominal wall to the inferior vena cava. This is called the

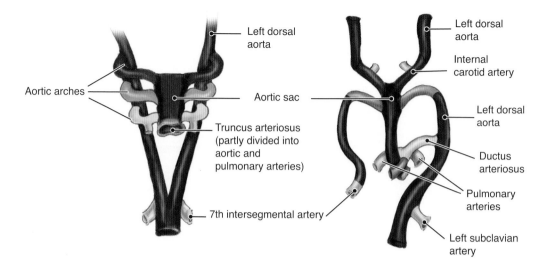

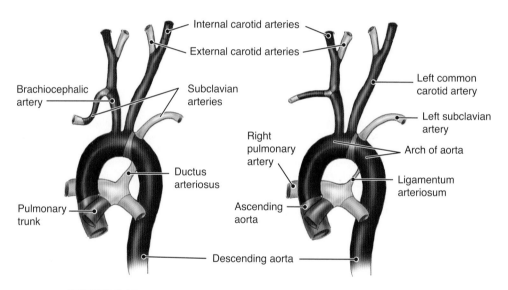

FIGURE 2.11   **Transformation of the aortic arches.**

This schematic shows how the original outflow tube of the heart septates and then transforms its vertebrate arch pattern into a mammalian pattern. Despite this complicated transformation, developmental mistakes are rare—certainly more rare than are congenital heart defects.

round ligament of the liver, because it appears to go from the inside of the umbilicus right into the crack between the two liver lobes (Fig. 2.13).

For this umbilical vein to reach the ductus venosus, it must deal with the **ventral mesentery** of the foregut, which would appear to present a curtain-like barrier against anything trying to reach the back of the abdominal wall (where the inferior vena cava is located) from the front. Indeed, the very existence of the ventral mesentery is what permits this vital connection between mother and fetus. The mesentery is a double layer of peritoneal membrane, with a potential space between the two. The left umbilical vein travels in that potential space, and when it withers at birth, it forms a cord-like ligament that defines the lower border of the mature mesentery.

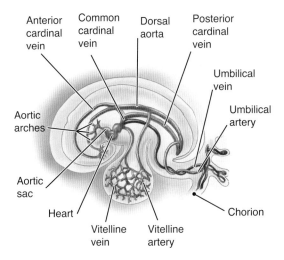

A

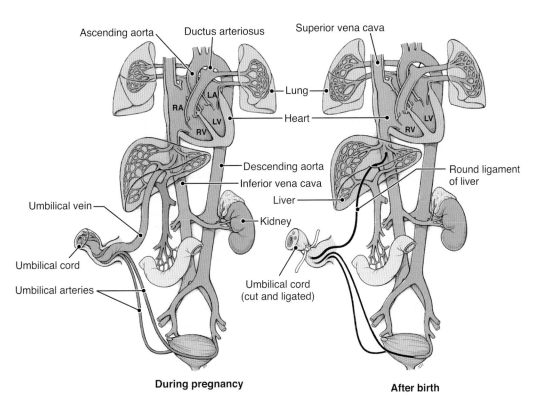

B

FIGURE 2.12   Circulatory routes during gestation (A) and changes at birth (B).

At birth, the connections between mother and fetus are severed, literally. The umbilical arteries and veins wither into ligamentous cords. By that time, the yolk sac has diminished to a trivial unit, and portions of the vitelline vessels transform into parts of other major vessels. The introduction of atmospheric oxygen to the newborn lung leads to mechanical closure of the foramen ovale and withering of the shunt between the pulmonary trunk and the aorta. LA = left atrium; LV = left ventricle; RA = right atrium; RV = right ventricle. (From Sadler TW. Langman's Medical Embryology, 10th Edition. Baltimore: Lippincott Williams & Wilkins, 2006. Figures 12.46, p.190, and 12.47, p. 192.)

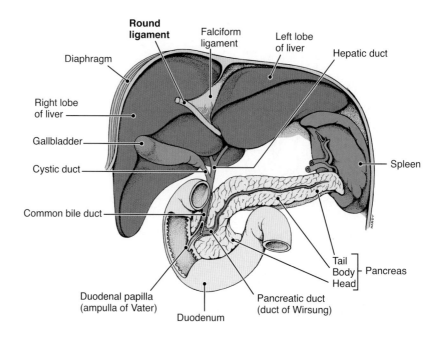

FIGURE 2.13   **Fetal circulation remnants.**

In the adult state, the ventral mesentery reflects off of the liver and to the anterior wall of the abdomen; this is shown at the very top of this picture. The "bottom" of this ventral mesentery is a round cord of fibrofatty tissue, called the round ligament of the liver, that is the remnant of the left umbilical vein. The fetal circulatory system is dynamic, true to mesodermal tissue planes, and persistent in the adult body—even if in withered form. (From Neil O.Hardy, Westport, CT. *Stedman's Medical Dictionary*, 28th Edition. Baltimore: Lippincott Williams & Wilkins, 2006.)

As the yolk sac is exhausted, the vitelline veins become absorbed, in part, in the substance of the liver, and the left vitelline vein loses its connection to the heart. The right vitelline vein persists as an important "last few centimeters" of the **inferior vena cava** between the liver and the heart. It also persists below the liver as a gathering vein for the vessels that drain the gut tube. This is important, because it becomes the only route for the venous blood of the gut tube to reach the heart. Thus, it carries everything that the gut tube has absorbed from the outside world. Before reaching the heart, this blood should go through a toxicity screen. The **right vitelline vein** below the liver becomes the **portal vein**, the critical shunt from the gut tube to the liver for the processing of absorbed compounds before the blood reaches the heart.

The closed system of circulation is centered by a "self-contracting" pump of cardiac muscle called the **heart**. The original outflow direction tube branches into a series of arteries and then capillaries, which release their nutrient content through diffusion of blood across tissue membranes. Pools of spent fluid are drawn into complementary capillary networks that steadily converge into larger and larger caliber veins, which by definition carry blood back toward the heart (the original inflow direction parts of the tube).

THE ADULT HEART

The heart is a remarkable muscle for an organ—and a remarkable organ for a muscle. Entire fields of medicine are devoted to studying and caring for something that is preprogrammed to run the same way for decades and that is nearly impossible to fix when it breaks. The gross anatomy is conceptually very simple but is visually intricate. The heart also is one of the most individual structures of the body, which is to say that it looks, relatively, quite different from person to person. You can study one or two examples of the biceps brachii muscle and get a good command of its gross anatomy, but the heart is different. Use the time in laboratory to study all the hearts in the room.

As noted above, the heart is the muscular bulge of the central part of the original circulating tube. It buds off a piece of itself to be the "middle man" of the oxygenating cycle (the pulmonary circulation) and, thus, completes growth as a two-sided, four-chambered, rhythmically contracting muscle-pipe. The chambers are familiar: two atria for receiving blood and two ventricles for ejecting blood. The right atrium receives blood from the body and plops it into the right ventricle, which pumps it out to the lungs via the pulmonary trunk and arteries. From the lungs, blood returns to the heart via the pulmonary veins. It collects in the left atrium, which plops it into the left ventricle, which powerfully pumps it out of the heart through the aorta and then on through the entire body (the systemic circulation).

Anatomically, then, what should we expect? Not much from the atria, which seem to be merely swellings in the transition from tubular vessels to the contracting pump in the ventricles. Solid muscularity should be found in the ventricles, because the force of their contraction must be enough to send blood off to distant tissues. And something of a gateway should exist between the different sections of the system—between the atrium and ventricle (an **atrioventricular valve**), and between the ventricle and its arterial barrel (a **pulmonary valve** and an **aortic valve**). These gateways should prevent blood from flowing "backward" when tempted by fatigue, gravity, malfunction, or blockage somewhere in this closed tubular system. We also should expect a route for the heart muscle itself to receive nutrient blood and to return depleted blood, because it is working at least as hard as any other part of the body.

The atria fulfill our expectations. The right atrium is so possessed by the incoming venous ports that it is barely more than a sac in which blood pools before falling into the right ventricle (Fig. 2.14). A **superior vena cava** connects in from above, bringing blood from the head, neck, "axis" (the vertebrae and ribs), and upper extremities. Its complement from below is the **inferior vena cava**, bringing blood from almost the entire body inferior to the heart proper. Only the heart itself remains. The venous drainage of the heart ultimately collects into a wraparound vein called the **coronary sinus**, which empties into the right atrium along its lower margin near the entry of the inferior vena cava.

When you cut into the right atrium and peel back its wall, you will see the smooth surfaces that surround where these veins connect (see Fig. 2.14). You also will see a small bit of surface marked by treads, or cord-like muscle ridges. These ridges are called **pectinate muscles,** and they constitute the remnants of the original atrium that came over to the right side as the heart developed. The right atrium shows two other gross anatomies. One is the remnant depression in the wall between it and the left atrium, which during the fetal period was a two-flap flow-through called the **foramen ovale**. This shallow depression is called the **fossa ovalis**. The other notable gross anatomy is the orifice between the right atrium and the right ventricle. This is called the **right atrioventricular orifice**, and the three tissue flaps that close over it constitute a **tricuspid valve**.

The right ventricle has one large input hole (the **atrioventricular orifice**) and one large output barrel (the **pulmonary trunk**). The rest of it is a thickly-muscled squeeze-box (Fig. 2.14). Here, the muscle ridge network is called **trabeculae carnae** rather than pectinate, and one of the trabeculae is noticeably thick and located along the septum between the right and left ventricles. This is called the **septomarginal trabecula**, and it supplies key electrical impulse–conducting fibers to the ventricle (Fig. 2.15).

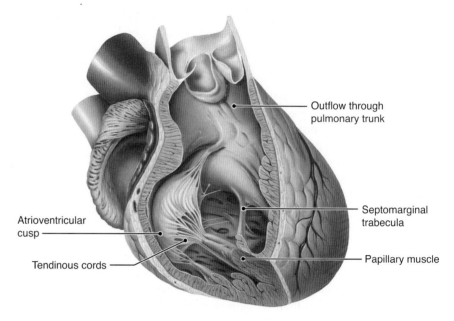

FIGURE 2.14   Interior view of right side of heart.

The atrioventricular orifice recalls a "trapdoor" design in which blood that has accumulated in the atrium "drops through" the opening. The valves are arranged to prevent the flow of blood back into the atrium when the ventricle contracts, not to release blood from the atrium into the ventricle. (Image provided by Anatomical Chart Co.)

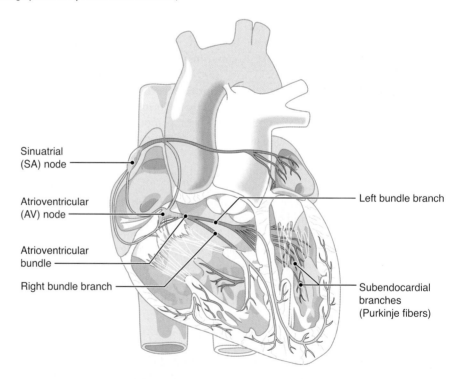

FIGURE 2.15   Conducting bundles of the heart.

Moving parts in any mechanical system usually are the ones that suffer wear and tear and break down. The heart is no exception. The moving parts are the cusps of the valves leading into and out of the chambers, and they suffer collapse and prolapse. Following the direction of blood flow, the first one will be the right atrioventricular valve. Recall that it has three cusps, which are named **posterior**, **septal**, and **anterior**, roughly according to how they fit relative to one another in a standing person. They mesh together well, and because of their intrinsic muscle tone, they maintain a good passive closure of the orifice. When blood drops from the right atrium to the right ventricle, it usually is a matter of too much volume on top of a passive trapdoor. The ventricle side of the valve, however, is much more developed.

The atrioventricular orifice is a liability for the right ventricle when it contracts to propel blood through the pulmonary trunk barrel. This contraction increases pressure in the ventricle tremendously, which means that blood could very easily regurgitate back through the tricuspid valve and into the right atrium. Within the right ventricle, the "underside" of the tricuspid valve cusps is connected to the ventricular wall by muscular strings called tendinous cords, or **chordae tendinae**, and the muscular bulge in the wall of the ventricle where they anchor is called a **papillary muscle**. This design resembles a parachute, in which the chute itself is the valve, the parachute strings are the chordae tendinae, and the parachutist (where all the strings converge) is the papillary muscle (Fig. 2.16). This tether apparatus actually pulls down on the tricuspid valve cusps during ventricular contraction or, at the very least, prevents the cusps from prolapsing up into the right atrium as pressure builds in the contracting right ventricle.

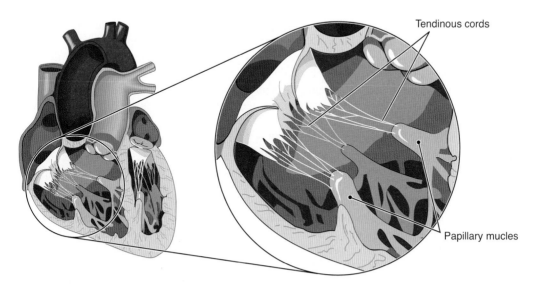

FIGURE 2.16 **Functional anatomy of the tricuspid valve.**

Drawings of the internal heart always make it difficult to appreciate how the papillary muscle and tendinous cords work to keep the atrioventricular valves from blowing back into the atrium when blood is forcibly expelled from the ventricles through either the pulmonary trunk or the aorta. It actually is an elegant design, and one that is amazingly resilient given the number of times that your heart beats in your lifetime. In the cadaver lab, students will see how fragile these valves and cords appear, and yet the design works for, literally, a lifetime. (LifeART image copyright © 2007 Lippincott Williams & Wilkins. All rights reserved.)

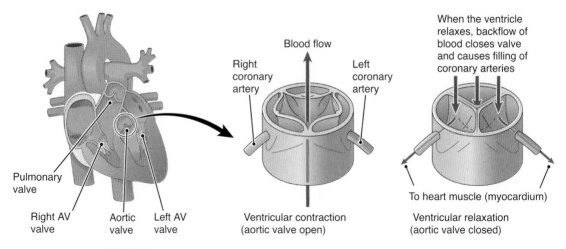

FIGURE 2.17   **Outflow dynamics in the aorta and pulmonary trunk.**

The aortic and pulmonary valves accomplish the task of preventing reflux differently than the atrioventricular (AV) valves do. Blood easily shoots through the gates from below, but once through, it has a hard time leaking back down into the ventricles. The blood pools in the small wells between the flaps of the gate and the wall of the vessel, and the weight of these pools acts to keep the central meeting point of the flaps tightly appressed. Weighted nodules in the very center of the flaps help to "flop" the flaps back downward after the pulse of blood, thus prepositioning them for the welling of blood that seeps back down the vessel. (From Cohen BJ. Memmler's Human Body in Health and Disease, 10th Edition. Baltimore: Lippincott Williams & Wilkins, 2005.)

The **pulmonary orifice**, of course, is designed to be blown open by the very same contraction. It also has three cusps—**anterior**, **right**, and **left**—that offer no resistance to the gusher of blood leaving the right ventricle and destined for the lungs. This orifice, however, must somehow prevent that blood from trickling back down the pulmonary trunk and "leaking" back into the right ventricle. The concavity/convexity of these cusps produces a "cupping" type of closure (as seen from above). This effectively prevents backflow of blood without the need for a papillary muscle system in the wall of the pulmonary trunk (Fig. 2.17).

Blood returning to the lungs collects in four **pulmonary veins**, two from each lung. These four veins plug directly into the left atrium and, as described above, actually become most of the wall of the left atrium. Like the right atrium, the left atrium retains some of the original muscular surface, which also is called **pectinate muscle** here and is found in the **auricle** portion of the atrium. No other veins provide input to the left atrium, and pooled blood soon overpowers the resistance of the valve covering the **left atrioventricular orifice**. This valve has only two cusps (**bicuspid**), compared with three on the right side of the heart (Fig. 2.18). It usually is called the **mitral valve** (in reference to the shape of certain religious hats and turbans called miters).

The mitral valve, like the tricuspid valve, is tethered to the wall of the ventricle below it. This would be the left ventricle, which is the thickest and most powerful quadrant of the heart. Because of the extraordinary pressure that can build up in the left ventricle, particularly in hearts that have to work very hard, this valve endures substantial wear and tear. If the cusps of the valve do not meet in perfect alignment, as appears to be the case in a small percentage of the population, **mitral valve prolapse** (a relatively common heart problem) may result.

The left ventricle, thus, presents the same basic design as the right ventricle: tendinous cords and papillary muscles to secure the atrioventricular valve, muscular ridges to accentuate contraction of the ventricular wall, and a large barrel outflow (in this

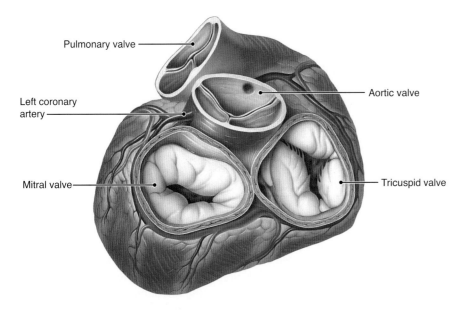

Pulmonary valve

Left coronary artery

Mitral valve

Aortic valve

Tricuspid valve

FIGURE 2.18   **Superior view of the ventricular ports.**

This is an artistic, but not very anatomic, look at the two atrioventricular orifices (in the lower part of drawing) and the blood vessel orifices leaving the heart (the upper two holes). The left atrioventricular orifice is protected by a valve with two cusps instead of three. Clinicians refer to this overworked cusp as the bicuspid valve, or mitral valve. (Image provided by Anatomical Chart Co.)

case, the aorta). The **aortic valve** is a three-cusp valve: **right**, **left**, and **posterior**. Like the valve leading into the pulmonary trunk, these cusps maintain a good passive closure because of their cup-like design.

Irregular heartbeats bring patients to the clinic. A part of every routine physical is to listen to the sounds of the heart chambers and valves through a stethoscope. Indeed, the anatomic position of the heart behind the bony sternum and rib cage limits where valve sounds can be heard to very specific locations. Because sound travels in the direction of the blood flow, these specific locations are in the spaces between ribs that lie in the direction of blood flow from each valve (Fig. 2.19). Now

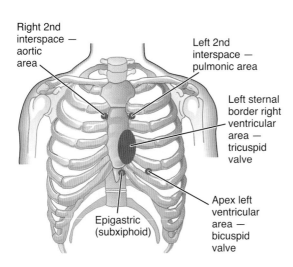

Right 2nd interspace — aortic area

Left 2nd interspace — pulmonic area

Left sternal border right ventricular area — tricuspid valve

Epigastric (subxiphoid)

Apex left ventricular area — bicuspid valve

FIGURE 2.19   **Areas of referred heart sounds on the chest wall.**

The thoracic cage complicates efforts to listen to heart sounds where they are made. Sound carries along the pathway of the blood, so zones of auscultation for detecting the heart sounds reflect where that sound can be heard best between the ribs and alongside the sternum. (From Bickley LS, Szilagyi P. Bates' Guide to Physical Examination and History Taking, 8th Edition. Philadelphia: Lippincott Williams & Wilkins, 2003.)

is the time to learn why the sounds are heard in these locations. Listening skills will come with practice.

Buried in the well of the right cusp and the left cusp are holes that lead to small arteries. These are the **right coronary artery** and the **left coronary artery** (Fig. 2.20). They begin at the very base of the aorta, and they branch out in a variety of patterns to serve the surface of the heart. They are small in diameter—absurdly small compared to the diameter of the base of the aorta. Because of the high pressure of blood flow that they must tap, and aggravated by the incessant demands of the heart muscle for oxygen, these arteries are vulnerable to rupture. If one of them does rupture, then oxygenated blood will be denied to a part of the heart muscle. This condition is known as a **myocardial infarct** (MI) and is commonly called a heart attack. Blockage of the coronary arteries by plaque or atherosclerosis requires that a surgeon redirect blood (a **bypass operation**) from the aorta to the areas supplied by the affected artery. If a bypass involves more than one channel of a coronary artery, it is called a double bypass, triple bypass, quadruple bypass, and so on. The ability of the heart to withstand an infarct and to weather both the failure of an artery and its surgical repair is truly remarkable.

The coronary arteries mark the first possible diversion of oxygenated blood once it leaves the heart through the aorta. Our account of the rest of the **systemic circulation** will follow the successive other possible diversions, and their diversions, and so on, until the branches are too small to register in a course on gross anatomy. The goal is to give you a sense of how the trunk (the aorta) "branches" and "twigs" its way to reach the major structures of the body (Fig. 2.21). Along the way, you will learn the importance of **anastomosis**, which is a kind of end-to-end connection of different arteries that enables blood to reach a target from more than one approach. Anastomosis is like an intersection of arteries so that in the event of a block in one channel, blood can back up and travel around the block by using the connection afforded by the intersection, or anastomosis.

Aorta

Consider first the complete aorta. Anatomists describe the aorta as having regions or sections: **ascending**, directly off the heart; an **arch**, as it bends backward and toward the left to run alongside the vertebral column; **descending**, which describes the entire rest of its length; and along the descending aorta, a **thoracic** section above the diaphragm and an **abdominal** section below the diaphragm. The end of what we call the aorta is found just above the pelvis, where it appears to divide into two large arteries, one for each leg (Fig. 2.22). In this case, each half of the division is called a **common iliac artery**, from which will spring an **internal iliac branch** to serve the cavity of the pelvis and an **external iliac branch** to continue the central line into the leg proper.

Branches of the Arch of the Aorta

As the aorta bends to reach the vertebral column, it is as close to the head as it will ever get. For the most part, arteries take the most conservative route that development allows, so it is safe to assume that branches of the arch of the aorta will be destined to serve the nearby head, neck, and upper limb. Indeed, the first branch of the arch (as the blood flows, or from proximal to distal along the tube) is called the **brachiocephalic trunk**. This name, although long in letters, explains exactly where the branch is headed (no pun intended)—to the arm (*brachium* is a root word referring to the arm) and to the head (*cephalic*, from ceph, for head).

The brachiocephalic trunk exists because the arch of the aorta is moving from right to left as well as from front to back. The arch must send a big shunt over the right side

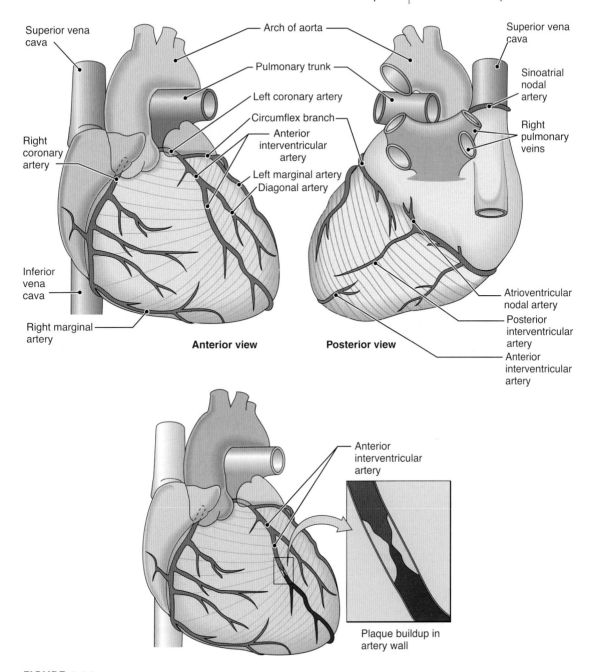

Superior vena cava

Arch of aorta

Superior vena cava

Pulmonary trunk

Sinoatrial nodal artery

Left coronary artery

Circumflex branch

Right pulmonary veins

Right coronary artery

Anterior interventricular artery

Left marginal artery

Diagonal artery

Inferior vena cava

Atrioventricular nodal artery

Posterior interventricular artery

Right marginal artery

Anterior view

Posterior view

Anterior interventricular artery

Anterior interventricular artery

Plaque buildup in artery wall

FIGURE 2.20   **Coronary arteries.**

The right and left coronary arteries arise at the very base of the aorta. They serve the heart muscle as functional end arteries (vessels without adequate "backup"). As a result, plaque formation can lead to starvation of muscle tissue (ischemia), tissue death (necrosis), and heart attack (myocardial infarction). (From Willis MC. Medical Terminology: A Programmed Learning Approach to the Language of Health Care. Baltimore: Lippincott Williams & Wilkins, 2002.)

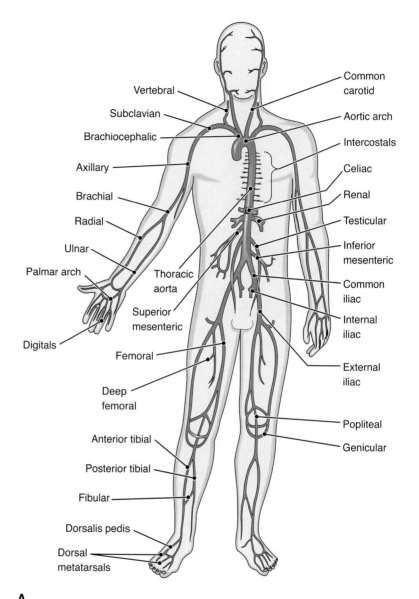

A

FIGURE 2.21   **The central route of arterial flow, with major named branchings.**

(From Cohen, BJ, Taylor JJ. Memmler's Human Body in Health and Disease, 10th Edition. Baltimore: Lippincott Williams & Wilkins, 2005.)

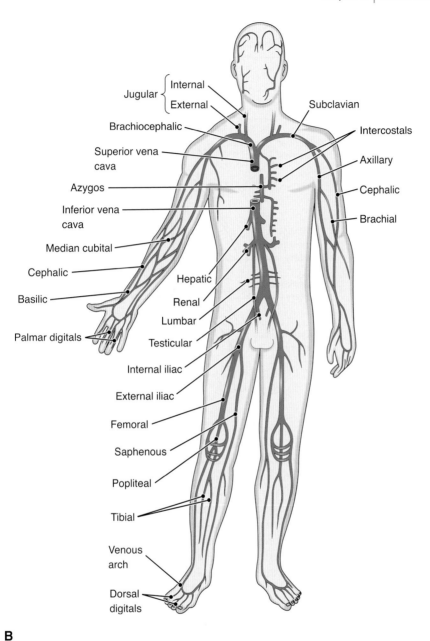

B

FIGURE 2.21 (*Continued*).   **The central route of venous return, with major named branchings.**

FIGURE 2.22   **The aorta below the diaphragm.**

From this position, the aorta directly serves the elongated gut tube, the kidneys, the gonads, the lower extremity, and the surrounding body wall. (Modified from LifeART image copyright © 2007 Lippincott Williams & Wilkins. All rights reserved.)

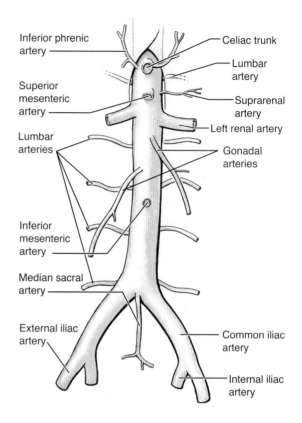

Inferior phrenic artery

Celiac trunk

Lumbar artery

Superior mesenteric artery

Suprarenal artery

Left renal artery

Lumbar arteries

Gonadal arteries

Inferior mesenteric artery

Median sacral artery

External iliac artery

Common iliac artery

Internal iliac artery

until it is lined up sufficiently under the right side of the head and neck to give a dedicated branch to the head and a dedicated branch to the arm. Because the arch is skewed to the left side of the trunk, it can give, on that side, a direct branch to the head (**left common carotid**) and a direct branch to the left arm (**left subclavian**). On the right, these two branches are merged into a common trunk (**brachiocephalic trunk**) to anchor back into the aorta, which can be seen as a more conservative design than keeping two separate but parallel, side-by-side branches spanning that distance in the upper chest.

The brachiocephalic trunk divides into a **right common carotid artery** and a **right subclavian artery**. The carotid artery runs up the side of the neck and will branch into many other arteries serving the neck, head, and brain. The subclavian artery is named because it begins deep to the clavicle bone in the root of the neck. We will return to it after we color in the many branches of the carotid.

The common carotid is called common because it carries blood to both the "outside" portions of the head (the face, neck, and cranium) and the "inside" portions of the head (the brain). The two carotid pathways separate soon into an **external carotid branch** and an **internal carotid branch** (Fig. 2.23). The internal carotid divides no further until it actually enters the cranial cavity and serves the brain. The external carotid, however, blooms into several smaller arteries that blanket the head and neck. They are described here in the typical order of branching, but you should think of them in terms of the logical regions of the head and neck that must be served.

The first branch of the external carotid is called the **superior thyroid artery**. Its name indicates two things: first, that is serves the **thyroid gland** and that general area of the neck, and second, that somewhere, there must be an inferior thyroid artery (because anatomic tradition requires complementary descriptors). The next branch is called the **ascending pharyngeal artery**, a small and deeply diving branch rarely seen

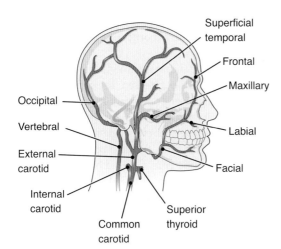

Superficial temporal

Frontal

Maxillary

Occipital

Vertebral

Labial

External carotid

Facial

Internal carotid

Common carotid

Superior thyroid

FIGURE 2.23   Carotid circulation.

Blood supply to the head and neck travels mostly in the carotid system, first through a common carotid artery and then through an internal carotid artery to the brain and an external carotid artery to everything else. (From Cohen, BJ, Taylor JJ. Memmler's Human Body in Health and Disease, 10th Edition. Baltimore: Lippincott Williams & Wilkins, 2005.)

in gross anatomy courses. It serves the pharynx muscle sleeve. A larger and more evident branch of the external carotid is called the **lingual artery**, which has the bed of the tongue for its territory. The next branch is the prominent **facial artery**, which lies across the bone of the lower jaw to snake up the edges of the mouth and nose and into the corner of the eye, where it finally dissipates. As its name implies, the facial artery must serve most of what you can touch below the eyes and above the jaw line.

The "latter half" of the external carotid begins with the **occipital branch**, a long artery that must wind its way around to the back of the head to serve the superficial structures there. A tiny branch of the external carotid, the **posterior auricular artery**, is next. It is dedicated to the junction of the earlobe and the head, a duty it shares with smaller branches of the other external carotid branches. This leaves two more direct branches of the external carotid. Whenever an artery "terminates" as two branches, these branches can be described as the "continuations" of the artery. In this case. we have two regions of the head that have not yet been served: the region behind the zygomatic and mandible bones, and the top and front of the braincase (the "temple" and "forehead" regions). The two terminal branches of the external carotid are the **maxillary** and the **superficial temporal**. The maxillary dives into the space behind the side of the lower jaw and ramifies into all the deeper spaces beyond that. Ultimately, branches of it will serve the nasal passages and fit through a small hole into the braincase to serve the meningeal coverings of the brain. The superficial temporal wiggles up the side of the head in front of the ear and spreads out to serve the scalp, from as far back as where the occipital artery leaves off to as far anterior as the forehead.

The **internal carotid** artery does not branch until it enters the braincase (through a series of holes and canals that force it into a few right-angle turns). Once it lies in contact with the brain, however, it provides one branch to serve an extension of the brain (the eyeball) and then participates in a vital anastomotic ring around the base of the brain (known as the circle of Willis, or the **circulus ateriosus**). The branch that serves the eyeball is called the **ophthalmic artery**. This makes perfect sense, because the eyeball is an extension of the brain for detection of the outside world. The ophthalmic artery sends a dedicated branch, called the **central artery of the retina**, into the dural sheath of the optic nerve. This is a true end artery, not connected to any other route, so blockage of it results in irreversible necrosis of the retina.

The ophthalmic artery also serves the structures that develop to move the eyeball, so it is considered to be the principal artery of the orbit. It ends by traveling through a hole in the frontal bone and spreading out over the eyebrows, where it anastomoses with terminal branches of the superficial temporal branch of the external carotid.

Study closely the termination of the internal carotid. It is a major source of blood supply to the brain, and as such, its branches often are the source of **cerebral vascular accidents** (CVAs), or strokes. The design of branches formed by the internal carotids and the **vertebral arteries** (see below) is called the **circulus arteriosus**, or circle of Willis. The internal carotids contribute the circle by dividing into **anterior cerebral arteries** and **posterior communicating arteries**. As the name of the composite implies, the circulus arteriosus is quite anastomotic (Fig. 2.24). This helps in the case of cerebrovascular accidents, most of which result from blood that is under too much pressure in a larger source artery trying to squeeze into a smaller branch artery headed away from the circle. (See Clinical Anatomy Box 2.4).

The **right subclavian artery** carries the rest of the blood from the brachiocephalic trunk, and the **left subclavian artery** is a direct branch of the arch of the aorta. The subclavian arteries deliver blood to the upper limb. Because they must travel under the clavicle and through the armpit to get there, however, they are the perfect choice for accessory arteries to complete the service to the neck and head. Another way to think

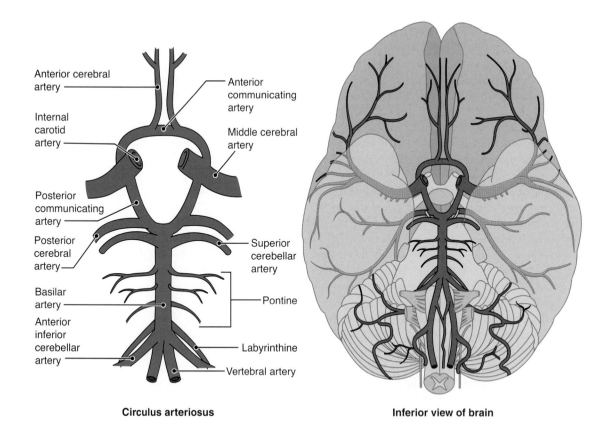

Circulus arteriosus   Inferior view of brain

FIGURE 2.24   **Division of the internal carotid.**

The internal carotid begins to branch out once it enters the cranial cavity and achieves the underside of the brain. After sending an ophthalmic branch forward into the orbit, the artery divides into a large middle cerebral and a small anterior cerebral branch as part of the circle of Willis that serves the entire brain. (Modified from LifeART image copyright © 2007 Lippincott Williams & Wilkins. All rights reserved.)

CLINICAL ANATOMY

Box 2.4

ANEURYSMS AND STROKE

When internal carotid circulation fails, blood is denied to brain tissue, and neurologic deficits can be immediate, profound, and irreversible. An aneurysm (A) results from dilation of the arterial wall, rupture of which denies blood to downstream targets, and the buildup of blood against brain tissue (hematoma). A dislodged plaque from atherosclerotic buildup in the common carotid can lodge in a smaller-caliber branch (B). This leads to necrosis of brain tissue, because blood is stopped at the plug, or rupture of the smaller vessel from the force of the blood behind the plaque (also leading to a hematoma; see C). Disruptions of blood supply to the brain are informally called strokes.

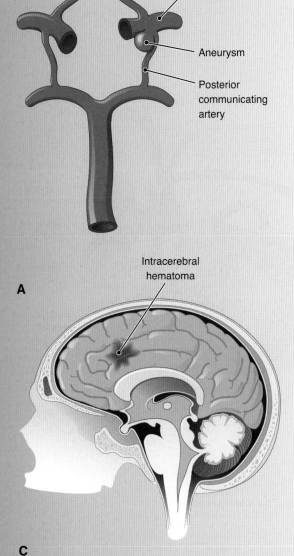

Middle cerebral artery

Aneurysm

Posterior communicating artery

Intracerebral hematoma

A

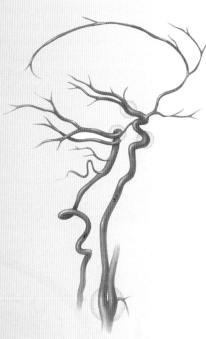

B

Cerebral vascular accidents. (A from Porth CM. Pathophysiology, 6th Edition. Philadelphia: Lippincott Williams & Wilkins, 2002; B provided by by Anatomical Chart Company; C from Cohen BJ. Medical Terminology, 4th Edition. Philadelphia: Lippincott Williams & Wilkins, 2003.)

C

about this is that they provide branches that anastomose with the route of the carotids. They also provide one unusual branch, the **internal thoracic**, that carries blood down the inside of the chest wall.

The branches of the subclavian are, in sequence, the **vertebral**, **thyrocervical trunk**, **internal thoracic**, and **costocervical trunk**. They supply the brain, the deeper parts of the lower neck, the upper surface of the rib cage, and the chest wall (Fig. 2.25). The subclavian changes its name to the **axillary** after it emerges from beneath the clavicle and dives into the axilla, or armpit.

The **vertebral artery** is the most direct of the four branches. After arising from the subclavian, it shoots up to the brain via the holes in the transverse processes of the cervical vertebrae. When it runs out of cervical vertebrae, it snakes around to the foramen magnum and rides alongside the brainstem into the cranial cavity. The two vertebral arteries then merge in the middle to form the **basilar artery**, which is a major root of the circulus arteriosus. It anastomoses with the internal carotid circulation through its **posterior cerebral branches**, which connect to the **posterior communicating arteries**. Small but very important branches of the vertebral artery are the **anterior spinal artery** and the **posterior spinal artery**, which provide blood to the entire length of the spinal cord (with help from other arteries).

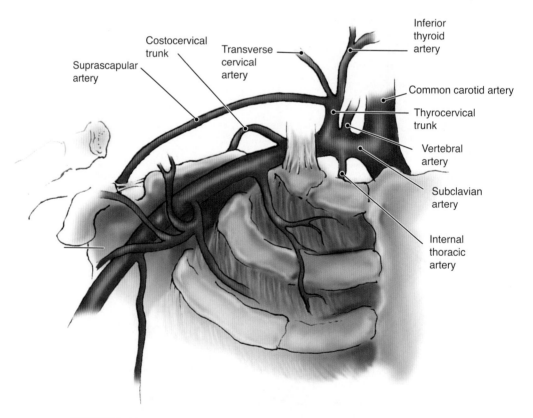

FIGURE 2.25   **The pathway of the subclavian artery.**

From here spring the branches that feed the deep neck, shoulder, chest wall, vertebral column, and brain.

As its name implies, the **thyrocervical trunk** delivers blood to the thyroid gland and to the neck. It reaches the thyroid gland by its **inferior thyroid branch** (thus complementing—and anastomosing with—the superior thyroid branch of the external carotid). It serves the neck through two branches: a **transverse cervical artery** and a **suprascapular artery**. The suprascapular artery is destined for the scapula and will participate there in a major anastomosis. The **internal thoracic artery** has nothing to do with the neck or the upper limb, which makes it an unusual branch of the subclavian artery. As the name implies, it travels along the inside of the thoracic (or chest) wall, but it does much more than that. It is a source artery for the many **anterior intercostal branches** that run around the chest wall parallel to the ribs. This makes it a kind of surrogate aorta for the front part of the trunk (Fig. 2.26). At the bottom of the sternum it divides into a branch that follows the arc of the rib cage down to the side (the **musculophrenic branch**) and then continues along the inside of the abdominal wall (as a **superior epigastric artery**). The internal thoracic artery thus provides numerous connecting possibilities between blood that routes along the subclavian and blood that routes through the thoracic and abdominal aorta, and by passing near the heart along the deep surface of the sternum, the internal thoracic is nicely positioned to be used as a bypass artery to repair circulation to the heart. Indeed, between the vertebral artery service to the head and the internal thoracic artery service to the body, the stretch of main artery called the subclavian supports much more than just a pipeline of blood to the upper limb.

The **costocervical trunk** is the least conspicuous of the subclavian branches. Through its **deep cervical branch**, it provides one route of anastomosis with the occipital branch of the external carotid. Because of its position relative to the first rib, it also provides the first and second **posterior intercostal arteries**. The descending aorta provides all the others (as a result of its location next to the vertebral column from which the ribs commence); however, because of the arch of the aorta, the costocervical trunk is closer to the route of the highest two.

Branches of the Axillary Artery

Once it emerges from under the clavicle, the tube that carries blood from the aorta to the upper limb changes names from subclavian to **axillary**. Before it enters the dangling upper limb, it has several opportunities to send blood out to the edge of the trunk, the armpit, and across the first major joint space to be encountered—the shoulder joint. The axillary artery reaches out to these possible targets through six typical branches (Fig. 2.27).

The first branch is the highest thoracic artery, or **supreme thoracic artery**. Like the costocervical trunk, it serves the first intercostal space, and it is the branch you are least likely to find when dissecting a cadaver. A larger and more apparent branch is the **lateral thoracic artery**, which laces over the side of the rib cage and, along the way, provides a source of blood to the mammary gland. A conspicuous **thoracoacromial trunk** sticks up out of the axillary artery like a fireplug, providing a bloom of branches to serve the big muscles that bracket this area: the pectoralis major and minor muscles, and the deltoid muscle. The final three branches are found in the armpit itself. A **subscapular artery** becomes a **thoracodorsal branch** and a **circumflex scapular branch** that will wind around the bottom of the scapula (as the suprascapular branch of the thyrocervical trunk did in the upper part). Two **circumflex humeral branches** (**anterior** and **posterior**) will lasso the shaft of the humerus bone just below the shoulder joint to form a simple anastomosis. After the departure of the circumflex humerals, the tube continuing into the arm is called the **brachial artery**.

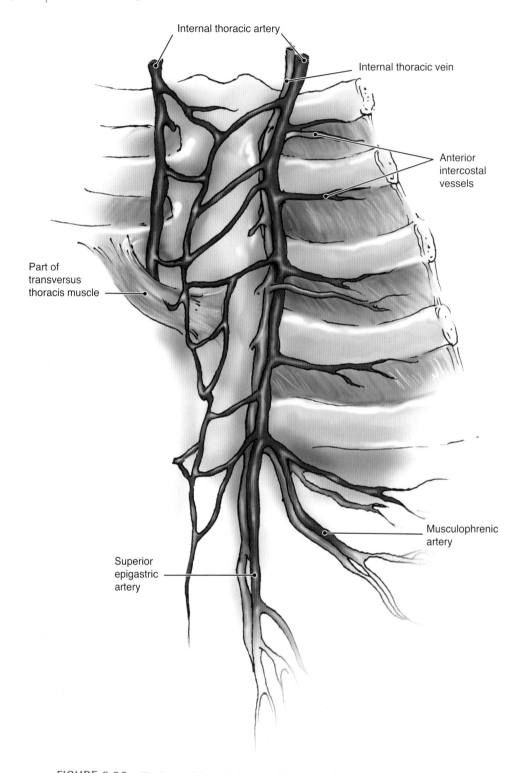

Internal thoracic artery

Internal thoracic vein

Anterior intercostal vessels

Part of transversus thoracis muscle

Musculophrenic artery

Superior epigastric artery

FIGURE 2.26   **The internal thoracic branch of the subclavian artery.**

This route serves the anterior chest wall and can form a nice anastomosis with intercostal arteries of the chest wall that come directly off of the thoracic aorta. It terminates as musculophrenic and superior epigastric arteries that serve the abdominal wall.

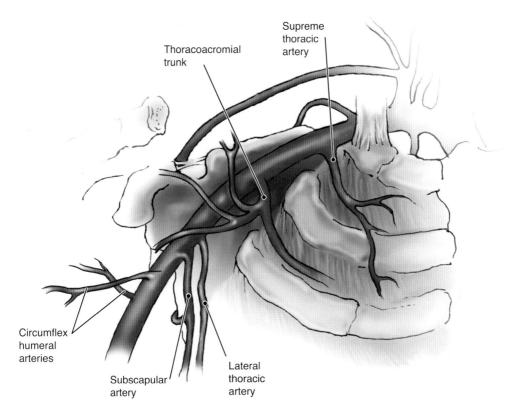

FIGURE 2.27   **The axillary artery.**

The axillary segment of the central line of circulation continues from the subclavian segment and leads to the brachial segment. Branches of the axillary artery serve the shoulder, armpit, upper extremity, breast, and chest wall.

The nature of blood vessels to fan out around a joint is a common pattern in the body and merits more study. Most joints in the body allow a tight flexion or extension around the joint. A position like this might pinch off a big vessel trying to cross the joint to serve more distal structures. To compensate, blood vessels do two things. First, they tend to travel across the most concave part of the joint so that they stretch as little as possible, and second, they tend to fan out into many smaller vessels around the joint as a hedge against the stress.

We now continue to follow the trajectory of the subclavian artery. We have just identified the six branches of the axillary component of the tube. Now called the **brachial artery**, the tube has entered the part of the upper limb that hangs from the body (the part below the shoulder joint), normally called the **arm**. From here, by necessity, the artery parallels the shaft of the humerus and stays quite close to it. A **deep humeral** (or **profunda brachii**) **artery** branches off midway down the upper arm and becomes a principal artery for the musculature "behind," or posterior to, the humerus. Across the elbow joint, the brachial artery sprouts a few bypass, or collateral, arteries before dividing into prominent and parallel **radial and ulnar branches** (Fig. 2.28). The radial artery is familiar because its pulse is felt just "above," or proximal to, the base of the thumb.

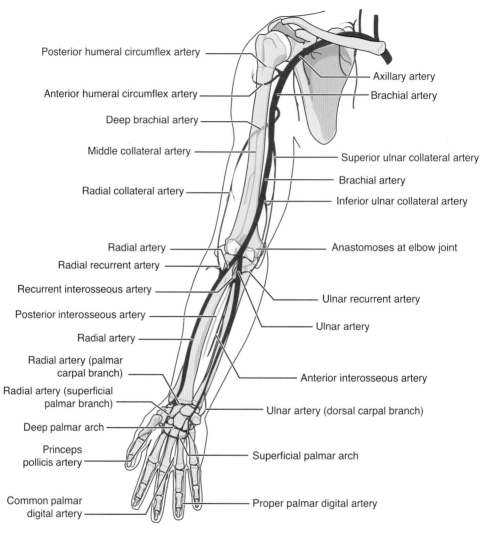

Posterior humeral circumflex artery

Anterior humeral circumflex artery

Deep brachial artery

Middle collateral artery

Radial collateral artery

Radial artery

Radial recurrent artery

Recurrent interosseous artery

Posterior interosseous artery

Radial artery

Radial artery (palmar carpal branch)

Radial artery (superficial palmar branch)

Deep palmar arch

Princeps pollicis artery

Common palmar digital artery

Axillary artery

Brachial artery

Superior ulnar collateral artery

Brachial artery

Inferior ulnar collateral artery

Anastomoses at elbow joint

Ulnar recurrent artery

Ulnar artery

Anterior interosseous artery

Ulnar artery (dorsal carpal branch)

Superficial palmar arch

Proper palmar digital artery

FIGURE 2.28   Arterial supply to the arm, forearm, and hand.

Once across the shoulder joint, the arterial pathway mirrors the bony framework, with dense networks around the joints and a "cul-de-sac" looping at the end in the palm of the hand. (Modified from LifeART image copyright © 2007 Lippincott Williams & Wilkins. All rights reserved.)

These arteries, however, are heading rapidly toward a dead end. Where will they go after reaching the fingers? Instead of these two arteries routing directly into the fingers as dead ends, they reach over to each other in the palm of the hand and form two arcades, or arches (Fig. 2.29). The ulnar artery takes the lead role in the **superficial palmar arch**, and the radial takes the lead role in the **deep palmar arch**. And so ends the subclavian detour from the central line of systemic circulation.

Descending Aorta

Within approximately 10 cm of leaving the heart, the aorta yields all the blood necessary to feed the head, neck, and upper limbs. The descending aorta must supply the trunk and its contents before dividing to serve the lower limbs. Because the thorax and

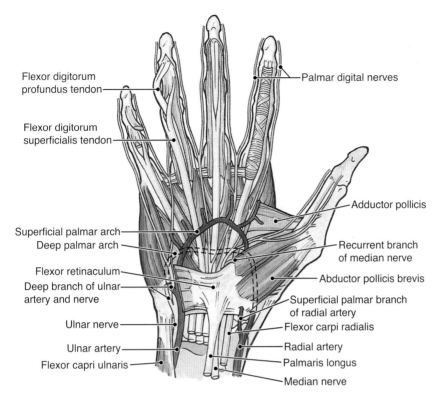

Flexor digitorum profundus tendon

Flexor digitorum superficialis tendon

Palmar digital nerves

Adductor pollicis

Superficial palmar arch
Deep palmar arch

Recurrent branch of median nerve

Flexor retinaculum
Deep branch of ulnar artery and nerve

Abductor pollicis brevis

Superficial palmar branch of radial artery
Flexor carpi radialis

Ulnar nerve

Ulnar artery

Radial artery
Palmaris longus

Flexor capri ulnaris

Median nerve

FIGURE 2.29   **Arterial anastomoses of the hand.**

The radial and ulnar arteries connect to each other through two loops: a superficial palmar arch and a deep palmar arch. This ensures adequate perfusion in the event of lacerations, which are common injuries to the fingers. (From Moore KL, Agur AM. Essential Clinical Anatomy, 3rd Edition. Baltimore: Lippincott Williams & Wilkins, 2007.)

abdomen seem to be so discrete from one another in the adult, anatomists typically refer to a **thoracic aorta** and an **abdominal aorta**, but this distinction is purely spatial. The thoracic aorta serves the lungs and the body wall as defined by the rib cage. It does not serve the heart muscle directly, because this was the very first obligation of the ascending aorta via the **coronary arteries**, and, in truth, its service to the lungs seems relatively minor. Tiny **bronchial arteries** track out from the thoracic aorta or from one of its somatic branches and follow the bronchi into the lung architecture. The size of the lungs compared to the tiny size of these arteries seems absurd until you realize that the lungs are all about oxygenating a large volume of blood delivered by the pulmonary arteries. A fair amount of direct diffusion of oxygen compensates for the small volume of oxygenated blood carried in the aortic branches to the lungs. Other visceral branches of the thoracic aorta, such as the esophageal branches, also are so small that you are unlikely to discover them when dissecting a cadaver.

The major diversions of the thoracic aorta are the segmental **posterior intercostal arteries** (Fig. 2.30). Beginning at the third intercostal space, the aorta releases branches at a right angle to run out along the grooved underside of each rib. These intercostal arteries will branch out to serve all the associated structures of the body wall, such as the breast. They also form one of the more obvious anastomoses in the body. As the posterior intercostal arteries course around the rib margin, they connect

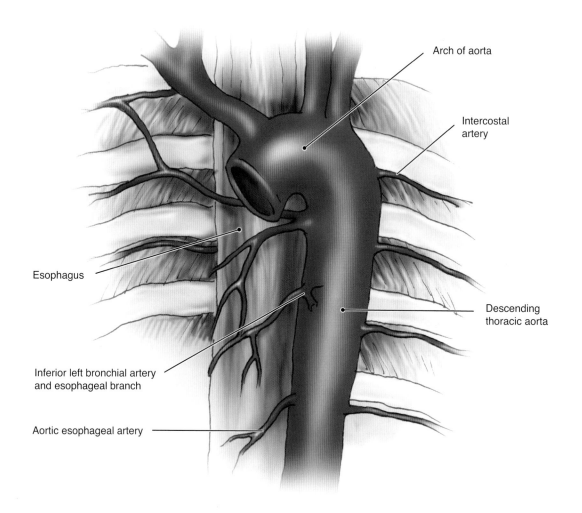

Arch of aorta

Intercostal
artery

Esophagus

Descending
thoracic aorta

Inferior left bronchial artery
and esophageal branch

Aortic esophageal artery

FIGURE 2.30   **The thoracic aorta.**

After blood has passed diversions to the head, neck, and upper extremity, the aorta carries it through the thorax. The segmental organization of the trunk is in full evidence here—as the aorta descends, it gives intercostal branches to each vertebral level.

to **anterior intercostal arteries**, which are branches of the internal thoracic branch of the subclavian artery. Indeed, it is easier to think of the internal thoracic and the thoracic aorta as being directly linked by intercostal arteries that parallel the rib cage. This is an extensive anastomosis that can play an important role in getting blood to the lower half of the body in the event of a congenital constriction in the top of the thoracic aorta (**coarctation of the aorta**).

The muscular diaphragm marks the boundary between the thoracic and abdominal cavities. Because the aorta passes behind it, we should expect that some branches will serve it. A small **superior phrenic artery** passes from the thoracic aorta to the upper surface of the diaphragm, and a small **inferior phrenic artery** passes from the abdominal aorta to the lower surface of the diaphragm. Much of the rest of the diaphragm is served by one of the terminal branches of the internal thoracic, the **musculophrenic artery**.

The abdominal aorta must serve a greater "amount" of viscera considering the length of the gut tube and its large derivatives (e.g., the liver). Its most prominent branches now are the visceral ones, which can be divided into those that are paired (one on each side) and those that are single, midline trunks. The paired visceral branches are dedicated to the organ structures that are not digestive (the kidneys and gonads). The unpaired midline visceral trunks are dedicated to the unpaired midline gut tube and its derivatives, and they include one trunk from the abdominal aorta for each developmental "region" of the gut tube: the foregut, the midgut, and the hindgut (see related discussion of the gut tube below).

The foregut artery, the **celiac trunk**, emerges from the front surface of the aorta just below where the diaphragm crosses. To serve all the foregut derivatives, it quickly splits into three segments (Fig. 2.31). One departure is the **left gastric artery**, which is

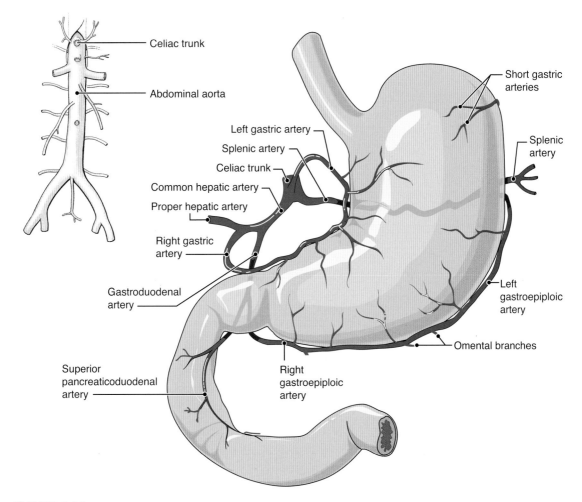

FIGURE 2.31   **The abdominal aorta and supply of the foregut organs.**

The aorta below the diaphragm serves the gut tube through three midline arteries. The first, which runs to the derivatives of the foregut, is the celiac trunk. It divides almost immediately into a small branch for part of the stomach, a large branch for the spleen, and a large branch for the liver, gallbladder, duodenum, and rest of the stomach. (Modified from LifeART image copyright © 2007 Lippincott Williams & Wilkins. All rights reserved.)

responsible for the upper region of the big, swollen stomach part of the tube. Another departure is the **common hepatic artery**, which is responsible for that other enormous part of the foregut, the liver. Along the way, it will feed a major portion of the stomach as well. The third departure is the **splenic artery**, which travels to the far left side of the body to serve the spleen. Along the way, the splenic artery lies against the substance of the pancreas and provides branches to it.

As a first approach to learning the names of the gut tube arteries, consider the logic of what they do. The stomach is a bloated cylinder. The arteries wrap around it like a primitive fishnet, with sources at each of the three celiac branches (left gastric, splenic, and common hepatic). The liver, however, is more like a sponge in construct. As such, it receives a single big artery in its gateway, or port; this is the **proper hepatic branch** of the common hepatic artery. The associated gallbladder gets an associated artery (the **cystic artery**) of the one serving the liver. This leaves the derivatives that are either retroperitoneal (behind the peritoneum) or nearly so: the proximal duodenum and the pancreas. These derivatives pick up supply from nearby twigs of the common hepatic and splenic arteries. The three branches of the celiac trunk anastomose with each other extensively, and the sub-branches that serve the "final" part of the foregut will anastomose with the sub-branches of the midgut artery that serve the "beginning" parts of the midgut.

The **superior mesenteric artery** of the midgut emerges from the aorta approximately 1 or 2 cm below the celiac trunk (Fig. 2.32). Its distal design is much different, however, because it is serving a single, linear expansion of the gut tube. It serves the rest of the duodenum, the jejunum, and the ileum of the small bowel as well as the cecum, ascending colon, and part of the transverse colon of the large bowel. This means that it covers several meters of tube, so it approaches the task very economically. Staying within the **dorsal mesentery** of the midgut, the superior mesenteric artery simply fans out a series of branches to reach sequential segments until it anastomoses along the border of the transverse colon. Because the pattern of the inferior mesenteric artery of the hindgut is very similar, the anastomosis between the superior and inferior mesenteric is seamless along the border of the transverse colon.

The different major spokes of the fan-like wheel of arteries that serve the midgut begin with the **pancreaticoduodenal branches** that anastomose with similar branches of the celiac trunk serving the duodenum and pancreas. Remember that although the regions of the gut tube correspond to dedicated arteries, the rule of anastomosis overwhelms any tendency for parts of the tube to maintain exclusive routes of blood supply. Thus, the earliest branches of the artery of the midgut anastomose with the last branches of the artery of the foregut.

The names of the spokes that follow the superior mesenteric fan of branches are **jejunal**, **ileal**, **ileocolic**, **right colic**, and **middle colic**, and they reveal the portions of the gut tube that their descendant branches serve. The ileocolic spoke is responsible for the key transition from the narrow ileum to the dilated cecum, which also is the region of the **appendix**. The right colic assumes the ascending colon, and the middle colic logically covers the transverse colon, at least until the range of the inferior mesenteric spoke invades the same arterial arcade from the region of the left colic flexure (bend where the transverse colon becomes the descending colon).

The **inferior mesenteric** departs well below the other two gut tube arteries and is not exactly in the midline of the aorta (Fig. 2.33). This reflects the fact that most of what it serves is on the left side of the abdominal cavity: the left half of the transverse colon, the descending colon, the sigmoid colon, and finally, the midline rectum. Its method of reaching these parts of the tube is similar to that of the superior mesenteric—it sends a spoke-and-arcade branch sequence out through the dorsal mesentery. The spokes typically are a **left colic** (that reaches back across the transverse colon to anastomose with the middle colic), **sigmoid**, and **superior rectal**.

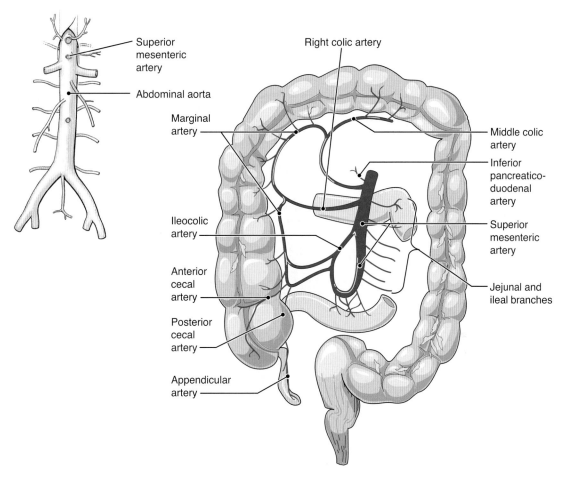

FIGURE 2.32   **The superior mesenteric artery serves the midgut derivatives.**

This tube is longer than the celiac trunk and typically includes primary branches for the pancreas, duodenum, ileocecal junction, ascending colon, and transverse colon. The long jejunum and ileum receive a battery of primary branches from the left side of the superior mesenteric. (Modified from LifeART image copyright © 2007 Lippincott Williams & Wilkins. All rights reserved.)

The **superior rectal branch** is the final extent of the inferior mesenteric artery, but it does not serve the very end of the rectum. This is an area in which the gut tube arteries anastomose with arteries that serve the body wall. As described later, the exit of the hindgut is a combination of the end of the endoderm and an "in-pocketing," or invagination, of the ectoderm. The terminal part of the anal canal (below the end of the endodermal part of the tube) is served by **middle rectal artery** and the **inferior rectal artery**, which branch off of the bifurcated aorta. The veins that accompany the middle and inferior rectal arteries drain back to the heart without going through the liver. The veins accompanying the superior rectal artery drain back through the liver and, thus, are subject to swelling if the portal system is blocked. The rectal varices that can result are commonly called **hemorrhoids**.

Now that we have supplied blood to the abdominal gut tube, let's go back to the beginning of the abdominal aorta and consider what else it has to serve, such as the abdominal wall (both front and back) and the organs that are not part of the gut tube. The abdominal aorta does not provide branches that directly serve the front of the

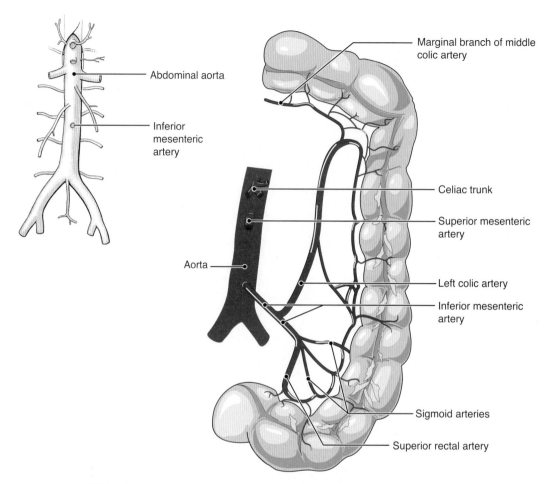

Labels on figure:
- Abdominal aorta
- Inferior mesenteric artery
- Marginal branch of middle colic artery
- Aorta
- Celiac trunk
- Superior mesenteric artery
- Left colic artery
- Inferior mesenteric artery
- Sigmoid arteries
- Superior rectal artery

FIGURE 2.33   **The inferior mesenteric artery serves the hindgut derivatives.**

The inferior mesenteric artery begins with anastomotic service to the transverse colon and ends with a superior rectal branch to the rectum. It typically is smaller in caliber than the other two gut arteries, and it can be compromised by abdominal aortic aneurysms, which typically occur just below the renal arteries. (Modified from LifeART image copyright © 2007 Lippincott Williams & Wilkins. All rights reserved.)

abdominal wall. Recall that the internal thoracic branch of the subclavian artery travels alongside the inner surface of the sternum, then divides into a **musculophrenic branch** and a **superior epigastric branch**. The superior epigastric branch runs the length of the abdominal wall, on either side of the umbilicus and deep to the muscle layer. Ultimately, it anastomoses with an **inferior epigastric artery**, but this is a branch of the **external iliac** continuation of the aorta.

The abdominal aorta serves the back of the abdominal wall in a manner identical to the service of the back of the thorax. At each vertebral level, the aorta sends a branch out at a right angle to itself (see Fig. 2.22). In the lumbar region of the vertebral column, however, there are no ribs to guide the path of the arteries. Instead, the lumbar arteries sandwich themselves between two layers of abdominal wall muscle, then spread out to cover the back and sides of the abdominal wall. Their branches will anastomose with branches of the superior and inferior epigastric arteries, thus completing the circuit around the wall.

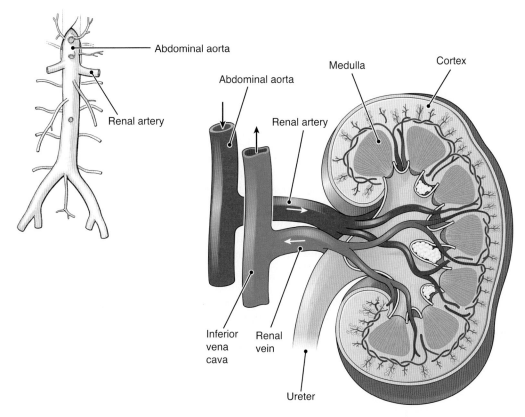

FIGURE 2.34   **Arterial supply of the kidneys.**

The renal arteries depart the abdominal aorta at an approximately 90° angle. They are wide-caliber arteries that pump the entire bloodstream through the kidneys in a short period of time. Also departing directly from the abdominal aorta are gonadal branches, which track the migration of the testis or the ovary, and segmental lumbar branches, which run to the body wall musculature. (From Cohen BJ. Memmler's Human Body in Health and Disease, 10th Edition. Baltimore: Lippincott Williams & Wilkins, 2005.)

The nondigestive organs that are found along the back of the abdominal wall include the suprarenal glands, the kidneys, and the gonads (before their migration). The abdominal aorta feeds each one of them with dedicated direct branches. The suprarenal glands on each side receive a **middle suprarenal artery**. They also receive multiple small superior suprarenal arteries that detour down from the inferior phrenic and an inferior suprarenal that detours up from the renal artery. The small suprarenal gland is highly vascularized.

By far, the largest branches of the abdominal aorta are the **renal arteries**, which typically are found just below the junction of the first and second lumbar vertebrae (Fig. 2.34). Because the aorta is positioned slightly to the left of midline, the right renal artery is longer and must cross over the vertebral bodies to get to the right side. The renal artery divides into a dedicated branch for each of the five segments of the kidney, and this is one area of the body where anastomoses are lacking (i.e., the five branches of the renal artery do not anastomose with one another). As just mentioned above, the renal artery will give an inferior suprarenal branch to the suprarenal gland, and it will give small branches to the renal pelvis and the upper part of the ureter that drains the kidney.

One of the most unusual arteries in the body is the **gonadal artery**, which is the final direct visceral branch of the aorta. The gonadal artery is unusual because it is a narrow-diameter branch directly off of the very-large-diameter aorta. It also is unusual because it leaves the aorta in the middle of the lumbar region and travels a great distance to reach its target. The male gonad, or the **testis**, lies far away in the scrotal pouch. The female gonad, or the **ovary**, is dangling just inside the rim of the pelvis. This unusual arrangement makes perfect sense, however, because the gonads originated along the back of the abdominal wall where their arteries first appear. The gonads then migrate and, in doing so, take the arteries with them. In the male, the artery is called the **testicular artery**, and in the female, it is called the **ovarian artery**. The clinical significance of this blood supply is that the migration takes the arteries across some other sensitive structures, such as the ureter, which passes deep to the arteries, and the iliac arteries. On the left side, the vessels will cross the sigmoid mesocolon (a sleeve of tissue that supports the sigmoid part of the large intestine). The mesocolon is subject to twisting, which may require surgery; therefore, surgeons must take care to secure the gonadal arteries before reducing the **sigmoid volvulus**.

Only one direct branch of the abdominal aorta remains. At the very end of the aorta, where it bifurcates to surf the pelvis on its way to the lower limb, the aorta must divide into right and left **common iliac arteries**. Trickling down from this bifurcation will be the **median sacral artery**, so named because it is unpaired and (usually) in the midline. It travels along the "front," or ventral, surface of the sacrum bone and provides one final anastomosis between the abdominal aorta and the branches of its branches.

Beyond the Aorta

The best route to the lower limb is actually over the top of the pelvic bones, not through the pelvic cavity. Therefore, the aorta divides at approximately the level of the L4 vertebra, well before it has descended into the pelvic cavity. The aorta divides into arteries called **common iliac arteries**, which, in this case, means that the blood they carry is a common supply to the internal aspect and the external aspect of the ilium. To put it another way, the common iliacs carry blood to both the pelvic cavity inside the arc of the ilium and to the lower limb that buds off of its outer limit. The common iliacs head toward the path of least resistance around the curvature of the ilium, much like a race car taking the inside track along a tight turn.

Because this continuation of the aorta must serve the organs of the pelvic cavity, now is a good time for that dedicated branch to leave the circuit. The **internal iliac artery** departs from the common iliac early in its tour around the pelvic curvature (Fig. 2.35). This artery drops over the precipice of the pelvic brim and scatters itself to every structure it can find. The spatial arrangement of the branches is very complex and highly variable. Dissecting the artery in a cadaver is cumbersome, and to save time, many courses use prosected cadavers (or even skip the exercise entirely). The best strategy may be to consider what structures must be served and to study an illustration of a "typical" internal iliac artery. The contents of the cavity are well-perfused and rarely subject to ischemia, so mastering the exact configuration of the internal iliac is less clinically relevant than in other areas of the body.

The organs of the pelvic cavity also must be served. Both sexes have a bladder, so one early branch of the internal iliac should serve the bladder. The **umbilical artery** branches immediately off of the internal iliac, then swoops just over the bladder on its way to withering into a fibrous **lateral umbilical ligament** on each side of the body. As

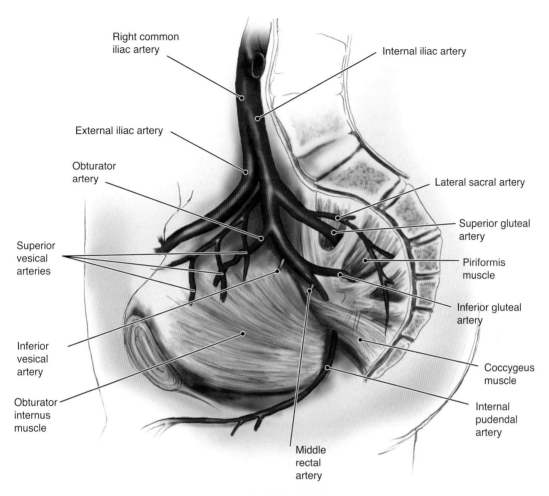

Right common
iliac artery

Internal iliac artery

External iliac artery

Obturator
artery

Lateral sacral artery

Superior
vesical
arteries

Superior gluteal
artery

Piriformis
muscle

Inferior
vesical
artery

Inferior gluteal
artery

Obturator
internus
muscle

Coccygeus
muscle

Internal
pudendal
artery

Middle
rectal
artery

FIGURE 2.35   **Bifurcation of the aorta and branches of the internal iliac artery.**

The aorta bifurcates into an external iliac artery for service to the limb and an internal iliac artery for service to the pelvic cavity and genitalia.

it passes over the bladder, it sends a **superior vesical branch** to its broad upper surface. The reproductive tract in both sexes must be served as well. In males this consists of the **prostate, ductus deferens**, and the **seminal vesicles**. Because these structures port into the urinary system, their blood supply comes from the **inferior vesical branch** of the internal iliac that also serves the lower bladder. In the female, a much larger organ system must be served. For the **uterus** and **vagina**, a network of arteries (sourced as the uterine and vaginal branches of the internal iliac) cooperate. In addition, both sexes have a lower rectum, which is served by a **middle rectal artery**. Note that this most inferior part of the digestive system is fed by arteries that are not part of the gut tube trio described above; likewise, venous drainage from here will route back to the heart without going through the liver.

It is logical to assume that branches of the internal iliac will serve the externalization of the pelvic cavity organs, and this is partially true. Because a substantial amount of skin is involved in these same structures, however, the blood supply is shared between branches of the internal and external iliac. The **internal pudendal artery**

branch of the internal iliac is the major source of blood to the outer limit of the anus and to the external genitalia (Fig. 2.36). However, just as there is a muscular diaphragm separating the thoracic cavity from the abdominal cavity, a similar diaphragm stretches across the lower part of the pelvic cavity that helps to suspend the contents of the abdominal cavity in place. For a branch of the internal iliac to reach the **perineal** structures, it must either pierce this diaphragm or go around it, and it chooses the latter.

To reach the perineal structures, a branch of the internal iliac ducks out of the pelvic cavity through the greater sciatic foramen, then spins around toward the front along the outer surface of the pelvic diaphragm. It gives off the third key artery to serve the end of the rectum, the **inferior rectal artery**. Once around to the front of

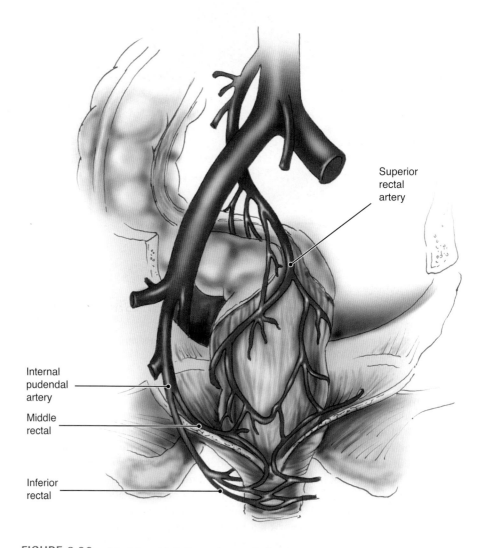

Superior
rectal
artery

Internal
pudendal
artery

Middle
rectal

Inferior
rectal

FIGURE 2.36   **Arterial supply to the rectum, posterior view.**

The rectal branches of the internal iliac artery complete the vascular service to the rectum that began with the superior rectal branch of the inferior mesenteric artery. Thus, the proximal rectum is served by gut tube arteries, and the distal rectum/anus is served by somatic branches. Venous drainage likewise will follow different paths back to the heart.

the body, it branches out to serve the urogenital structures and achieves a minor anastomosis with the **external pudendal artery** that comes off the nearby **femoral artery**.

The fact that smaller arteries can leave the pelvic cavity helps to explain the other branches of the internal iliac artery. All around the pelvic cavity are avenues toward muscular compartments of the lower limb. Through the front of the cavity is the medial, or adductor, compartment of the thigh. Through the back of the cavity, where the internal pudendal artery exits, is the gluteal region of the lower limb. Accordingly, an **obturator branch** of the internal iliac sneaks out under the pubic bone and supplies the adductor muscles, and the **superior gluteal artery** and **inferior gluteal artery** turn outward through the greater sciatic foramen to serve the buttock muscles.

The obturator artery, curiously enough, is the source artery for the one and only "twig" that serves the head of the femur inside the hip joint cavity. It is not up to the task (see the discussion of avascular necrosis of the femoral head below). The final two branches of the internal iliac artery play out the role of body wall service that the aorta left behind. One branch is the **iliolumbar artery**, which snakes up along the sacroiliac joint and anastomoses with the lowest lumbar arteries. The other branch is the **lateral sacral artery**, which reaches inward along the surface of the sacrum and anastomoses with the median sacral artery.

By definition, the **external iliac artery** begins where the internal iliac begins (Fig. 2.37). A fair amount of the external iliac is a branchless extension of the aortic pathway along the pelvic brim. As it nears the front of the pelvis, it must ramp over the pubis bone but under the inguinal ligament overpass, after which it just drops into the lower limb in anatomic free fall. Before it crosses under the inguinal ligament and changes its name to the **femoral artery**, it gives off a major branch to the front of the abdominal wall (the **inferior epigastric artery**) and a minor branch to the side of the abdominal wall (the **deep circumflex iliac**). Remember that the inferior epigastric joins the superior epigastric head-to-head somewhere near the umbilicus to complete a powerful anastomosis between the subclavian circulation and the lower aorta circulation. In the event of a radical obstruction in the abdominal aorta, blood can reach the lower extremity through this subclavian–internal thoracic–superior epigastric—inferior epigastric detour.

An even more important clinical reason to master the anatomy of the inferior epigastric artery is to diagnose the common condition of an **inguinal hernia**. One diagnostic difference between an **indirect** inguinal hernia and a **direct** inguinal hernia is its position relative to the course of the inferior epigastric artery. The artery marks a sort of boundary line such that lateral to the artery, a loop of bowel may enter the inguinal canal itself (an **indirect hernia**). Medial to the artery, however, it must push out or push through the muscle of the abdominal wall (a **direct hernia**). Other factors will help you to determine which type of hernia you need to repair, but the anatomy of the artery remains a key diagnostic trait.

Once past the inguinal ligament, the continuation of the central line of circulation is called the **femoral artery** (Fig. 2.38). The rest of our description of the arterial supply now refers to the lower limb. In some ways, the knowledge of this limb is more applicable to clinical care than is the knowledge of the upper limb (because of circulatory problems in the elderly and morbidly overweight). The toes are farther away from the heart and more difficult to self-elevate above the heart, so peripheral vascular disease and the risk of thrombus formation are more likely in the lower limb.

We have seen that independent arteries service the inner thigh and the gluteal region. Branches of the femoral artery will anastomose with them, but before that, the

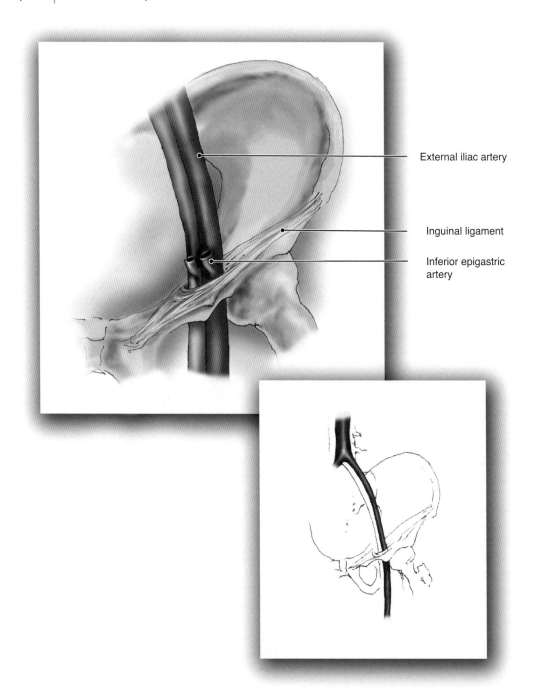

External iliac artery

Inguinal ligament

Inferior epigastric artery

FIGURE 2.37   **The external iliac pathway.**

As the external iliac slides under the inguinal ligament to reach the lower limb, it provides an inferior epigastric branch that travels back up the abdominal wall to link with the superior epigastric termination of the internal thoracic artery. In addition, the path of the inferior epigastric branch marks the boundary between an indirect inguinal hernia (lateral to the artery) and a direct inguinal hernia (medial to the artery).

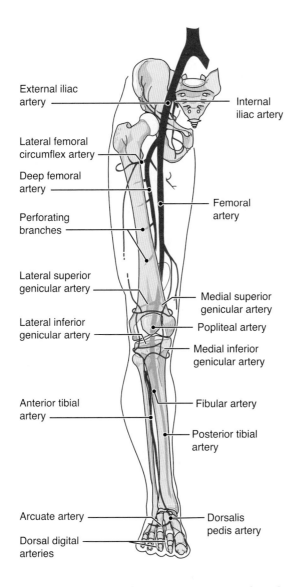

External iliac artery

Internal iliac artery

Lateral femoral circumflex artery

Deep femoral artery

Perforating branches

Femoral artery

Lateral superior genicular artery

Medial superior genicular artery

Lateral inferior genicular artery

Popliteal artery

Medial inferior genicular artery

Anterior tibial artery

Fibular artery

Posterior tibial artery

Arcuate artery

Dorsalis pedis artery

Dorsal digital arteries

FIGURE 2.38   **The femoral artery.**

The femoral artery is exposed close to the skin, just below the inguinal ligament, which puts it at danger during trauma but convenient for access during clinical procedures, such as catheter placement. It sends blood around the hip joint and to the muscular thigh via deep femoral and circumflex femoral branches. (Modified from LifeART image copyright © 2007 Lippincott Williams & Wilkins. All rights reserved.)

femoral gives some minor complementary arteries, such as the **superficial circumflex iliac** (to match a branch of the external iliac) and the **external pudendals** (usually a superficial and a deep) to serve peripheral areas of the external genitalia.

Following the pattern of the upper limb, the first major branch of the femoral artery will run parallel to it and serve a different component of the big cylinder of the thigh. This would be the **deep femoral artery** (*profunda femoris*), and it branches off very soon after the femoral artery begins. This large branch will run along the margin of a large muscle in the inner thigh (the adductor magnus) and send branches of its own boring through the muscle to reach the posterior compartment of the thigh (the perforating branches). Another way to think of it is that the posterior compartment of the thigh (the hamstring compartment) does not have a dedicated longitudinal artery of its own.

In most cases, the deep femoral artery will give off two other major branches just after it arises from the femoral. These are the **medial circumflex femoral** and **lateral circumflex femoral**, and they play much the same role as their analogs in the arm (the anterior and posterior circumflex humerals). In some cases, one or both of the circumflex femorals branch directly off of the femoral, or they branch off as a singular division of the deep femoral and then subdivide later. However, they also do much more. The lateral circumflex femoral drops a large branch down the outer part of the thigh just before it makes its final ascent to the hip joint. This is the **descending branch**, and it provides a fair amount of blood to the muscular anterior compartment and even participates in the extensive anastomosis around the knee joint. The medial circumflex femoral supplies a large amount of the circulation inside the hip joint capsule, which in general is not well-supplied collaterally. **Avascular necrosis** of the femoral head is an unfortunate, irreversible condition that can result from traumatic shearing of this artery, such as in a football tackle or motor-vehicle accident.

The large femoral artery then gradually spirals down the thigh under cover of the sartorius muscle. Just as in the arm, the major artery must avoid getting pinched off when the joints that it crosses are in a locked position. For the femoral artery, the key joint is the knee joint, and the safe position to be in is behind it, not in front of it (where the femoral artery begins in the thigh). The course of the femoral displays its need to get to the back of the knee joint. It waits until the last possible opportunity to spin around, and just above the medial epicondyle of the femur, it drops back through a gap in the adductor magnus muscle called the **adductor hiatus**. As it does, it gives off a small **descending genicular artery** that participates in the knee joint anastomosis.

The femoral artery must now get between the epicondyles so that it can drop straight down between them, along the back surface of the knee joint capsule. At this point, it is called the **popliteal artery** because it is found in the popliteal fossa. And so the story of the femoral is complete: key branches occurring early and then a direct path down the thigh and around the knee.

The **popliteal artery** provides several other branches that circumscribe the knee joint and link up with the femoral branches mentioned above (Fig. 2.39). The popliteal branches are logically named the **superior genicular artery** and the **inferior genicular artery** (*genu* is a root term for knee), and each one has a medial and a lateral component. In between them all is the small **middle genicular artery**, which heads into the knee joint capsule itself. Once past the knee joint, the popliteal artery gives rise to important **sural arteries** that serve the heads of the gastrocnemius muscle.

FIGURE 2.39   Arterial routes and the knee joint.

The popliteal artery continuation of the femoral artery sends branches around the knee joint to support flow in any leg posture. The joint is well perfused by this thorough network. (Modified from LifeART image copyright © 2007 Lippincott Williams & Wilkins. All rights reserved.)

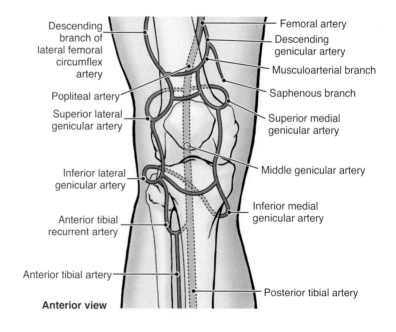

Descending branch of lateral femoral circumflex artery
Popliteal artery
Superior lateral genicular artery
Inferior lateral genicular artery
Anterior tibial recurrent artery
Anterior tibial artery

Femoral artery
Descending genicular artery
Musculoarterial branch
Saphenous branch
Superior medial genicular artery
Middle genicular artery
Inferior medial genicular artery
Posterior tibial artery

Anterior view

These arteries are important because, by some accounts, they are virtually end arteries unto themselves. If avulsed or blocked, the head of the gastrocnemius muscle can necrose and die; this risk is elevated in people who play contact sports, such as football, lacrosse, and rugby.

The central line has now reached the leg proper. Just as the brachial artery divided to form parallel radial and ulnar arteries, the popliteal typically divides at this point to form the parallel **anterior tibial artery** and **posterior tibial artery** (Fig. 2.40). The posterior tibial artery is larger, because most of the muscle mass in the leg is situated "behind" the large tibia bone. Let's begin with the anterior artery.

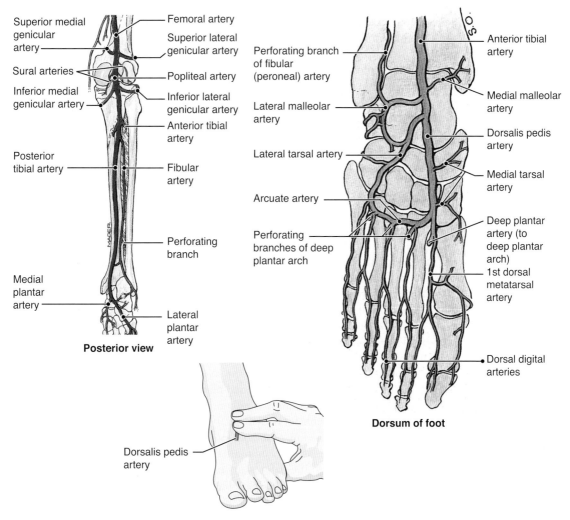

FIGURE 2.40   Arterial supply of the leg.

The popliteal artery continues down the calf musculature as the posterior tibial artery. The anterior tibial artery reaches the front of the leg and crosses the ankle joint on the top of the foot as the dorsalis pedis artery. A pulse may be taken here as a measure of the integrity of peripheral blood flow. (From Moore KL, Agur AM. Essential Clinical Anatomy, 3rd Edition. Baltimore: Lippincott Williams & Wilkins, 2007. Inset from Bickley LS, Szilagyi P. Bates' Guide to Physical Examination and History Taking, 8th Edition. Philadelphia: Lippincott Williams & Wilkins, 2003.)

A small anterior muscular compartment fills the front part of the outside part of the calf. These muscles draw the toes up toward the knee (**dorsiflexion**) and assist in rolling the inside of the foot upward (**inversion**). These muscles are served by the **anterior tibial artery**, which reaches them by traveling through an interosseous membrane between the tibia and fibula. As it does, it provides an anterior tibial recurrent branch to the knee joint anastomosis. Just as the anterior compartment leg muscles lead onto the top of the foot (the dorsum of the foot), the anterior tibial artery crosses the ankle joint and terminates in a loop among them. As it approaches the ankle joint from above, it closely follows the course of the tibialis anterior muscle. Once across the ankle joint, its continuation is called the **dorsalis pedis artery**, and the pulse of this artery is palpable just inside the large tendon of the tibialis anterior (see Fig. 2.40).

The dorsalis pedis artery terminates by sending an arcuate loop across the bases of the lesser toes and by continuing as the first dorsal metatarsal artery next to the big toe. This is an important branch, because it provides a "twig" that dives deep into the substance of the foot and anastomoses with the extensive circulation of the sole of the foot.

Meanwhile, the **posterior tibial artery** must cover a much more extensive set of muscles. To meet this challenge, it sends off a parallel artery called the **fibular artery** to the outside of the calf. Together, these supply the posterior and lateral muscular compartments, respectively. Of the two, the posterior tibial continues into the sole of the foot as the primary blood supply to the tissue layers that comprise this complement to the palm of the hand.

The **fibular artery** provides blood to the two muscles of the lateral compartment, and it terminates around the ankle joint by providing anastomoses to both the anterior and the posterior tibial. It may be the only significant artery of the lower limb that does not participate in the knee joint anastomosis.

The posterior tibial artery lies deep within the beefy posterior muscular compartment of the calf. It will follow a few tendons around the medial side of the ankle joint and under the big arch in the foot to reach the muscle layers of the sole of the foot. These are the tendons that provide powerful flexion to the toes. Together with the posterior tibial artery and the tibial nerve, they run a well-protected route alongside the ankle joint to reach the plantar surface of the foot. Along the way, the posterior tibial sends a small branch to the calcaneus bone that it is leaving behind and to the ankle joint that it has just passed.

Balance and locomotion overwhelmingly depend on the big toe; the other toes are called "lesser toes" for a reason. Once into the sole of the foot, then, it is no surprise that the posterior tibial artery divides into a **medial plantar artery** and a **lateral plantar artery** (Fig. 2.41). The medial plantar artery is responsible chiefly for the big toe, and the lateral planter artery is responsible for virtually everything else. The medial plantar basically runs a straight path along the line of the big toe, and it sends an "exit ramp" over to the plantar arch formed by the lateral plantar artery at the bases of the big toes, thus completing a loop very similar to the palmar arches of the hand. This plantar arch sends a communicating artery up through the space between the first and second toes to anastomose with the dorsalis pedis artery, thus completing an arch-to-arch communication reminiscent of the connections between the superficial and deep plantar arches.

Once the popliteal artery parents the arteries of the leg, which, in turn, service the foot, the central line of systemic circulation is exhausted. You should now be able to deduce how blood reaches a given structure in the event that a major part of the route is blocked or needs to be blocked to conduct a procedure. You should use a sense of anatomy to understand why some arteries are at greater risk of injury than others. And you should apply a sense of development to understand why the heart looks the way that it does and why the tube that led away from it branches when and where it does.

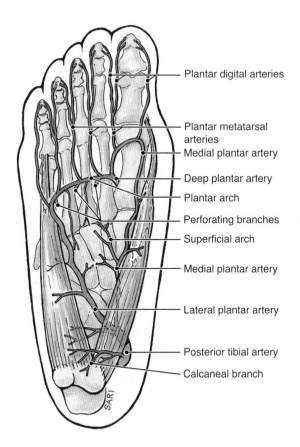

Plantar digital arteries

Plantar metatarsal arteries

Medial plantar artery

Deep plantar artery

Plantar arch

Perforating branches

Superficial arch

Medial plantar artery

Lateral plantar artery

Posterior tibial artery

Calcaneal branch

FIGURE 2.41 **Arterial supply of the plantar surface of the foot.**

The final stop for lower-limb circulation is the sole of the foot, where the posterior tibial artery splits into a small medial plantar artery dedicated to the big toe and a large lateral plantar artery for the lesser toes. The sole of the foot lacks the same arching connectivity of the palm of the hand, but penetrating branches of the plantar arteries do connect to the dorsal arcade off of the dorsalis pedis artery. (From Moore KL, Agur AM. Essential Clinical Anatomy, 3rd Edition. Baltimore: Lippincott Williams & Wilkins, 2007.)

The remaining half of circulation is the venous system, which tends to develop opportunistically and less programmatically, and so is described in much less detail.

Venous Return to the Heart

Think now about the route that blood takes to get back to the heart. From microscopic capillary networks, veins progressively coalesce into larger and larger channels of blood flow until the gross structure of a vein is formed. The vein itself does not drain a region of tissue; rather, it simply transports collected blood to a larger vein, then to an even larger vein, and so on, until it reaches one of the main tributaries to the heart. Recall that venous blood enters the heart through one of three ports: the **superior vena cava**, the **inferior vena cava**, or the **coronary sinus** that drains the heart muscle itself. This section is the story of how the veins come to be and which ones deserve a careful study.

Veins vary quite a bit from person to person, which confounds the efforts of gross anatomists to name them reliably. Only the major veins of the body form a regular pattern, so our emphasis will be on the major routes back to the heart. The surgical risk of cutting into a person without knowing where their veins are is mitigated by the fact that most veins lack a smooth muscle layer that keeps them open in the absence of blood pressure. If a vein near the skin is cut, blood will escape. However, the vein can be cauterized (permanently) in the same step, and blood will find an alternate route back toward the heart. It makes little sense to talk about anastomoses in the venous system, because the system itself is almost reflexively anastomotic. In other words, very few venous routes are linear, and most areas of the body are extensively served by venous networks and plexuses.

The somewhat passive venous return system relies heavily on posture, muscle contraction, and fluid balance to work effectively. After drawing blood into venules through capillary action, the only means of continuing that flow through larger and larger channels (often against gravity) is to "squeeze" it toward the heart through contraction of the adjacent muscles. Indeed, physical activity is essential for adequate venous return and is why invalid and postoperative patients must be attended with pressurized stockings, raisable beds, and physical therapy.

Veins are found chiefly in two areas of the body: just under the skin (**superficial**) and in the company of large deep arteries (**venae comitantes** or **accompanying veins**). The veins near the surface of the body help to regulate internal temperature by bringing the blood close enough to the atmosphere for temperature diffusion to occur. These veins also can deliver blood when body position or internal blockage pinches off the route of the deeper venae comitantes. The deep veins are well-protected and enjoy the support provided by the muscle masses that they drain and travel beside. Some veins are even large enough to contain valves to resist backflow.

Like the arteries, veins are best learned in the direction of blood flow, so we will reverse our coverage of the body, beginning with the lower limb and finishing with how blood of the head and neck reaches the heart. This is not as daunting as it seems, however, because in most areas, the veins are intimately adjacent to the arteries and are named the same. Therefore, by learning the arterial routes, you can ascertain the routes of venous return. In areas of major significance, the veins tend to have names of their own, so they cannot be learned simply by calling to mind the nearby artery. Veins form "opportunistically," which means that they often take the shortest route to a larger vein instead of completely backtracking along the course of the artery that they accompany. For this reason, the venous system is substantially more asymmetric than the arterial system.

Formation of the Inferior Vena Cava

Blood from the body below the diaphragm drains back to the heart via, ultimately, the inferior vena cava. This includes the drainage of the gut tube, which is significant, because this blood must first go through a strict filtration in the liver. In many ways, the formation of the inferior vena cava resembles the disassembling of the abdominal aorta, and that makes our survey of it relatively concise.

Beginning in the foot are two important venous channels, one superficial and one deep, as previewed above. The deep channel accompanies the medial and lateral plantar arteries and leads to the deep vein of the lower extremity, with names identical to the artery names of the central line (**posterior tibial**, **popliteal**, **femoral**, **external iliac**, **common iliac**, and **inferior vena cava**). Its tributaries include the veins that accompany the branches of the femoral artery, such as the **deep femoral**.

The superficial channel is, in some ways, of greater clinical significance. It begins as a **dorsal venous arch** across the base of the toes, similar in design to the arterial arch that resulted from the anterior tibial artery. The dorsal venous arch heads back across the ankle joint on both the medial and lateral sides. The lateral passage becomes the **small saphenous vein**, also superficial, along the back of the calf. The medial passage becomes one of the most important veins in the body, the **great saphenous vein**.

The great saphenous vein commences just anterior to the big knob on the inside of the ankle joint, the medial malleolus (Fig. 2.42). By some accounts, this is the most regularly occurring vein location in the body, which makes it a last resort target for

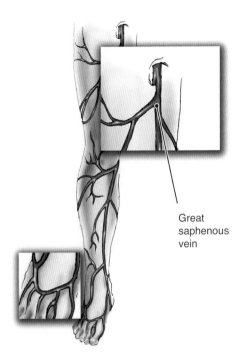

FIGURE 2.42   **The great saphenous vein.**

The long journey back to the heart for venous blood begins in the foot, where superficial veins traffic more blood than the deep veins that accompany the central arteries. Just anterior to the medial malleolus of the tibia is the beginning of the largest vein in the body, the great saphenous vein, which uses muscle contraction against the skin as a "pump" to keep blood flowing against gravity and toward the heart. This vein is so large and thick that it can be used as an artery in bypass surgery.

Great saphenous vein

venipuncture if no others can be found. From this beginning, the great saphenous vein remains superficial and medial as it courses up the leg, past the inner surface of the knee, and up the thigh atop the adductor compartment muscles until it dives into the **femoral vein** in the heart of the region known as the **femoral triangle** (Fig. 2.43). The great saphenous vein becomes "great" by drawing almost all the superficial drainage of the lower limb. The small saphenous vein long ago dove into the popliteal vein, leaving much of the calf and all of the thigh to its great saphenous partner.

The great saphenous vein is the longest continuous vein in the body, which may seem disadvantageous considering that it also is as far from the heart as any other vein. The body struggles at times to keep enough venous pressure to secure good drainage within the great saphenous and into the femoral, and if it loses this struggle, the uncomfortable conditions of venous insufficiency and **varicose veins** can result. Regular exercise is the best prophylactic against this form of edema. Sometimes, however, even a healthy saphenous vein has to be removed—but for the good purpose of being a surrogate artery in a bypass operation. The great saphenous is so large and durable that it makes an excellent graft in vascular surgeries. The procedure is common enough to be called, simply, a "saphenous cutdown."

Once the great saphenous drains into the femoral vein, the system has almost reached the inguinal ligament. In this position, the large femoral vein is vulnerable, because no muscle comes between it and the skin surface. Also in this position, it lies medial, or to the inside, of the femoral artery. This is an unusual orientation for large veins and arteries. The femoral artery is vulnerable here as well, and the reason is developmental. The lower limb rotated during development so that you can stand effectively on a fully extended limb, with the result that the "armpit" of the lower limb, the femoral triangle, is exposed and faces forward (see Fig. 2.43).

As the femoral vein "limbos" under the inguinal ligament and into the pelvic cavity, its name changes to the **external iliac vein**. The external iliac vein draws returning blood from veins that accompany the deep circumflex iliac and inferior epigastric arteries. It

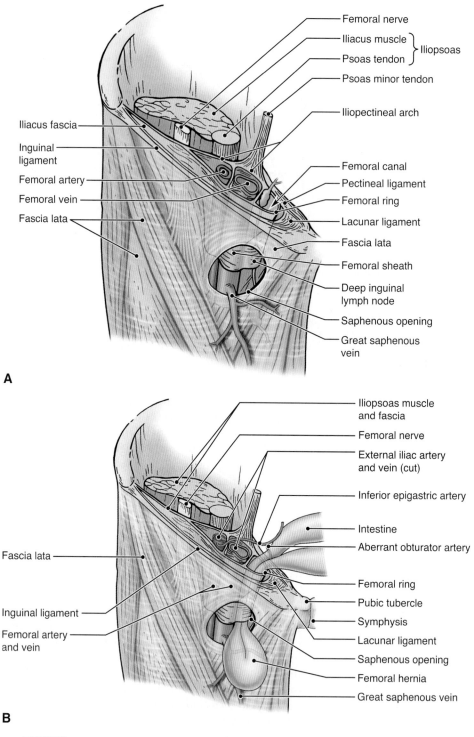

FIGURE 2.43 **The femoral vein and triangle.**

The great saphenous vein empties into the deep vein network at the top of the thigh, but by this time, it is so large that it cannot do so cryptically. Instead, it enters through a large gap in the deep fascia called the saphenous opening (**A**). Indeed, the femoral triangle around the great vessels is susceptible to herniation, although less so than the inguinal region. Medial to the femoral vein is a channel of space that is loosely packed with fat and lymph nodes, through which the gut tube may protrude from undue abdominal pressure (**B**). (From Moore KL, Dalley AF. Clinically Oriented Anatomy, 5th Edition. Baltimore: Lippincott Williams & Wilkins, 2006.)

soon joins with the **internal iliac vein** to form the **common iliac vein** parallel to the artery of the same name. The internal iliac vein mirrors the internal iliac artery almost completely, in the sense that every named branch of the artery has a corresponding vein draining back toward the internal iliac; one exception is the **iliolumbar vein**, for reasons explained below. A few tributaries of the internal iliac merit special mention.

Recall that the internal iliac artery, via its internal pudendal branch, supplies the external genitalia. Venous return from these structures therefore should end up in the internal iliac vein, and for the most part, it does. A key vein in this route is the **deep dorsal vein** of the clitoris in the female or the penis in the male (Fig. 2.44). This vein ultimately drains into the channel that accompanies the internal pudendal vein. The state of erection that is a key part of the response to sexual stimulation is the result of a large volume of blood entering a spongy connective tissue and getting trapped. Its venous exit must be blocked for the tissue to become turgid, or "erect." Successful (natural) clamping of the deep dorsal vein is necessary achieve this state.

Another tributary of the internal iliac is clinically significant in general practice. The **inferior rectal veins** that accompany the inferior rectal arteries along the lowest parts of the rectum are implicated in the painful condition of **hemorrhoids**. Venous return from the lowest one-third of the anal canal does not pass through the liver. It enters the **middle rectal vein** and **inferior rectal vein**, both of which drain into the internal iliac and, therefore, directly into the **inferior vena cava** (Chapter 3, page 139). The practical significance of this observation is that the tissue being served is supplied with the same very sensitive nerve endings that reach the rest of the skin. Tissues that drain to the portal vein do not sense general pain, touch, or temperature.

We are now very close to the beginning of the inferior vena cava. The external and internal iliac veins join together to form the short but stout common iliac vein. The artery of the same name has no small branches, but the vein does pick up a small tributary. The nearby iliolumbar vein ports directly into the common iliac vein rather than running down into the pelvic cavity to link up with the internal iliac. This is an example of the recurring theme of "opportunistic" design in the venous network. The

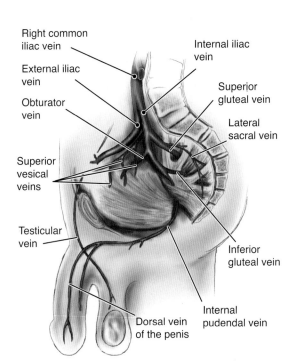

FIGURE 2.44   Venous return from the pelvis and perineum.

Pelvic and perineal drainage parallels the arterial structure, including the veins that drain the genitalia. These are important veins for maintaining states of erection, which are the result of engorging tissues with blood and then suppressing venous return from them for a short period of time.

Right common iliac vein

Internal iliac vein

External iliac vein

Obturator vein

Superior gluteal vein

Lateral sacral vein

Superior vesical veins

Testicular vein

Inferior gluteal vein

Internal pudendal vein

Dorsal vein of the penis

iliolumbar vein finds the larger and closer common iliac, and a merger is induced. To bring blood back down into the pelvic cavity only to have it ascend out again to reach the common iliac vein would be inefficient. Arteries, in contrast to veins, are governed in their formation by a more fixed blueprint of how their target organs develop.

Because the **inferior vena cava** lies just to the right of the midline (in conjunction with the aorta, which lies just to the left), the left common iliac vein must stretch across the midline to reach it (Fig. 2.45). This puts the left common iliac in the most opportunistic position to pick up the **median sacral vein**, which it usually does. The formation of the inferior vena cava is at the L4–L5 vertebral junction, slightly below the bifurcation of the aorta. The right common iliac artery typically crosses over, or anterior to, the converging common iliac veins.

The inferior vena cava is a huge vessel. It begins as the single chute for all venous blood from the pelvis and lower limbs. As it climbs the abdominal cavity, it picks up the venous drainage of the body wall and the kidneys. It is spared the substantial drainage of the gut tube, however, which first goes through the **portal system** of veins into the liver, but only temporarily. In the hidden recess behind the liver and just under the diaphragm, the inferior vena cava will receive two large-caliber **hepatic veins** that carry the treated gut tube drainage.

Some of the veins that accompany the segmental lumbar arteries of the abdomen drain directly into the inferior vena cava as it ascends the vertebral column. The upper **lumbar veins** initiate a separate route to the heart by forming the beginning of the **azygos network** of veins (see below). In parallel with the large renal arteries, the large

FIGURE 2.45 **Formation of the inferior vena cava.**

Venous return from the lower limb, pelvis, and body wall forms the "big river" of the inferior vena cava, just right of midline and slightly inferior to the bifurcation of the aorta. Renal veins also deliver directly to the inferior vena cava. Remember that venous channels are opportunistic—they form locally instead of programmatically. This is why the gonadal vein on the left side ports into the nearby renal vein instead of crossing midline to the get directly to the inferior vena cava. Note that no venous drainage of gut tub is part of this system; that blood drains separately into the liver before entering the inferior vena cava through short but stout hepatic veins (top of the figure).

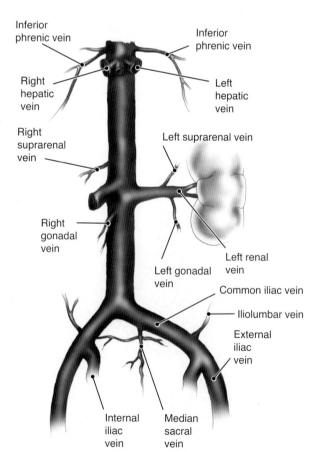

Inferior phrenic vein

Inferior phrenic vein

Right hepatic vein

Left hepatic vein

Right suprarenal vein

Left suprarenal vein

Right gonadal vein

Left gonadal vein

Left renal vein

Common iliac vein

Iliolumbar vein

External iliac vein

Internal iliac vein

Median sacral vein

renal veins run sideways, directly into the inferior vena cava. The left renal vein is longer than the right, so it lies in a more direct position to receive some other expected veins. For example, the **gonadal veins**, which in theory should drain directly into the inferior vena cava, because the gonadal arteries are direct branches of the aorta, actually empty into the inferior vena cava on the right side but into the renal vein on the left. Likewise, the **suprarenal vein** on the right side runs the short distance directly back to the inferior vena cava, but the left suprarenal vein drops into the closer left renal vein. Indeed, the venous system is a virtual "catch as catch can" operation.

The inferior vena cava terminates by running through a dedicated caval opening in the central tendon of the diaphragm and plugging into the right atrium of the heart just beyond. The final veins to empty into the inferior vena cava are the **hepatic veins**, which are so short that they are barely vessels at all. A large right hepatic vein and a left hepatic vein deliver treated blood from most of the liver tissue, and a middle hepatic vein typically delivers blood from the liver's **caudate lobe**. Smaller and more numerous veins may reach into the inferior vena cava below these major veins as an opportunistic connection between it and the adjacent right and caudate lobes.

The liver, of course, serves the vital function of processing the material that the body has absorbed into the bloodstream from the outside world. Most of this material is the desired nutrient matter that you have ingested (the food that you like to eat), but some of it is inappropriate, unkind, or toxic to the tissues. As a result, all the venous drainage from the beginning of the stomach to near the end of the rectum is routed to the liver. The network of veins formed along the way is called the **portal system**, and you should study the anatomy of this system very closely.

The Portal System of Venous Return

Keep in mind that vein formation is highly variable, and the typical portal venous system described below is only that—typical. It does not match the arterial supply to the gut tube very well, which makes it slightly more complicated to learn. The basic separation of foregut, midgut, and hindgut routes applies to the veins, but the names and interconnections are different. The foregut structures, for example, drain into a large **splenic vein** that accompanies the splenic artery across the back of the abdomen. Along the way, the splenic vein receives many smaller veins that service the stomach, but some of the gastric veins reach directly to the terminal vein of the system (the **portal vein**). The **left gastric vein** and the veins of the lesser (concave) curvature of the stomach sometimes will shunt directly to the portal vein (Fig. 2.46).

Remember that the splenic vein is on the left side of the body. The hindgut portion of the gut tube also is mostly on the left side of the body, so it is no surprise that the **inferior mesenteric vein** drains directly into the splenic vein instead of into the more distant portal vein. Remember also that the inferior mesenteric vein drains the gut tube almost, but not quite, to the end of the rectum. The last tributary to the inferior mesenteric vein is the **superior rectal vein**, which indicates that the middle and inferior parts of the rectum drain somewhere else (see Chapter 3).

The midgut drains into the **superior mesenteric vein**, which is exactly like its arterial partner in coverage. As the tributaries close together, the diameter of the superior mesenteric vein becomes quite large, and in the dissection field, it appears to be a direct line leading to the portal vein and the liver. The **portal vein** is the combination of the superior mesenteric vein and the splenic vein, and it occupies a key position in the mesentery of the abdomen as it approaches the liver. We now consider that position more closely.

As described in detail later, much of the gut tube is suspended in a dorsal mesentery. The liver buds away from the gut tube anteriorly, or ventrally, and is suspended in the ventral mesentery that is particular to the foregut only. At the foregut/midgut transition, the ventral mesentery ends, leaving a kind of lower, free edge to the curtain of mesodermal tissue. Because the stomach rotates so much during development, this free edge begins, logically, in the transverse plane, but it rotates up and to the right so that it finishes more in a vertical plane facing the right side of the body. As with other soft-tissue connections in the body, this underfold of the ventral mesentery is called a ligament (the **hepatoduodenal ligament**). Three major items travel to and from the liver within the protective sleeve of the hepatoduodenal ligament: the **common hepatic artery** feeding the liver, a bile duct delivering output from the liver to the intestine, and a very big vein (the **portal vein**) delivering blood to the liver for processing.

This combination of structures is called the **portal triad**, and its arrangement within the hepatoduodenal ligament is a critical piece of clinical knowledge. Surgical removal of the gallbladder requires that the cystic duct leading from the gallbladder to join the bile duct be cut; however, the surgeon must be very careful not to cut the nearby artery and portal vein. The typical arrangement in space has the bile duct dis-

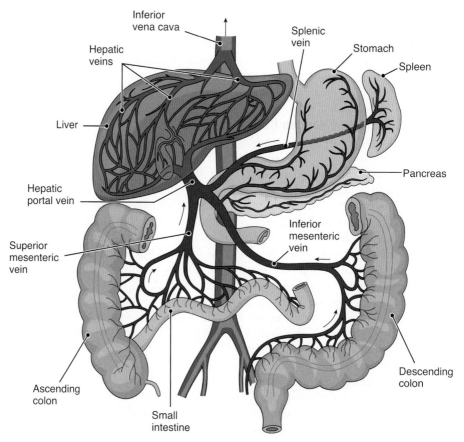

FIGURE 2.46   The hepatic portal system of venous drainage of the gut tube.

Venous drainage of the gut tube and associated organs first routes to the liver before returning to the heart. Problems in the liver can cause a "traffic jam" of blood trying to get there, which leads to problems at the periphery, where veins are small. (From Cohen, BJ, Taylor JJ. Memmler's Human Body in Health and Disease, 10th Edition. Baltimore: Lippincott Williams & Wilkins, 2005.)

posed to the right, the proper hepatic artery disposed to the left, and the big portal vein disposed posteriorly (behind them).

Once the portal vein reaches the liver, it deconstructs into capillaries once again so that portal blood can soak the liver tissue (hepatic parenchyma). Once processed, blood in the sinusoids is drawn into a venous capillary bed that recombines into larger (but short) veins. The recollection of blood and reconstruction of veins becomes the multiplex called the **hepatic veins**. This architecture is called a portal system in general, so the proper designation for the gut tube drainage is really the **hepatic portal system**.

Smooth functioning of the hepatic portal system depends heavily on the vigor of the liver. A damaged liver cannot process the inflow and outflow adequately, so parts of the system located both before and after suffer. The body carries more toxins, and blood backs up in the portal vein and its tributaries. **Portal hypertension** is one of the more common clinical conditions in the developed world. Aside from the major complications associated with an incompetent liver, portal hypertension also has anatomic consequences. Pressure backs up blood all the way to the very limits of the gut tube drainage. These are found at the top end (the **gastroesophageal junction**), at the bottom end (the **rectum**), and oddly enough, at the umbilicus. Pressure in the portal system will tend to force portal blood into the systemic veins that drain the esophagus and the lower part of the rectum. These produce varices and/or hemorrhoids.

The umbilicus is involved because it includes the remnant of the vascular connection between mother and infant. Although the **umbilical vein** of the fetus has withered into the **round ligament**, a series of small, paraumbilical veins still connect the abdominal wall to the former connections of the umbilical vein, including the nearby portal vein. Obstruction or high pressure in the portal system can cause these paraumbilical veins to swell, creating a marked and diagnostic condition around the belly button known as **caput medusae** (in reference to the snake-like hair cords of the Greek mythological figure Medusa) (Fig. 2.47).

Formation of the Superior Vena Cava

The rest of the body ultimately drains into a large but short channel called the **superior vena cava**. The body wall tends to drain independently of the arms, which, in turn, are independent of the head and neck The story of the superior vena cava is the story of the **azygos system** of veins from the body wall (Fig. 2.48), the **subclavian system** of

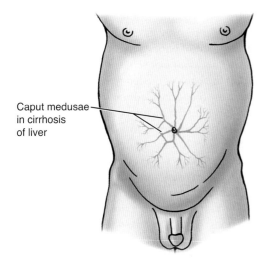

Caput medusae in cirrhosis of liver

FIGURE 2.47   Portal hypertension.

Portal hypertension results in bulging and potential rupture of veins at the periphery of the hepatic portal system. Typical presentations include rupture of the gastroesophageal veins, rectal hemorrhoids, and a snake-like pattern of bulging veins around the umbilicus called a "caput Medusae" (shown here). (From Moore KL, Dalley AF. Clinically Oriented Anatomy, 5th Edition. Baltimore: Lippincott Williams & Wilkins, 2006.)

FIGURE 2.48   **The azygos vein system.**

The chest wall, heart, lungs, upper limb, and head drain into the superior vena cava. The last region to connect is the chest wall through the azygos vein. This unpaired vein also is important because it links the inferior vena cava and the superior vena cava and, thus, can be used as an alternate route to the heart from below the diaphragm.

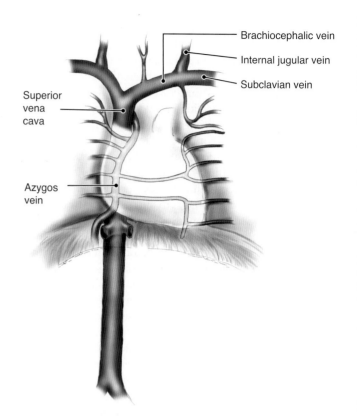

Brachiocephalic vein

Internal jugular vein

Subclavian vein

Superior vena cava

Azygos vein

veins from the upper limb, and the **jugular system** of veins from the head and neck. Because the superior vena cava is just to the right of the midline, we also must expect some vessels from the left-side versions of these veins to cross the midline en route.

The **azygos system** reflects two primary objectives of venous system design. One is to provide multiple routes for blood to return. Another is to take the least complicated course from the tissue source to the "vein of passage," or the vein that moves back to the heart as opposed to the vein that drains tissue directly. The analogy of the American highway system may be useful here. Neighborhoods (tissues) are served by grids of roads with many small drives and streets and intersections (small, irregular, nameless veins). One road leads out of the neighborhood and toward the highway (big vein, or vein of passage). The highway has a few entry ramps (tributary veins) from other neighborhoods, but for the most part, it is an expressway toward the city (the heart).

The azygos system arises from two large veins of passage in the abdominal region. On the right side of the body, it typically begins as an exit vein from the inferior vena cava. On the left side, it typically arises from the back of the left renal vein. In this way, the azygos system provides a minor detour for blood headed toward the heart in the giant abdominal veins of passage. On the right side, the incipient vein is called the **azygos vein**, and on the left side, it is called the **hemiazygos vein**.

From this beginning, the azygos system flows toward the heart along the sides of the vertebral bodies, where it lies in perfect position to collect the segmental veins that drain the body wall and run alongside the intercostal and lumbar arteries. Indeed, from a variable point along the lumbar vertebrae, the segmental spaces begin to empty into the azygos and hemiazygos veins rather than into the inferior vena cava, in keeping with the primary objective of the venous system to take the least complicated course to the nearest vein of passage. Ascending lumbar veins also may connect the iliolumbar veins of the internal iliac system with the azygos system, further extending the azygos network.

On the left side of the body, the hemiazygos vein ascends into the thorax through the substance of the left leg of the diaphragm to approximately the level of the eighth thoracic vertebra. At this point, it turns sideways under the aorta, around the vertebral body, and over to the right side, where it empties into the azygos vein. This leaves unaccounted the upper intercostal spaces on the left side. An **accessory hemiazygos vein** forms in approximately the fourth intercostal space. The intercostal vein there simply turns inferiorly when it reaches the vertebral body. It picks up the remaining intercostal veins down to the level of the hemiazgyos vein, where it then crosses over the vertebrae in parallel and empties into the azygos vein. The uppermost intercostal veins, however, drain into more nearby veins, such as the **brachiocephalic** (see below).

On the right side of the body, the azygos vein ascends uninterrupted from its modest beginning in the upper lumbar region of the inferior vena cava until it passes behind the root of the lung and reaches the level of the right atrium (see Fig. 2.48). It passes behind the diaphragm alongside the aorta very near to the midline of the body. At this point, the inferior vena cava is pulled forward into the region of the central tendon of the diaphragm thanks to the draw of the liver and the position of the right atrium of the heart. After the azygos vein has passed behind the root of the lung, it receives a tributary vein from some of the intercostal spaces above the root of the lung. Then, it shoots sideways by 90° to climb up the vertebral body and plugs into the superior vena cava just before the superior vena cava itself reaches the top of the right atrium. The azygos system, thus, provides a minor route for some blood in the inferior vena cava system to reach the heart and a more opportunistic route for blood from the body wall to reach a larger vein of passage.

The **subclavian system** routes blood back from the upper limb to the heart. Just as the subclavian artery feeds the adjacent neck and chest wall structures en route to the arm, the subclavian vein draws venous return from all nearby trunk structures as it connects the arm drainage to the superior vena cava. Beginning distally, in the fingers, are superficial and deep networks of veins, just as in the foot. The deep network is anatomically unremarkable, because it accompanies in space and in name the branches of the radial, ulnar, brachial, and axillary segments of the central line of circulation. The accompaniment is so complete, in fact, that for much of the route up the arm, the vein network forms true venae comitantes, or parallel paired veins on either side of the artery. This pairing accompaniment typically coalesces into a single vein in the uppermost part of the arm (a **brachial vein**) or in the armpit (an **axillary vein**).

The superficial network of veins in the upper limb is more interesting anatomically. The network on the palmar side of the hand is minor compared to that on the dorsal side, as you can readily see from your own hands. As early as the wrist level, you can detect two major superficial vein channels from the **dorsal venous plexus** that run up the length of the pronated forearm (Fig. 2.49). A smaller one (both typically and relatively) on the pinky-finger side (the medial side, in standard anatomic position) is called the **basilic vein**, and a larger one (both typically and relatively) on the thumb side (the lateral side) is called the **cephalic vein**. The cephalic vein will be continuous all the way up the limb and across the front of the shoulder (where it is still called the cephalic vein). At that point, it runs superficially in the distinct groove between the deltoid muscle and the pectoralis major muscle. It traffics a significant amount of blood in the upper limb, much like the great saphenous vein in the lower limb, and it ends by diving into the **axillary vein** just before it hits the clavicle bone.

The superficial network of veins in the upper limb is important clinically for the procedure of drawing blood (**venipuncture**). The superficial veins in the cubital fossa

FIGURE 2.49 Venous drainage of the upper limb.

The upper limb drains like the lower limb, in the sense that a large amount of venous blood travels in the superficial veins. From a prominent arch on the back of your hand, you can trace a channel up the radial side of your forearm into the cubital fossa, where the median cubital, basilic, and cephalic veins usually are visible and available for venipuncture. The cephalic vein, which receives most of the blood in this system, empties into the deep veins that accompany the arteries. At this point, the deep veins have coalesced into a single, large brachial vein, which is called the axillary vein when it sidles next to the artery of the same name. (LifeART image copyright © 2007 Lippincott Williams & Wilkins. All rights reserved.)

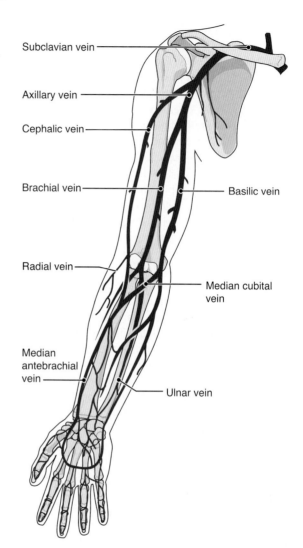

Subclavian vein

Axillary vein

Cephalic vein

Brachial vein

Basilic vein

Radial vein

Median cubital vein

Median antebrachial vein

Ulnar vein

(the "inside" or "cup" of the elbow) usually are the first choice for routine venipuncture. At this point, the cephalic and basilic veins are connected by an oblique **median cubital vein** that often is the most visible one under the skin and, therefore, of interest to phlebotomists.

The **axillary vein** typically is the first unpaired deep vein. It is formed as a continuation of the brachial vein and it receives the superficial network. Unlike the cephalic vein, the basilic vein took a more subtle route earlier along the biceps brachii muscle, where it slid slightly deeper until it ramped into the beginning of the axillary vein. The axillary vein also draws blood from the starburst of veins accompanying the arteries that branched off in the axilla. Blood from the shoulder complex, the lateral side of the body wall, the pectoral muscles, and very importantly, the breast collects in veins (**circumflex scapular vein**, **lateral thoracic vein**, and **thoracoacromial vein**) that route back to the axillary.

The axillary vein changes its name to the **subclavian vein** at approximately the outer border of the first rib. Its course underneath the clavicle is important to understand for the insertion of central line catheters. The subclavian joins the **internal jugular vein** to form the **brachiocephalic vein** behind the medial end of the clavicle.

Between its beginning and its end, it draws chiefly from one tributary, the **external jugular vein**. Indeed, the veins that accompany the branches of the subclavian artery (**vertebral, thyrocervical trunk, internal thoracic,** and **costocervical trunk**) drain to other nearby vessels, such as the external jugular veins and the brachiocephalic veins (Fig. 2.50).

As the other main tributary of the subclavian vein, the **external jugular vein** delivers blood from a wide territory of the superficial head and neck. In general, it drains blood from areas that are served by the external carotid artery, but unlike that artery, it can be small or absent. In these cases, the **internal jugular vein** is larger. Venous networks in the head are extensive, as you can sense when you are embarrassed or overexerted. No reliable, "typical" pattern exists to describe, but certain tributary veins are more regular than others. The veins of the scalp typically join together to form a **superficial temporal vein** that corresponds to the artery and is the stereotypic throbbing vein of the temple in caricatures of irate people. This vein picks up drainage from the **maxillary vein** (accompanying the maxillary artery) as it descends along the side of the head. Based on its position at this point, it is called the **retromandibular vein** and, in effect, is the source of the external jugular. Variation is common.

The other major drainage route of the outer structures of the head is the route of the **facial vein**, which parallels the course of the facial artery. As the facial vein crosses down over the edge of the mandible, it may send some blood to the external jugular via a bridge between it and the retromandibular vein. Once conjoined, the external jugular vein is at full charge down the side of the neck superficial to the large sternocleidomastoid muscle. The prominent vein is made even more prominent in this position under muscle strain. The external jugular dives deep to the clavicle just to the side of where the sternocleidomastoid muscle inserts, and in this position it empties into the subclavian vein.

To form the superior vena cava, then, all that is left is the blood from the central nervous system and nearby structures from the head. The internal carotid artery is dedicated to the central nervous system. Some of its delivery reaches peripheral tissues around the eye, but the vast majority of its service is to the brain. The veins that drain the same tissue are not quite as exclusive to the central nervous system, in keeping with the nature of venous drainage to be opportunistic. The **internal jugular vein** will drain the brain, but it also will drain nearby tissues of the face and neck on its way to the chest. Its commencement is very interesting anatomically.

The brain is highly vascularized. It contains a thorough network of typical, vein-like vessels that draw from the ventricles of cerebrospinal fluid that are found nearby. These

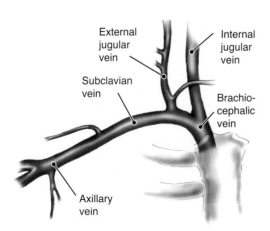

External jugular vein

Internal jugular vein

Subclavian vein

Brachio-cephalic vein

Axillary vein

FIGURE 2.50 Axillary, external jugular, and subclavian veins.

Blood from the upper limb, neck, and face will drain into the axillary and external jugular veins, respectively. The continuation of the axillary toward the heart is called the subclavian, in keeping with the companion artery.

veins drain from the "inside" region of the brain to the "outside" region of the brain, meaning that blood moves toward the surface of the brain and the interface between the neural tissue and the meninges (specifically, the **dura mater**). The **cranial venous sinuses** are fixed shunts, sleeved by dura mater, that receive the brain drain and flush it around the inner circumference of the cranial vault like a roulette ball (Fig. 2.51).

The venous sinuses that are apparent in gross anatomy are the **straight sinus**, the **superior sagittal sinus**, the **inferior sagittal sinus**, the **sigmoid sinus**, the **petrosal sinuses**, the **cavernous sinus**, and the **transverse sinus**. They connect with and/or become one another and, ultimately, take the blood toward a bony gap, the **jugular foramen**, near the foramen magnum. Here, like a collecting bag, the endothelial tissue of a true vein begins as a "hang-down" from the jugular foramen. This is the commencement of the internal jugular vein, and it lies very close to the course and entry point for the internal carotid artery. Study of the sinus impressions on the bones of the skull is a tradition in gross anatomy courses.

The unpaired sinuses begin with the superior sagittal sinus at the very front of the cranial cavity. This sinus grooves the midline of the cranium where the dura mater folds in on itself to fit into the space between the two hemispheres of the brain. This fold of dura mater is called the **falx cerebri**. The superior sagittal sinus ends in the back of the cranium by becoming the right transverse sinus at a point of the occipital bone known, logically, as the confluence of the sinuses. A smaller midline sinus is the inferior sagittal sinus, which runs in the lower sling of the falx cerebri. It ends toward the back of the brain by becoming the straight sinus, a continuation of the dural sleeve concept in the union line between the falx cerebri and the **tentorium cerebelli**. This route usually ends in the left transverse sinus.

The remaining gross sinuses are paired. The cavernous sinuses are located in the traffic-way between the brain and the organs of sight and smell in the face. Technically, these sinuses are lifts of dura on either side of the body of the sphenoid bone, but practically, they are perilously close to the surfaces of the eyes and nose. Infection can drain from the nose into the cavernous sinus, which then puts it in direct contact with the circulation of the brain. The risk here is that a thrombosis in a facial vein may pass backward into the large, open channel of the cavernous sinus, then lodge in a tinier tributary vein from the brain. The internal carotid artery swims right through the cavernous sinus itself like an underwater cable.

The sinuses continue backward from the superior orbital fissure and body of sphenoid as the petrosal sinuses (superior and inferior), which straddle the rock-hard bone house of the inner ear. The superior petrosal sinus leads to the final piece of the transverse sinus, whereas the inferior petrosal sinus leads, as if by gravity, directly down to the jugular foramen.

The transverse sinuses, as named, run transversely along the parietal and occipital bones. Each begins at the central confluence of sinuses at the posterior limit of the cranium and routes blood forward to the petrous portion of the temporal bone. There, the transverse sinus receives the superior petrosal sinus and drops, in a wiggle, down to the jugular foramen as the sigmoid sinus. In concept, this is not unlike the way that rain is routed through gutters and drainpipes on its way to an underground sewer.

The sinuses also receive blood from emissary veins that drain the bones of the cranium and connect to the superficial veins of the scalp. Likewise, nearby tributaries of the external jugular system are connected to the sinuses by shunts and minor veins.

On its way to the base of the neck, the **internal jugular vein** accompanies the common carotid artery and the **vagus nerve** (see below) in a sheath of protective connective tissue. The internal jugular may receive small tributaries from the lingual vein of the tongue, and in its course through the neck, it typically receives flow from the

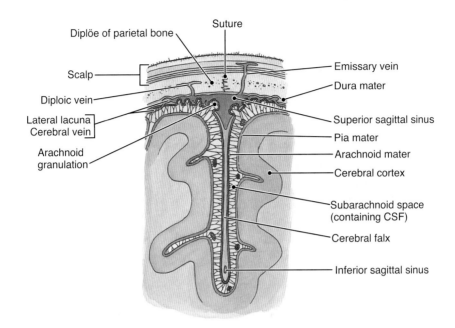

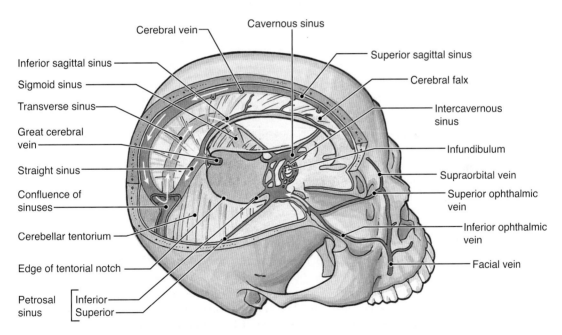

FIGURE 2.51   **Venous drainage of the brain.**

Blood from the brain drains differently than blood elsewhere in the body. Vein networks in the sub-arachnoid space drain directly into sleeves of the dura mater called dural sinuses (e.g., sagittal sinus, top). The dural sinuses act like a peripheral plumbing system by routing blood back toward the con-fluence of sinuses and then around the bowl the braincase until it all pours through the jugular fora-men, much like the drain in the bottom of a sink (bottom). CSF = cerebrospinal fluid. (From Moore KL, Agur AM. Essential Clinical Anatomy, 3rd Edition. Baltimore: Lippincott Williams & Wilkins, 2007.)

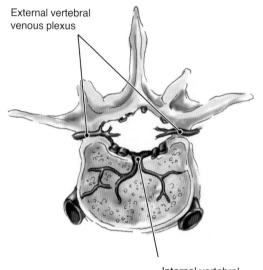

External vertebral
venous plexus

Internal vertebral
venous plexus

**FIGURE 2.52   Venous
drainage of the spinal cord and
vertebrae.**

Blood draining the spinal cord
mixes with blood draining the vertebral column, which is a potential
source of infection spread into the
central nervous system. The route
from here back to the heart obeys
"vein tradition"—via the nearest
large vein, which in the case of the
vertebral column could be the vertebral vein in the neck, the azygos
vein in the chest, or the inferior
vena cava below the diaphragm.

facial vein network. It terminates by joining the subclavian vein behind the medial end of the clavicle. This same arrangement applies to both sides of the body, so the union vein is called the **brachiocephalic vein** (literally, from the arm and the head). The two **brachiocephalic veins** merge (somewhat unequally;, see below) to form the **superior vena cava** (see Fig. 2.48).

The brachiocephalic vein is too conveniently positioned to be ignored by regional tissues. The span from the medial end of the clavicle to the lower border of the first rib on the right side puts the brachiocephalic vein in good position to receive smaller veins. The right brachiocephalic vein typically receives the **internal thoracic vein**, the **vertebral vein**, the **highest intercostal vein**, and sometimes, an **inferior thyroid vein**. The same is true for the left brachiocephalic vein, which then must also cross the midline to reach its right-side termination.

Now consider the vertebral vein more closely, because it also helps to drain the central nervous system. It accompanies the pathway of the vertebral artery, frequently as true venae comitantes. As it descends through the transverse foramina of the cervical vertebrae, it participates in the "open-gate" system of veins that serve the spinal cord and vertebral column. The spinal cord veins drain, in part, into an **internal vertebral plexus** of veins, which, in turn, drain into an **external vertebral plexus** that taps into the **vertebral vein** (Fig. 2.52). In other words, blood drains, in the true fashion of veins, by the most convenient local route. For the spinal cord, this means issuing blood out to the vertebral plexuses, where it drains into the nearest systemic vein, such as an intercostal, an azygos, or a vertebral vein. In turn, **this means that the venous drainage of the central nervous system is exposed to the body circulation, and vice versa.** Metastasis and spread of infection are facilitated by such a system.

THE LYMPHATIC SYSTEM

The heart, arteries and veins are most, but not all, of the anatomy of the circulatory system. The body also develops a clever network of tubes connected to the venous system that conduct an important fluid solution called **lymph**. Lymph is a Latin word for "clear springwater," and its purpose is to "keep the moving parts clean," something akin to the body's self-sustaining motor oil. Lymph maintains and exchanges fluid between the functioning cells of the body, and it captures and filters harmful or foreign proteins and cells. The anatomy of the system rarely is apparent in the cadaver of a gross anatomy course, but the understanding of its operation is critical for clinical medicine.

The body possesses three very important "filters" or "exchange stations" to maintain homeostasis, or chemical balance. The lungs exchange carbon dioxide for oxygen and, thus, resupply hemoglobin cells with a vital fuel source. The liver processes what you absorb from the outside world and renders, detoxifies, and discharges it via the venous system. The kidneys filter waste products, among other things, out of the bloodstream. These three hardworking organ complexes are critical for health and life. Even minor problems within them can lead to an acute and life-threatening disease state. To relieve some of their load and to attend to more local, on-site, minor fix-it needs, the lymphatic system roves everywhere that the circulation goes, provides a kind of "landfill" stationing of undesirable elements, and buffers or otherwise dilutes unfriendly compounds for permanent treatment by the liver and kidneys.

The anatomy of the lymphatic system will clarify (no pun intended!) these functions. Embryologists suspect, but are not sure, that this system of ducts, nodes, and channels derives directly from the tissue of the developing veins. This would be the logical, conservative hypothesis, because ultimately, lymphatic ducts empty into the venous system (Fig. 2.53). At the level of contact with cells, the system consists of tiny ductules. The ductules lead to **nodes**, which act as a kind of physical and chemical filter and are collections of lymphocytes, a type of white blood cell. Particles and substances that are not broken down by lymphatic fluid can be trapped by a node— potentially forever. In this way, the nodes can act like a "landfill" of nasty material. Lymph nodes around the lungs, for example, can trap the byproducts from smoking tobacco and very quickly become hardened black lumps. Lymph typically passes into a node via several incoming ductules, but it typically leaves the node through a single outflow, or efferent, ductule. All lymph generally passes through multiple nodes before entering the venous system.

Lymphatic concentration is not distributed evenly throughout the body. The central nervous system, for example, appears to be devoid of lymphatics. On the other hand, zones of high contact with the outside world, such as the dermis and mucous membranes, are networked with dense lymphatics. In some cases, the lymphatics do not form ducts and nodes, as in the case of the tonsillar tissue (tonsils) in the oral cavity; instead, they are self-contained hubs of active lymphocytes.

Some dense clusters of nodes are found in certain areas that act as "collecting zones," such as the root of the lung (**bronchomediastinal lymph nodes**), armpit (**axillary lymph nodes**), and along the armpit of the lower limb in the femoral triangle near the inguinal ligament (**inguinal lymph nodes**). Because the head has so many surfaces that interact with the outside world, lymphatic drainage there is especially important. Aside from the lymphoid tissues that prevail in the oral cavity, such as the tonsils, lymph from the head ultimately collects in palpable nodes along the large internal jugular vein. In clinical practice, you will closely examine the lymph nodes that are palpable through the skin. These nodes are critical sentinels of possible infections or spreading diseases. Part of every routine physical examination is a manual assessment of the key superficial lymph node plexuses—inguinal, jugular, and axillary—not to mention the familiar "Say AHHH" predicate to checking the tonsils. Their density and hardness reflect the effect of how infectious or pathogenic material has been transported to them from the primary affected tissue (e.g., the breast or lip or genitalia).

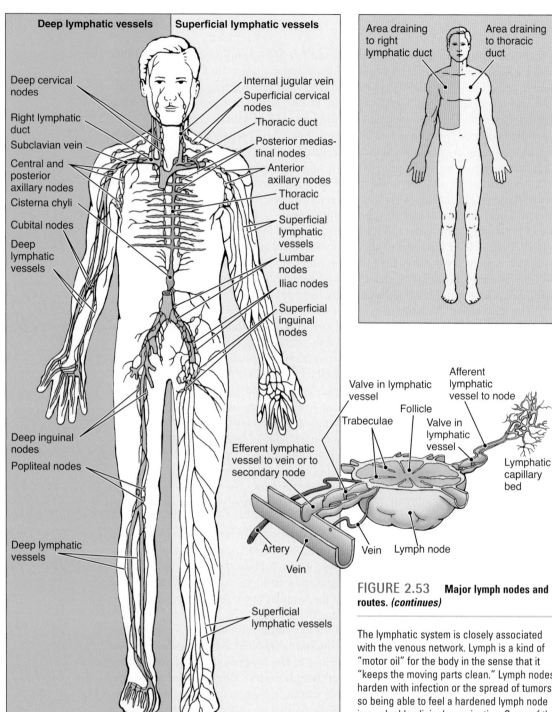

Deep lymphatic vessels | **Superficial lymphatic vessels**

Deep cervical nodes

Right lymphatic duct

Subclavian vein

Central and posterior axillary nodes

Cisterna chyli

Cubital nodes

Deep lymphatic vessels

Deep inguinal nodes

Popliteal nodes

Deep lymphatic vessels

Internal jugular vein
Superficial cervical nodes
Thoracic duct
Posterior mediastinal nodes
Anterior axillary nodes
Thoracic duct
Superficial lymphatic vessels
Lumbar nodes
Iliac nodes
Superficial inguinal nodes

Efferent lymphatic vessel to vein or to secondary node

Artery

Vein

Superficial lymphatic vessels

Area draining to right lymphatic duct

Area draining to thoracic duct

Valve in lymphatic vessel

Trabeculae

Follicle

Valve in lymphatic vessel

Afferent lymphatic vessel to node

Lymphatic capillary bed

Vein   Lymph node

FIGURE 2.53   **Major lymph nodes and routes. *(continues)***

The lymphatic system is closely associated with the venous network. Lymph is a kind of "motor oil" for the body in the sense that it "keeps the moving parts clean." Lymph nodes harden with infection or the spread of tumors, so being able to feel a hardened lymph node is a valuable clinical examination. Some of the nodes are close enough to the skin to be felt, particularly where the vein that they are traveling beside is also close to the skin (e.g., the inguinal region [femoral vein], the axilla [axillary vein], and the cervical region [external jugular vein]). (From Moore KL, Dalley AF. Clinically Oriented Anatomy, 4th Edition. Baltimore: Lippincott Williams & Wilkins, 1999; Cohen BJ, Taylor JJ. Memmler's Human Body in Health and Disease, 10th Edition. Baltimore: Lippincott Williams & Wilkins, 2005.)

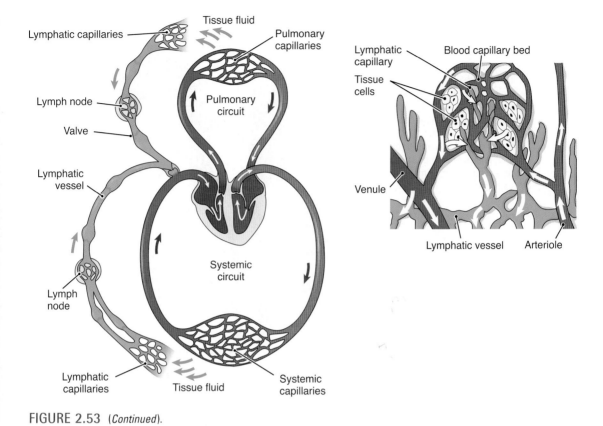

FIGURE 2.53 (*Continued*).

From the lower limbs and abdomen, lymph nodes drain into a deep sac in the upper lumbar region called the **cysterna chyli**. From this pool of captured fluid begins the **thoracic duct**, a definable, more or less central tube lying along the vertebral column. Nearby are the azygos vein, the esophagus, and the aorta. The thoracic duct tails off toward the left as it passes behind the heart and great vessels, and it empties into the very beginning of the left brachiocephalic vein (Fig. 2.54). Along the way, it collects lymph from the thorax, from the left arm, and from the left side of the head and neck. Lymph from the right side of the thorax, from the head and neck, and from the right arm collects into a much less noticeable **right lymphatic duct** that empties into the back of the right brachiocephalic vein.

Demands on the lymphatic system change with age. Growing children are more vulnerable than adults, so they need a more potent system of internal cleansing. For this purpose, a **thymus gland** develops in the neck region and stimulates development of the lymphatic system. The thymus gland grows until puberty, then diminishes in both size and function over the adult life span (see Chapter 6). Maintenance of interstitial fluid becomes more challenging with age. Obstruction within the venous system or the lymphatics can lead to excessive buildup of fluid, or **edema**. Peripheral edema is a sign of an inefficient or diseased circulatory system.

If the lymphatic system has anything like an organ of its own, that organ would be the **spleen**. As blood cells lose their utility or become polluted, they are "removed" by the circulatory system via lymphatic cannibalization as well as kidney and liver processing. They must be replaced, however, and as the body is growing, new cells must

FIGURE 2.54   **Thoracic duct.**

Lymph from almost everywhere in the body collects in the thoracic duct, which lies along the thoracic vertebrae before entering the venous system at the beginning of the left brachiocephalic vein. Lymph from the right lung, right side of the chest, right upper limb, and right side of the head collects in a complementary right lymphatic duct.

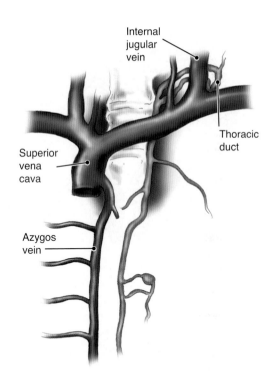

Internal jugular vein

Thoracic duct

Superior vena cava

Azygos vein

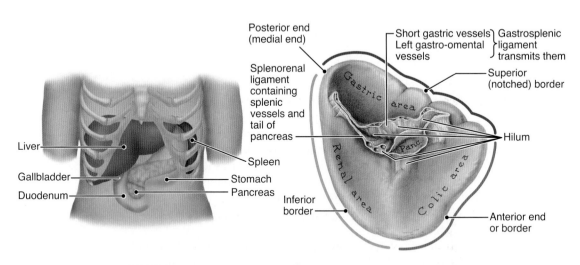

Posterior end (medial end)

Splenorenal ligament containing splenic vessels and tail of pancreas

Short gastric vessels
Left gastro-omental vessels
Gastrosplenic ligament transmits them

Superior (notched) border

Hilum

Gastric area

Renal area

Panc

Colic area

Anterior end or border

Inferior border

Liver

Gallbladder

Duodenum

Spleen

Stomach

Pancreas

FIGURE 2.55   **The spleen.**

The spleen is a lymphoid organ that monitors and filters blood from its rib-protected position in the upper left quadrant of the abdomen. An enlarged spleen can be palpated below the rib margin. It can be seen as a giant filtration plant at the end of the splenic artery and beginning of the splenic vein. (From Moore KL, Dalley AF. Clinically Oriented Anatomy, 4th Edition. Baltimore: Lippincott Williams & Wilkins, 1999.)

be produced to keep up, thus compounding the demand for new cells until adulthood. The spleen produces fresh blood cells, particularly in growing children. Its development is within the dorsal mesentery of the foregut, and its ultimate position in the adult body is of some clinical significance.

Mesoderm cells lodged in the dorsal mesentery of the foregut tube pull together and condense as the endodermal tube develops. These cells develop the classic capsule and parenchyma design that is typical of organs, but they never leave the comfortable sheath of the dorsal mesentery. Rather than get caught up in the extensive swiveling and drooping of the dorsal mesentery as the stomach expands and rotates, the spleen ducks back toward the posterior abdominal wall as the foregut matures (Fig. 2.55).

The spleen retreats into the recess behind the rotated stomach anterior to the left kidney and superior to the bend in the colon from transverse to descending colon (which is known as the **splenic flexure**). Its blood supply from the celiac trunk (the splenic artery) follows it and, thus, shoots across the back of the body wall at the level of the pancreas. This explains why a substantial part of the circulation of the pancreas comes from the splenic artery.

The spleen lacks a duct system of its own, so it has no complement to the ureter of the kidney or the bile duct of the liver. It pumps new blood cells into the bloodstream via the splenic vein, a major component of the portal system. The location of the spleen against the lower ribs in the "soft spot" on the left side of the abdominal wall makes it vulnerable to trauma, which can result in a "ruptured spleen" because of the organ's delicate capsule. In adults, the spleen may be removed in such cases with minimal consequence.

3

Digestive System

INTRODUCTION

At the top end of the endoderm (the oropharyngeal membrane), the ectoderm and mesoderm elaborate to protect the sensitive endoderm from direct contact with the outside world. Lips, teeth, and a large oral cavity grow as a kind of security post to guard the gut tube. They physically process what you acquire before you have to absorb it.

From this point on—or "down," as it were—the endoderm conforms to a tube, and it absorbs both beneficial and harmful things alike. Some parts of the tube are more receptive to certain compounds, such as proteins, than to others, and some parts mostly reclaim water that the body has added to the mix to prevent dehydration. Entire "organs" develop from the tube to assist with the complex task of breaking down molecules before the long and winding intestinal road of absorption.

The convoluted gut tube is suspended in the abdominal cavity in a sling of mesoderm, just as the early development of the embryo mandated. Like the lungs that derived from it, the gut tube presses against a closed sac—in this case, the peritoneum. The parietal peritoneum is highly sensitive, and it often bears the consequence of gut tube disorders or at least traffics pain referred by them. The diagnosis and treatment of disease states related to the gut tube, however, rely primarily on blood chemistry data, which limit the applications of basic gross anatomy. The primary objectives for learning gut tube anatomy should be to understand the relative position of organs for physical diagnosis and clinical imaging and to master the position and informative qualities of the peritoneal sac against which the tube and its accessory organs grow.

ABDOMINAL CAVITY

When we last tracked the endoderm, it had rolled into a continuous tube and was virtually surrounded by a layer of mesoderm (now called visceral, or splanchnic, mesoderm). This arrangement is best appreciated in cross-section (Fig. 3.1). The endoderm develops primarily into the **digestive system**, which includes the tube itself plus the organs that bud off of it. The tube will expand, convolute, bud organs, and rotate as it becomes the adult **gastrointestinal** (GI) **tract**. Its contact with the visceral mesoderm leads to formation of a smooth muscle wall around the endoderm cells, which gives

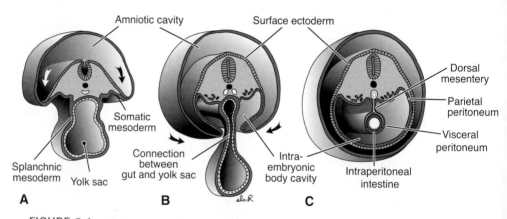

FIGURE 3.1   **The endoderm folds into a tube.**

This classic, cross-sectional view of the folding embryo shows how the endoderm layer of cells folds into a tube (**A**). As it becomes tubular, it maintains surface contact with the visceral layer of lateral plate mesoderm (**B**). The endodermal tube becomes "suspended" in a sling of visceral mesoderm. This sling is made up of two layers (one from each side of the body) and a potential space between them (**C**). Note how the aorta is positioned such that it can send a branch to the gut tube "between" the two layers of the mesoderm that sling the gut tube. This construct of mesoderm is called a mesentery. Because the one shown here reflects off of the "back" wall of the body, it is called the dorsal mesentery. Remember that the endoderm gives rise only to the epithelium of the gut tube, not to the smooth muscle that acts on it. That smooth muscle is a derivative of mesoderm. When it contracts, the tube is squeezed, and this action facilitates the peristaltic effect of moving food particles along the production line. (Adapted from Sadler T. Langman's Medical Embryology, 9th Edition Image Bank. Baltimore: Lippincott Williams & Wilkins, 2003.)

the gut tube a truly tubular appearance. It also enables a mechanical squeezing of the endodermal sleeve (peristalsis) that helps to move the processed food matter, or ingesta, along the system.

Part of the tube is found in the adult **thorax**, or **thoracic cavity**, and part is found in the **abdomen**, or **abdominal cavity**. These two cavities of the body are separated by the **diaphragm**, which, as you remember, was part of the transverse septum of mesoderm but became relocated during longitudinal folding. We should now finish the story of the cavities before we further examine the development of the tube itself.

The lateral folding of the embryo creates a captured cavity, the intraembryonic coelom. This merged cavity space is continuous from top to bottom until the transverse septum cuts the single cavity in half during the longitudinal fold (see Figs. 1.18 to 1.21). The upper half becomes the thoracic cavity, and the piece of the coelom that remains there looks like a drooping arch. The heart grows against the bend of the arch, and the lungs grow against the "limbs" of the arch. Below the diaphragm, the merged limbs of the coelom become the **peritoneal sac**. The layer of mesoderm that completely lines and, thus, constitutes the peritoneal cavity is now called the **peritoneum**. Some of it coats the wall of the body (**parietal peritoneum**), and some of it coats the gut tube (**visceral peritoneum**). The highly elongated and organ-sprouting gut tube pushes against the peritoneum so much that very little "cavity" is left in the sac. Thus, fluid accumulation within the sac (**ascites**) quickly leads to discomfort and provokes medical attention.

Now that we have established how the peritoneal sac is formed, we can proceed to describe the gross anatomy of the digestive system. This relatively simple structural system of the body is incredibly complex physiologically. The clinical spectrum of complications in this system is vast, because its structure is in contact with the outside world and all its impurities. Major pathophysiologies, such as diabetes, cirrhosis, and colitis, result from dysfunctional behavior of this system consequent, in some cases, to consumption behavior. The clinical anatomy of these diseases is less apparent, so in studying the gross anatomy of the digestive system, the objectives are to master the names of its parts, to understand their nerve and blood supply, and to position the tube relative to the body wall that surrounds it.

ESOPHAGUS AND FOREGUT

The first part of the tube to consider is the section that connects the input hole (the mouth, or oral cavity) with the processing unit (the stomach, intestines, etc.). This part is called the **esophagus**, and it is located in the thorax. This section of the endodermal tube changes very little from its initial appearance (Fig. 3.2). It remains a flaccid tube surrounded by muscle. The muscle arises from the visceral mesoderm that coated the gut tube after lateral folding (see Fig. 1.16). When the muscles of the esophagus contract, they "pulse" whatever is inside the esophagus downward. This **peristalsis** is governed by parasympathetic fibers of the **vagus nerve** (cranial nerve X). Dysfunction of this process is increasingly common and can lead to **gastroesophageal reflux disease** (GERD).

The esophagus passes "behind" the diaphragm, but it projects forward just enough that the diaphragm "collars" it. The extent to which the diaphragm squeezes the transition between the esophagus and stomach (gastroesophageal junction) may lead to indigestion, reflux of food, and/or "heartburn." Heartburn refers to the mistaken sense that the discomfort is in the nearby heart and not the esophagus, which, in turn, might lead the patient directly to the emergency room. The gastroesophageal junction also renders the diaphragm vulnerable to slackening, which could result in a herniation of the gut tube. A **sliding hiatal hernia** is one in which the entire junction and the upper

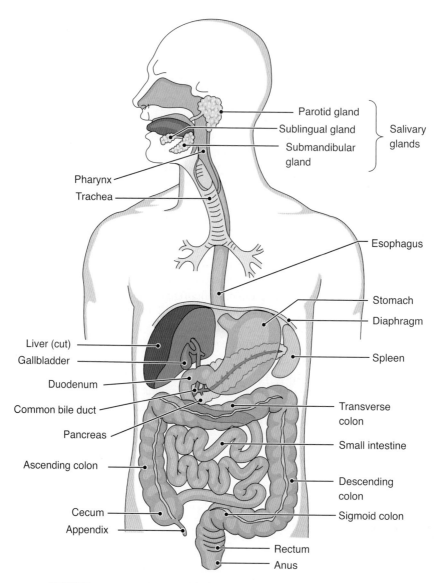

FIGURE 3.2   **The adult gut tube.**

The esophagus is an unmodified tube, just a conduit between where food is initially processed (oral cavity) and where it is digested (stomach and beyond). (From Cohen BJ, Wood DL. Memmler's The Human Body in Health and Disease, 10th Edition. Baltimore: Lippincott Williams & Wilkins, 2004.)

part of the stomach "slide up" through the hiatus, creating an uncomfortable "pinch" of the stomach sac (Fig. 3.3).

Anatomists describe the developing gut tube below the diaphragm as having three regions: a **foregut**, a **midgut**, and a **hindgut**. Each region draws a dedicated artery from the developing circulatory system, so this classification is somewhat logical. The foregut also is the part of the tube that buds off all the accessory organs, so the division of foregut and midgut is even more logical. The transition from midgut to hindgut is more arbitrary, in the sense that both have a similar function of absorption, their nerve supplies overlap, and the exact point at which the circulatory supply of one blends into the circulatory supply of the other is vague.

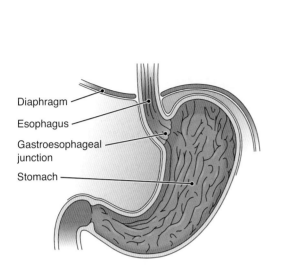
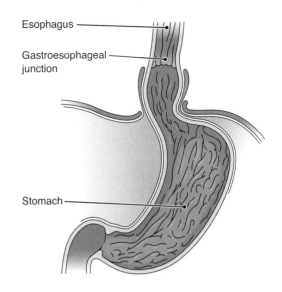

FIGURE 3.3   **Hiatal hernia.**

The relationship between the gut tube and the diaphragm is lax enough that the tube can herniate into the thorax, typically by "sliding" up the esophageal hiatus. (From Cohen BJ, Wood DL. Memmler's The Human Body in Health and Disease, 9th Edition. Philadelphia: Lippincott Williams & Wilkins, 2000.)

The foregut region becomes the stomach, the accessory organs of digestion and the first part of the duodenal portion of the small intestine. All this makes sense considering what the digestive system must accomplish once the ingesta finally gets below the diaphragm. The foregut is the domain of the **celiac trunk** of arteries (Fig. 3.4), the first of the midline branches of the **abdominal aorta**. The foregut has one more distinguishing feature. When the septum transversum arrived to divide the thorax from the abdomen, it actually bridged the space from the foregut to the ventral body wall. As the cranial portion of the septum transversum developed into the diaphragm, the caudal portion thinned into a **ventral mesentery**. Only the foregut has a ventral mesentery (Fig. 3.5). This ventral mesentery, which is exactly similar in design to the dorsal mesentery that runs the entire length of the gut tube, is available to sandwich anything that might bud off from the foregut.

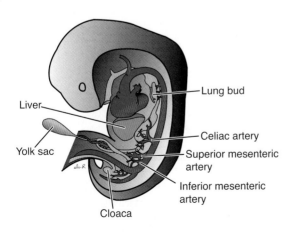

FIGURE 3.4   **A dedicated branch of the aorta serves each gut tube region.**

The celiac trunk serves the foregut region and the organs that bud from it. The superior mesenteric artery serves the midgut region, and the inferior mesenteric artery serves the hindgut region. Note that the term "mesenteric" is used here. This implies that the arteries are located within the mesentery between the body wall and the gut tube. (From Sadler TW. Langman's Essential Medical Embryology. Baltimore: Lippincott Williams & Wilkins, 2006. Figure 6.6A.)

FIGURE 3.5   **Formation of a ventral mesentery in the foregut region.**

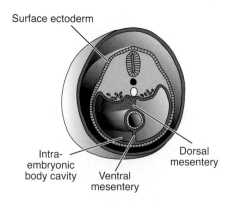

The accessory organs of digestion (liver, pancreas, and gallbladder) derive from the foregut only. Like the gut tube, they rest in a "sling" of mesoderm, but because the gut tube already occupies the dorsal mesentery, these organs need a mesentery of their own. The ventral mesentery appears to form from thinning of the overlying mesoderm of the septum transversum. (From Sadler TW. Langman's Medical Embryology, 9th Edition Image Bank. Baltimore: Lippincott Williams & Wilkins, 2004.)

The first task of the foregut is to store the ingesta, and the first structure of the foregut is an inflated part of the tube called the **stomach**. Structurally, the stomach is simply an expansion of the gut tube to form a larger pouch. Functionally, the stomach secretes a variety of strong acids to reduce the ingesta even more. These acids work effectively on protein compounds.

The stomach is not centered in the middle of the body, which is where it starts out as part of the endodermal gut tube. Indeed, the stomach rotates as it forms (Fig. 3.6). The dorsal border of the foregut expands first, creating a **greater curvature** along that border and a **lesser curvature** along the ventral border. At the same time, the tube spins 90° on its own axis because of the rapid growth of the liver (see below). This positions

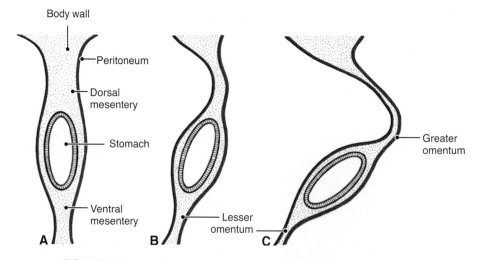

FIGURE 3.6   **The dorsal mesentery of the stomach warps.**

The stomach part of the gut tube balloons posteriorly but not anteriorly, resulting in a surface of greater curvature and a surface of lesser curvature. The stomach also rotates (**A**, **B**) to accommodate rapid growth of the neighboring liver (not shown). One result is a longer "apron" of dorsal mesentery, which is known as the greater omentum (**C**). (From Sadler TW. Langman's Medical Embryology, 10th Edition. Baltimore: Lippincott Williams & Wilkins, 2006. Figure 13.9A, p. 293.)

the greater curvature facing the left side. Eventually, this expanded greater curvature sags down so that it points inferiorly, and this is the final position of the normal stomach, the dominant organ in the left upper quadrant of the abdomen (Fig. 3.7).

Remember that like all parts of the gut tube, the foregut "suspends" from the vertebral column within the sling of dorsal mesentery created by the visceral layer of mesoderm. The expansion, twisting, and sagging of the stomach region affects this mesentery as well. It follows the position of the greater curvature such that it greatly elongates and folds down like an "apron" by the end of growth. This apron of mesentery is called the **greater omentum** (see Fig. 3.7).

Each gut tube region is served by a dedicated artery. The blood supply to the stomach must be from the artery of the foregut, the **celiac trunk**. A larger point, however, is at play here. Note that the gut tube began as a midline structure running parallel to,

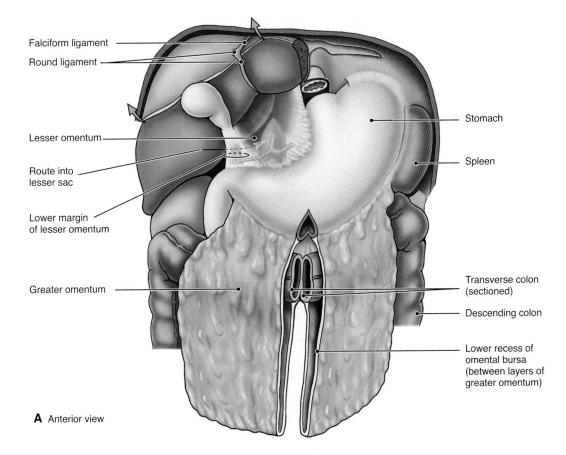

A Anterior view

FIGURE 3.7   **The stomach and its mesenteries. (*continues*)**

The dorsal mesentery persists as the remarkable greater omentum, a double-layer fold of fat-rich connective tissue (**A**). This unwieldy expanse of mesentery eventually incorporates the transverse part of the colon (**B**). It has been called the "abdominal policeman" because of its perceived role in defending the peritoneum by adhering to sites of inflammation, absorbing bacteria and other contaminants, and providing leukocytes for a local immune response. The ventral mesentery persists as the lesser omentum. It cordons a lesser part of the peritoneal sac posteriorly and ensheaths the ducts that connect the accessory organs back to the gut tube. (From Moore KL, Dalley AF. Clinically Oriented Anatomy, 5th Edition. Baltimore: Lippincott Williams & Wilkins, 2006. Figure 2.20, p. 237; from Cohen BJ, Wood DL. Memmler's The Human Body in Health and Disease, 10th Edition. Baltimore: Lippincott Williams & Wilkins, 2004.)

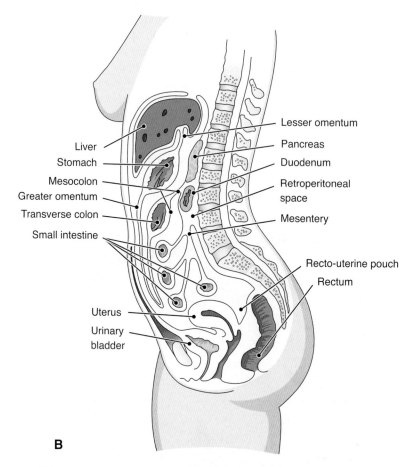

B

FIGURE 3.7   *(continued)* **The stomach and its mesenteries.**

but in front of, the vertebral column. The only structure between the two is the dorsal aorta. The shortest possible route for blood to reach the gut tube is as a direct branch of the aorta that runs between the two layers of mesoderm that droop off of the body wall to "sling" the gut tube (see Fig. 3.1). In the case of the stomach, the arteries are branches of the celiac trunk. However, because the dorsal mesentery of the stomach elongates so much as the foregut expands and rotates, it would not be economical for the blood supply to elongate and hang down like an apron as well. Instead, the blood supply to the stomach approaches from the top of the dorsal mesentery (to catch the very top of the greater and lesser curvatures), or it shuttles in at the bottom of the stomach expansion (to catch the bottom of the greater and lesser curvatures) (see Fig. 2.31).

The portion of foregut distal to the stomach will form the proximal part of the **duodenum** (Fig. 3.8). This C-shaped tube marks the transition toward the absorbing portion of the gut tube; it also marks the end of the accessory organs that are attached to the tube (see below). Developmentally, the part of the duodenum that forms from the foregut region of the tube is indicated by the persistence of a ventral mesentery (see Fig. 3.7). All subsequent parts of the tube have only a dorsal mesentery.

The duodenum demonstrates a key principle of digestive system anatomy. The gut tube greatly elongates during growth, reaching a linear distance of approximately 20 feet. To package all of that in the small volume of the adult abdominal cavity, the tube

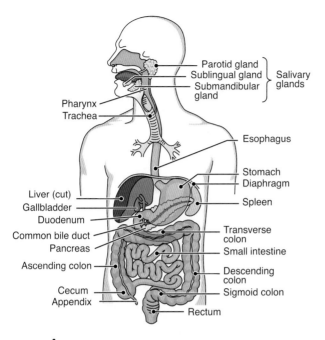

A

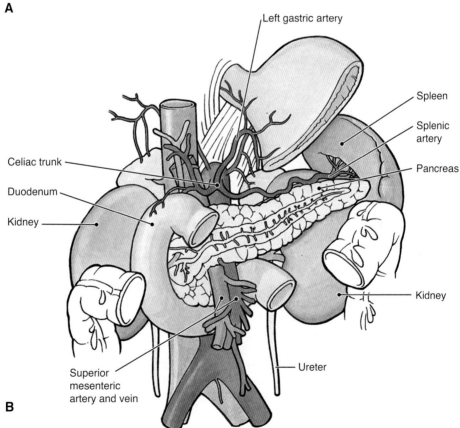

B

FIGURE 3.8 **Regional anatomy of the duodenum.**

The duodenum is the C-shaped continuation of the gut tube beyond the stomach (**A**). It rests in a key region of the abdomen, near each of the accessory organs of digestion and the kidneys, spleen, inferior vena cava, and aorta (**B**). (From Moore KL, Agur A. Essential Clinical Anatomy, 2nd Edition. Philadelphia: Lippincott Williams & Wilkins, 2002.)

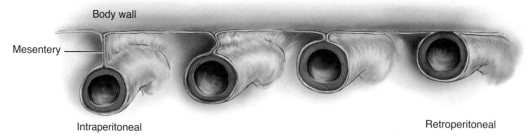

Body wall

Mesentery ———

Intraperitoneal

Retroperitoneal

FIGURE 3.9   **The tube pushes against the peritoneum to varying degrees.**

Because of cramped spacing in the abdominal cavity, the relationship of the gut tube to the dorsal mesentery distorts during growth. In some regions, the gut tube is pushed back against the body wall, effectively removing the dorsal mesentery. This condition is called "retroperitoneal," and the gut tube is essentially "fixed" in space against the back of the abdomen. In other regions the dorsal mesentery expands and twists dramatically to give the gut tube maximum flexibility and mobility.

must curl and "ball up," much like trying to put a long hose in a small box. All this accommodation distorts the relationship of the tube to the dorsal mesentery. The possible outcomes are illustrated in Figure 3.9.

Remember that the **mesentery** is really just two layers of mesoderm with a space between them. Part of this space is occupied by the gut tube, and part of it is empty except for the blood vessels and nerves that must serve the tube and its coating. Sometimes, the tube pulls farther away from the vertebral column, thus stretching the dorsal mesentery. This gives the tube the property of being very bendable and movable in the abdominal cavity, because it is "swinging" more freely from the support post of the vertebral column. The **jejunum** and **ileum** of the small intestine are examples of this condition. Because it appears as though the tube is completely surrounded by the visceral mesoderm, this condition is called **intraperitoneal**. The tube is not inside the peritoneal sac, but you will appreciate this best if you follow the developmental possibilities (see Fig. 3.9).

Parts of the tube are pushed back against the body wall by pressure from other organs. This condition is called **retroperitoneal**, because the whole tube appears to be behind the visceral mesoderm that forms the lining of the peritoneal sac. These parts of the tube are fixed in position, and they are only "blanketed" by the tangent peritoneal membrane. The duodenum has both an intraperitoneal part and a retroperitoneal part (Fig. 3.10). The first part of the duodenum, derived from the foregut, is intraperitoneal; the remaining two-thirds of the duodenum are retroperitoneal.

The duodenum is really at the mercy of the developing stomach and the large liver. This means that as the stomach spins on its long axis and sags to the left, the duodenum is "kicked up" to the right, and in the end, the convexity of the "C" in the C-shaped duodenum lies to the right of the vertebral column (see Fig. 3.10). The position of the duodenum across the level of the first few lumbar vertebrae will prove to be a very busy area of the abdominal cavity.

ACCESSORY ORGANS OF DIGESTION

Human dietary needs are broad. We require a wide variety of food types, many of which challenge the digestive system. Logically, the structures that help you to digest will be located at the top end rather than at the bottom end of the system. The acces-

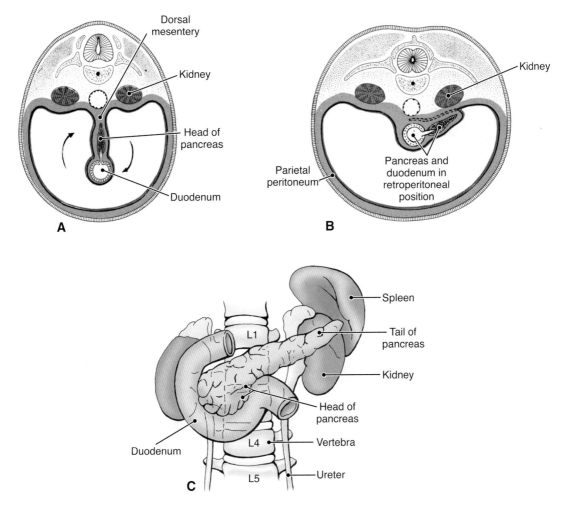

FIGURE 3.10   The duodenum is whipped around by the liver and stomach.

Like the tail of a dog or the end of a whip, the duodenum bends into a C-shape, cocks upward with ascension of the liver, and swivels back to the body wall. (**A–B**) It ends up at the level of the L1–L3 vertebrae (**C**) in a design that descends beside the vertebral bodies, then runs transversely across them before terminating as the jejunum. (Modified from Sadler TW. Langman's Essential Medical Embryology. Baltimore: Lippincott Williams & Wilkins, 2006. Figure 6.5N,O,P, p. 65.)

sory organs of digestion include the **liver**, the **gallbladder**, and the **pancreas**, each of which derives from the foregut. Moreover, they each bud off of the foregut within the other unique aspect of foregut anatomy—the **ventral mesentery**. The fact that the foregut is the only region containing both accessory organs of digestion and a ventral mesentery is no coincidence, of course.

Liver and Gallbladder

The liver begins to bud off of the foregut tube during the fourth week of embryonic growth. At this point, it is simply called the **hepatic diverticulum** (Fig. 3.11). The "top," or cranial, part of the diverticulum goes on to become the liver, which quickly becomes the largest organ in the fetus. Blood cell production is an early function of

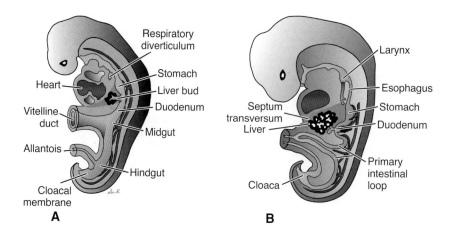

A

Respiratory diverticulum
Stomach
Heart
Liver bud
Vitelline duct
Duodenum
Allantois
Midgut
Cloacal membrane
Hindgut

B

Larynx
Esophagus
Septum transversum
Stomach
Liver
Duodenum
Cloaca
Primary intestinal loop

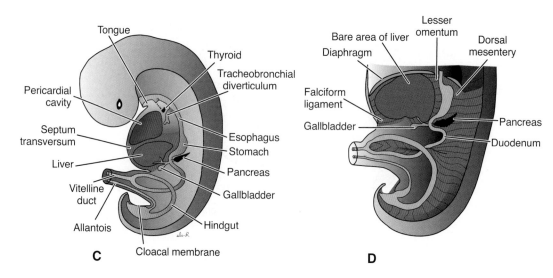

C

Tongue
Thyroid
Tracheobronchial diverticulum
Pericardial cavity
Septum transversum
Esophagus
Stomach
Liver
Pancreas
Vitelline duct
Gallbladder
Allantois
Hindgut
Cloacal membrane

D

Lesser omentum
Bare area of liver
Dorsal mesentery
Diaphragm
Falciform ligament
Gallbladder
Pancreas
Duodenum

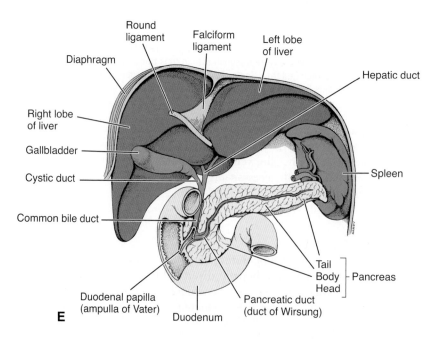

E

Round ligament
Falciform ligament
Left lobe of liver
Diaphragm
Hepatic duct
Right lobe of liver
Gallbladder
Spleen
Cystic duct
Common bile duct
Tail
Body
Head
Pancreas
Duodenal papilla (ampulla of Vater)
Pancreatic duct (duct of Wirsung)
Duodenum

FIGURE 3.11   **Origin of the accessory organs of digestion.**

The accessory organs of digestion (liver, gallbladder, and pancreas) first emerge as buds of the foregut tube in the space provided by the ventral mesentery. (**A–B**) As the organs enlarge and move, the foregut mesentery goes with them and persists in the same way that the dorsal mesentery does. (**C–E**) (From Sadler TW. Langman's Medical Embryology, 10th Edition. Baltimore: Lippincott Williams & Wilkins, 2006. Figures 14.14 and 14.15, p. 212; from Stedman's Medical Dictionary, 27th Edition. Baltimore: Lippincott Williams & Wilkins, 2000.)

the liver. The smaller, bottom part of the diverticulum becomes the **gallbladder**. Together, the liver and gallbladder lie within the ventral mesentery in the upper right quadrant, where the rapidly expanding liver has migrated as a result, in part, of the stomach expansion. This creates a dynamic in which the upper half of the abdominal cavity is dominated by a stomach on the left and a liver on the right, with a stretched ventral mesentery lying in between them (see Figs. 3.6 and 3.7).

The ventral mesentery continues beyond the liver to the anterior abdominal wall; in the adult, this film of tissue is called the **falciform ligament**. Remember that the mesenteric space (between the two layers of mesoderm that form it) is available as a route for nerves and blood vessels to travel through the abdominal cavity without puncturing or being inside the peritoneal sac. The falciform ligament provides just such an opportunity.

The liver grows so large that it impacts the diaphragm above it, much like a helium balloon that rises to the ceiling. This compression of the liver, coated by mesentery, against the diaphragm, likewise coated on its underside by the somatic layer of mesoderm, "erodes" the coatings and leaves the liver tissue in contact with the fascia of the diaphragm. This is called the **bare area** of the liver (Fig. 3.12). At the margins of the bare area of the liver, the mesoderm coating reflects onto the adjacent diaphragm. The peritoneal sac is still sealed shut along these reflections, but a number of blind pouches are left where fluid within the sac can accumulate.

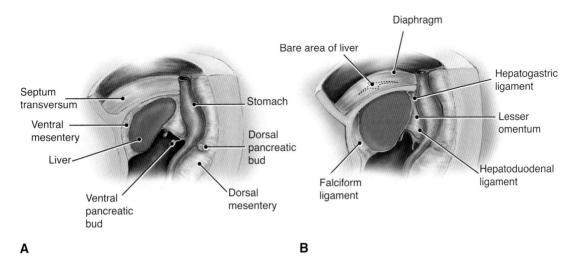

A   **B**

FIGURE 3.12   **The liver ascends during growth (A) and impacts the diaphragm (B).**

This impact pushes back ("reflects") the peritoneal coating of the liver and of the diaphragm, making a kind of "bare area" on the top of the liver. The liver essentially fuses to the diaphragm, which seals off the reflected arcs of peritoneum and keeps the peritoneal sac a closed space. (Adapted from Larsen WJ. Human Embryology, 1st Edition. New York: Churchill-Livingstone, 1993. Figure 9.8, p. 216.)

The **gallbladder** forms because the liver produces more bile than the body needs, and this bile must be stored somewhere. As the liver is expanding from the original bud off of the foregut tube, the connection that it maintains to the tube winnows into a narrow **bile duct**. A part of this duct pouches out to form the passive gallbladder and the **cystic duct** that connects it back to the bile duct (see Fig. 3.11D,E). Because gallbladder problems are common clinical presentations, the specific position and name of all the ducts and blood vessels near it are important to learn.

The liver and gallbladder bud off of the gut tube at virtually the lower, or distal, limit of the ventral mesentery. With the gut tube in its original, linear state, this lower limit of the ventral mesentery is shaped like the bottom of a sling, and it forms a sort of trough. After the stomach and liver have rotated, sagged, and risen, this lower limit of mesentery is oriented straight up and down, and it faces to the right (see Fig. 3.7A). It forms the perfect sling for transmission of the ducts that connect the liver and gallbladder back to the gut tube. Their ducts form an elegant, branching design before joining with the duct from the **pancreas** right before entering the proximal part of the duodenum (see Fig. 3.11E). These **hepatic** and **bile** ducts run within the sling at the distal end of the ventral mesentery, which in the adult is termed the **hepatoduodenal ligament**.

This ligament ensheaths three important, large structures related to the physiology and circulation of the gut tube: the **hepatic artery**, which serves the foregut organs; the **portal vein**, which delivers all gut tube venous blood to the liver; and the **bile duct**, which is the site of common clinical disorders (e.g., gallstones). These three structures are collectively called the **portal triad**, and recognizing their gross anatomy during mobilization or surgery of the bowel is a critical skill.

Pancreas

The pancreas is the final accessory organ of digestion that forms from the foregut tube. It actually begins as a separate **dorsal bud** and **ventral bud**, each with its own connecting duct to the foregut. The dorsal pancreatic bud generally is larger, and the ventral bud eventually rotates toward it (Fig. 3.13). As with many tissue structures that are similar to one another, once the ventral and dorsal buds come into contact, they functionally fuse. The fused pancreas stays connected to the duodenum through the **main pacreatic duct**, which also incorporates the bile duct. Thus, just before they enter the wall of the duodenum, the main pancreatic duct and the bile duct merge to form a

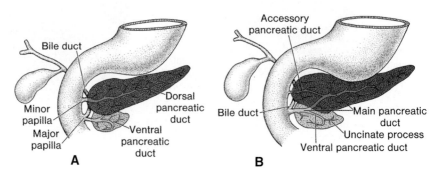

FIGURE 3.13   The pancreas forms from two buds.

The ventral bud, which is connected to the base of the bud that grows the liver, rotates in concert with the duodenum (**A**). When it merges with the dorsal bud (**B**), the main and accessory ducts usually merge as well. (From Sadler TW. Langman's Medical Embryology, 10th Edition. Baltimore: Lippincott Williams & Wilkins, 2006. Figure 14.21, p. 216.)

hepatopancreatic ampulla. The ampulla invades the wall of the duodenum at a location called the **major duodenal papilla**. Thus, all the efforts devoted to developing accessory organs of digestion converge into one small input line.

Of the accessory organs of digestion, the liver and gallbladder remain intraperitoneal, whereas the pancreas migrates to a retroperitoneal position. The liver and gallbladder receive all their arterial blood supply from branches of the celiac trunk, but the pancreas receives blood from both the artery of the foregut (**celiac trunk**) and the artery of the midgut (**superior mesenteric**) (see Fig. 3.8).

MIDGUT

The midgut includes the long run of bowel between the proximal duodenum and the transverse colon (Fig. 3.14). The great length of the midgut is achieved by an unusual growth process in which the gut tube is excused from the fetus through the umbilical hiatus and then, substantially elongated, is returned with significant rotation.

The adult parts of the gut tube that develop from the midgut are the rest of the **duodenum**, the **jejunum**, the **ileum**, the **cecum**, the **ascending colon**, and part of the **transverse colon**. You can think of the midgut as the length of the **small intestine** and part of the **large intestine**. Basic midgut function is simple—to squeeze the digested food matter against the inner, absorbing surface of a very long tube to extract nutrients that have been released by the digestion initiated in the foregut.

The midgut both elongates greatly and rotates during its development. It also remains tethered to the posterior abdominal wall by the dorsal mesentery all the while,

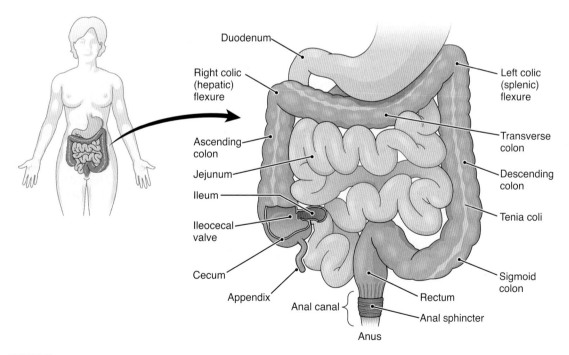

FIGURE 3.14   **Midgut derivatives.**

The midgut matures into the final third of the duodenum, the entire small bowel (jejunum and ileum), and the ascending and transverse portions of the colon. (From Cohen BJ, Wood DL. Memmler's The Human Body in Health and Disease, 10th Edition. Baltimore: Lippincott Williams & Wilkins, 2004.)

which explains why this mesentery comes to look like an opened Asian, or Oriental, fan. From the very beginning, it is supplied by the artery of the midgut, the **superior mesenteric artery** branch of the aorta (Fig. 3.15).

The first event during midgut development is elongation, which causes the tube to project ventrally, or toward the umbilicus of the embryo (Fig. 3.16). And it just keeps going. The midgut elongates so much that it actually herniates into the umbilical cord. This is considered to be a normal herniation, or a **physiological herniation**. The migration is so patterned, in fact, that a **cranial limb** and a **caudal limb** of the tube can be identified on opposite sides of an axis formed by the superior mesenteric artery that feeds the midgut (see Fig. 3.16A). The cranial limb superelongates and takes on the squiggly packing of the small intestine while it is herniated into the umbilical cord. The caudal limb, which will become the **cecum**, **appendix**, and **ascending colon**, expands less dramatically before it returns to the fetus.

While still in the umbilical cord, the midgut loop rotates 90° counterclockwise around the axis created by the superior mesenteric artery (as viewed from the front). This is the first of three such rotations before the tube finally settles into place during the tenth week of embryonic development. This may help to explain why the beginning of the large intestine is located on the lower right side of the abdominal cavity; it started out as the caudal limb of the midgut herniation. After 270° of counterclockwise rotation, it is banked against the right side of the body wall.

As the midgut tube is growing and rotating, a piece of the caudal limb does not grow at the same rate as the rest of the surrounding tissue—much like the tip of a long, skinny balloon as you inflate it. This pouch of slow growth is a **diverticulum** of the cecum portion of the midgut tube that becomes the adult **appendix** (see Fig. 3.15B,C). For many people, removal of the appendix is a first exposure to the world of doctors and hospitals. Finding the appendix beneath the skin of the abdomen during a physical examination is based on knowing how the gut tube rotates before birth; because the cecum ends up in the well of the right hip bone (see Fig. 3.15A), you can feel for the appendix between the hip bone and the umbilicus.

After the midgut has elongated, it returns to the abdominal cavity of the fetus in much the same way as you might suck in a strand of spaghetti through pursed lips. The cranial end returns first and collects in a giant squiggle in roughly the middle part of the lower abdomen. Technically, the mesentery that slings it begins at the **duodenojejunal junction**, or flexure, just to the left of the midline. The mesentery ends at the first part of the elongation to be retroperitoneal, which is the area of the cecum in the lower right quadrant. Thus, the dorsal mesentery of the intestines is rooted to the back of the abdominal wall along an oblique line that runs from upper left to lower right. It slings well over 10 feet of intestinal tube, despite a root that is closer to 10 inches in length. This is what gives the dorsal mesentery at this location a fan-like shape (much longer at its periphery than at its base).

The caudal end of the midgut loop returns to the fetal abdomen along the periphery, which is the only space left available because of the position of the small intestine.

FIGURE 3.15   **The small intestine suspends like a fan.**

The long tube of the small intestine includes a subtle transition from a jejunum to an ileum before emptying into the large cecum. The jejunal part is coiled into the upper quadrants of the abdomen (**A**) and typically transitions to the ileum in the left lower quadrant. The ileocecal junction (**B**) and the appendix are key features of the right lower quadrant. The arterial supply from the superior mesenteric arcades through the dorsal mesentery (**C**). (From Moore KL, Dalley AF. Clinically Oriented Anatomy, 5th Edition. Baltimore: Lippincott Williams & Wilkins, 2006. Figures 2.37, 2.38B, and 2.42B, p.265, 267, and 273, respectively.)

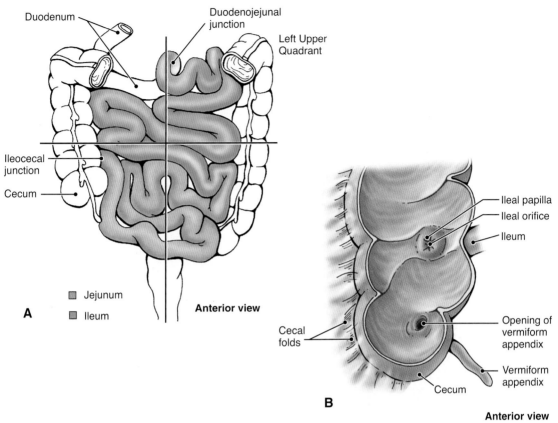

A

Duodenum

Duodenojejunal junction

Left Upper Quadrant

Ileocecal junction

Cecum

Jejunum
Ileum

Anterior view

Ileal papilla
Ileal orifice
Ileum

Cecal folds

Opening of vermiform appendix

Vermiform appendix

Cecum

B

Anterior view

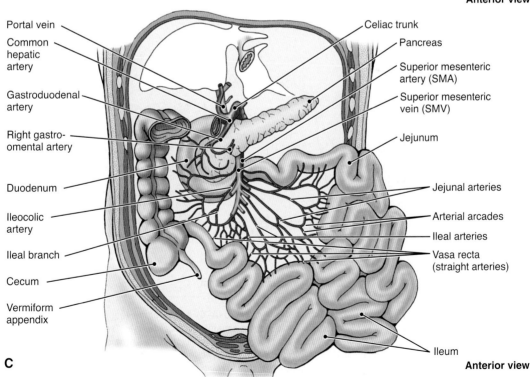

Portal vein

Common hepatic artery

Gastroduodenal artery

Right gastro-omental artery

Duodenum

Ileocolic artery

Ileal branch

Cecum

Vermiform appendix

Celiac trunk

Pancreas

Superior mesenteric artery (SMA)

Superior mesenteric vein (SMV)

Jejunum

Jejunal arteries

Arterial arcades

Ileal arteries

Vasa recta (straight arteries)

Ileum

C

Anterior view

Rotation of the Midgut

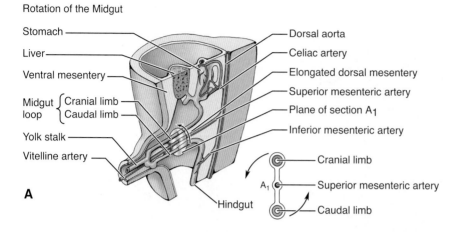

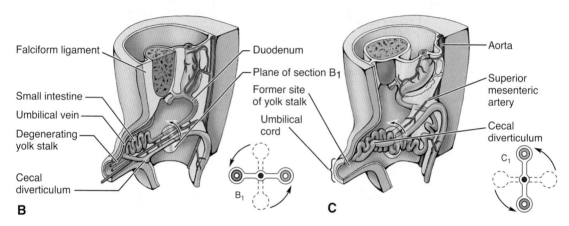

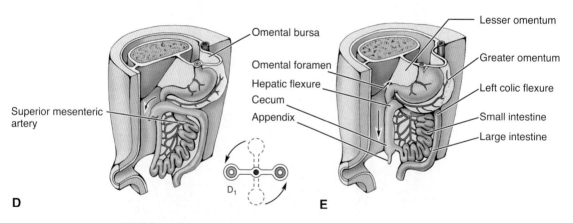

FIGURE 3.16   **Normal herniation of the midgut.**

As the midgut herniates into the umbilical cord (**A–C**), it also rotates (counterclockwise, as seen from the front). To pack more tube into the same amount of space, the tube "squiggles" into tight coils, which persist in the adult state as the coils of the small intestine. The midgut rotation completes its final turn, and the midgut loop returns to the fetal abdomen. The 270° rotation explains why the cecum ends up in the right lower quadrant (**D**). The herniation reduces as the tube returns to the fetal abdominal cavity (**E**). (From Moore KL, Dalley AF. Clinically Oriented Anatomy, 4th Edition. Baltimore: Lippincott Williams & Wilkins, 1999.)

Follow the gut tube from the cecum up the right side of the abdomen (**ascending colon**) to the liver, where it turns medially and runs across the abdomen as the **transverse colon**. The midgut portion of the tube transitions to the hindgut portion where the major source of blood supply to the transverse colon transitions from the **superior mesenteric artery** to the **inferior mesenteric artery**. This is a subtle transition in the sense that the morphology of the transverse colon shows no abrupt change; it merely turns inferiorly along the left side of the abdominal cavity (**descending colon**) in parallel to the cecum and ascending colon on the right.

HINDGUT

Compared to development of the midgut and foregut, development of the hindgut is simple. The hindgut must open to the outside world so that waste matter can be expelled, and this junction of the inner tube with the outer world is the focus of hindgut development. When the hindgut tube forms during lateral folding of the embryo, it opens to the outside world through an unmodified bottom end called a **cloaca** (Fig. 3.17A). Many animal species use this unmodified exit port to eliminate all forms of waste (both liquid and solid) and to expel eggs. Placental mammals modify the cloaca into separate tubes for solid and liquid waste and also make accommodations for the reproductive pathway. Concentrate on this aspect of embryology, because it explains the positional anatomy of the **perineal** region. Social norms discourage people from learning about this part of their own body despite its considerable clinical relevance. Knowing how it develops is the first step toward mastering its anatomy.

Division of the hindgut cloaca results from interference by mesoderm tissue. A mesoderm colony of cells termed the **urorectal septum** migrates from its formation point between the hindgut tube and the connecting stalk. Recall from Figures 1.23 and 3.11 that the **allantois** diverticulum is trapped up within the connecting stalk at this time, so the urorectal septum effectively sits between the blind pouch of the allantois and the hindgut tube proper. As its name implies, the urorectal septum will migrate toward the bottom end of the embryo, and in doing so, it will drive a wedge of mesoderm between the hindgut and the allantois (Fig. 3.17B,C).

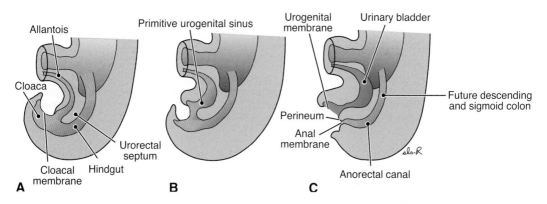

FIGURE 3.17   A wedge of mesoderm divides the hindgut.

Recall that the allantois diverticulum is trapped in the connecting stalk (**A**). A migrating urorectal septum of mesoderm pinches the base of the diverticulum off of the hindgut (**B** and **C**). This results in two portals to the outside world, one of which is still connected to the gut tube (anal) and one of which is a blind pouch (urogenital). (From Sadler TW. Langman's Medical Embryology, 10th Edition. Baltimore: Lippincott Williams & Wilkins, 2006. Figure 14.36, p. 225.)

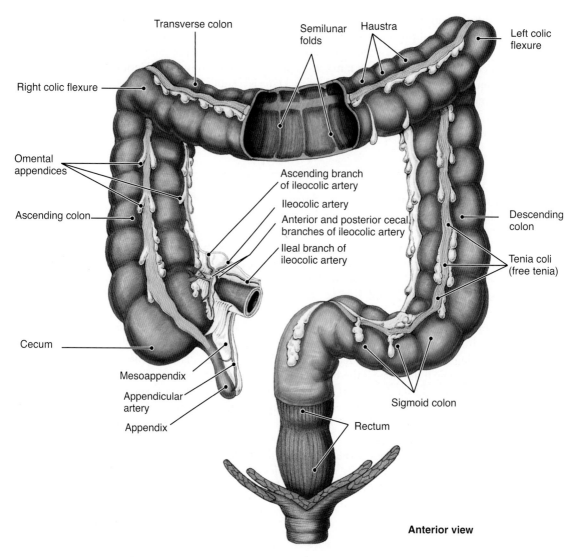

FIGURE 3.18   Hindgut derivatives.

The functional and structural transition between midgut and hindgut is subtle—along the distal portion of the transverse colon. The hindgut develops into the rest of the transverse colon, the descending colon, the sigmoid colon, and the rectum. (From Moore KL, Dalley AF. Clinically Oriented Anatomy,
5th Edition. Baltimore: Lippincott Williams & Wilkins, 2006. Figure 2.41, p. 272.)

To reach the bottom end of the embryo from this position, however, the septum
must push through the cloaca. The clump of mesoderm that drives through the endoderm of the cloaca and contacts the ectoderm is now called the **perineal body**. It divides
the former cloacal membrane into a rear part, for what is left of the hindgut, and a front
part, for the piece of the hindgut that is still connected to the allantois. This division now
gives the body a dedicated outflow track for solid waste (the hindgut) and a blind pouch
that terminates just "above" it as a **urogenital sinus** for fluid excretion and reproduction.
Obviously, more change is in order for this blind pouch (see Chapter 5).

The adult derivatives of the hindgut are the final portions of the large intestine and
the **rectum**. You have anticipated how the hindgut transitions from the transverse

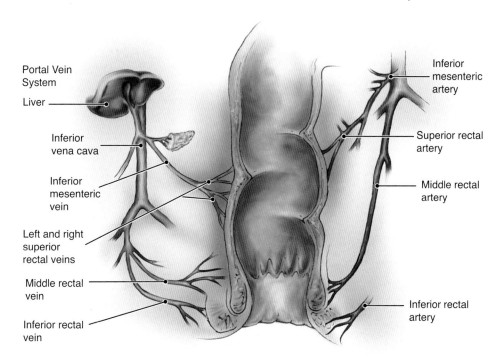

Portal Vein System

Liver

Inferior vena cava

Inferior mesenteric vein

Left and right superior rectal veins

Middle rectal vein

Inferior rectal vein

Inferior mesenteric artery

Superior rectal artery

Middle rectal artery

Inferior rectal artery

FIGURE 3.19   **The anal canal meets the outside world.**

The bottom of the gut tube is exposed to the outside world, but not without some protection. The ectodermal contact with the end of the tube curls inward, which pushes the endoderm approximately an inch superiorly into the anal canal. This enables voluntary sphincter muscles (see Chapter 7) to keep the anal orifice closed. In keeping with development, the endodermal portion of the anal canal is supplied by a gut tube artery and drains to the liver (via the inferior mesenteric vein), whereas the ectodermal portion is supplied by and drains back into the systemic circulation (via middle and inferior rectal vessels).

colon to the descending colon. As the descending colon reaches the well of the pelvis in the lower left quadrant of the abdomen, it actually "lifts off" the wall and is once again intraperitoneal. Think of it as laying a tube along the inside of a frame but ending up with more tube than frame. A relatively long stretch of tube must fit between the pelvic brim and the midline of the body, so it fans out just like the small intestine. This region is called the **sigmoid colon**, and it remains intraperitoneal (suspended by the **sigmoid mesocolon**) until it reaches the midline. Here, it falls back against the body wall and runs a straight course toward the outside world as the **rectum** (Fig. 3.18).

Development of the gut tube now is almost complete. The region that abuts (no pun intended) the bottom of the embryo will become the **anal canal**. This is the other region (besides the mouth) where endoderm meets ectoderm. As this junction develops, the part derived from ectoderm actually invaginates, or curls inward (Fig. 3.19). This protective step keeps the absorbent endodermal lining from constant exposure to the outside world. The bottom of the anal canal is, thus, composed of "in-turned" skin, which can press against itself through the action of sphincter muscles. This is one area in which shared venous drainage exists between vessels that lead back to the heart directly (**caval**) and those that lead back to the liver first (**portal**). The anal canal is, thus, said to be a region of "portal-caval anastomosis."

Respiratory System

INTRODUCTION

Life depends on absorbing energy, both gaseous and particulate energy, from the outside world. It makes perfect sense, then, that the anatomy for acquiring oxygen and transferring it to the body grows from the same tissue that absorbs particulate matter—the gut tube. The respiratory system is an elaboration of the endoderm layer that is modified to deal with a different kind of matter—gas as opposed to solid.

For expansion, the gut tube greatly elongates in the midgut region. This process increases the surface area of the extracting endoderm, so that the useful properties of what you ingest may be fully removed as the particles travel through the tube. We should also expect, therefore, that the part of the tube that is modified to extract oxygen from the air will greatly expand as well. The respiratory system expands as it develops, but in this case, expansion of the key parts—the terminal air sacs—occurs last. This is important because of the relationship between air sac maturity and viability in premature babies.

DEVELOPMENT

The first evidence of growth in the respiratory system is found along the part of the endodermal tube that will become the esophagus and that joins the floor of the **pharynx** region of the neck (more on neck development later). In this area, a **laryngotracheal groove** appears in the endoderm and grows caudally in the form of a laryngotracheal tube. This tube pouches out of the front of the future esophagus in the form of a **respiratory diverticulum**, or **lung bud** (Fig. 4.1). At some point, this outgrowth of the endodermal tube must separate from its origin, or you would have an open connection between the food pathway and the air pathway. This separation is accomplished by a migrating septum of tissue called, logically, the **tracheoesophageal septum**. Failure of this septum to complete its task leads to the most common developmental anomaly of the lower respiratory system—a **tracheoesophageal fistula** (Clinical Anatomy Box 4.1).

Just as the gut tube lies against a layer of mesoderm (the **visceral mesoderm**, or **peritoneal membrane**, in the abdominal region), so does the part of the gut tube that buds off to form the lungs. At all times, the lung bud is expanding against this same layer of visceral mesoderm, which in the chest region is called the **pleural membrane** rather than the peritoneal membrane (Fig. 4.2). Keep in mind the image of an organ (the lung) growing against a closed sac of tissue (the pleura). The pleura maintains a kind of "shrink wrap" against the lung surface as the lung expands (see Fig. 2.1). The pleural sac greatly reduces friction between the chest wall and the thin, delicate lining of the inflating air sacs.

As two major organ systems (lungs and heart) begin to form in the thoracic cavity, they induce a layer of somatic (lateral plate) mesoderm cells to migrate inward from each side, toward the midline. The cells form the **pleuropericardial folds** of tissue. The important thing to remember is that they merge with each other to "curtain off" the developing heart from the developing lungs (Fig. 4.3). The pleuropericardial folds

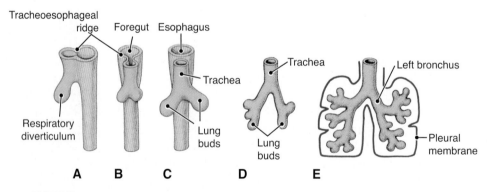

FIGURE 4.1   **The airway buds off of the gut tube.**

With only one tissue layer for absorbing the outside world, the separation of air absorption from food absorption takes place within this tissue at the top of the gut tube (**A**). The respiratory bud grows much like an inverted tree (**B–E**), with a trunk forming first, then branches, then smaller branches, and so on, as it grows toward the cavities on either side of the vertebral column in the thorax. (From Sadler TW. Langman's Medical Embryology, 10th Edition. Baltimore: Lippincott Williams & Wilkins, 2006. Figure 13.2a–c, p.196; from Sadler TW. Langman's Medical Embryology, 9th Edition Image Bank. Baltimore: Lippincott Williams & Wilkins, 2004. Figure 1205REV A & B.)

CLINICAL ANATOMY

Box 4.1

TRACHEOESOPHAGEAL FISTULA

The most common congenital anomaly of the lower respiratory system is tracheoesophageal fistula, in which the esophagus and trachea retain an open connection (A). Typically, the esophagus ends in a blind pouch (esophageal atresia (B)). Remember that the trachea and lungs form from a forward pouch of the gut tube. If the growth process fails to complete the emergence and separation of the trachea, then an abnormal connection with the esophagus will remain (A–C). Fetuses with esophageal atresia may be unable to swallow or absorb amniotic fluid. As a result, amniotic fluid builds up, leading to a condition called polyhydramnios (~1% of pregnancies). Polyhydramnios is linked to other congenital anomalies as well, which makes it a signal finding during prenatal care.

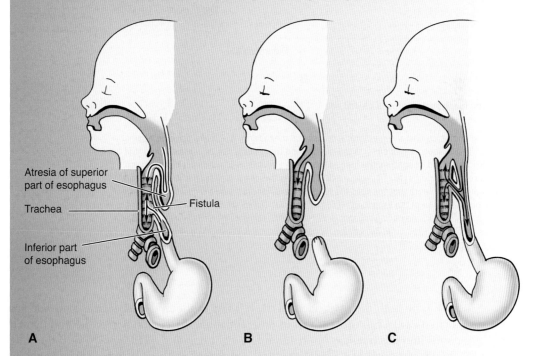

Tracheoesophageal fistula. (From Moore KL, Dalley AF. Clinically Oriented Anatomy, 4th Edition. Baltimore: Lippincott Williams & Wilkins, 1999.)

remain in the body as a physical barrier between the heart and lungs; in the adult, this barrier is called the **fibrous pericardium**.

FUNCTIONAL MATURITY OF RESPIRATION

Lung growth is pleasantly simple and logical. The original "bubble" of a diverticulum must greatly expand its surface area. The only space in which it can grow is toward the chest wall (from its starting point along the front of the esophagus). It can

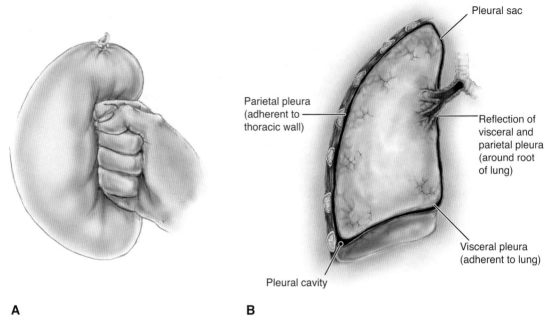

A

B

FIGURE 4.2   **The lungs push against a closed sac.**

Expansion of the lung comes against the membrane of visceral mesoderm, much like pushing against a closed balloon (**A**). The balloon, in this case, is the pleura, and the pleural sac becomes a potential space lined with a slippery fluid. It enables the lung to inflate and deflate without direct contact with the chest wall, thus reducing friction (**B**). The pleura that touches the chest wall (somatic, or parietal, pleura) is relatively thick; the pleura that touches the lung (visceral pleura) is so thin that it cannot be dissected from the outer surface of the lung itself. (From Moore KL, Dalley AF. Clinically Oriented Anatomy, 4th Edition. Baltimore: Lippincott Williams & Wilkins, 1999; adapted from Hall-Craggs ECB. Anatomy as a Basis for Clinical Medicine, 3rd Edition. London: Williams & Wilkins Waverly Europe, 1995. Figure 4.14, p.176.)

do this on both the right side and the left side of the midline because each side has a chest cavity. So, very early in its differentiation, the central part of the bud (which forms into the **trachea**) bifurcates into a right half and a left half. Now, if the lung simply expanded like a balloon into the chest cavity, then its surface area would be only as great as the surface area of the chest wall, and this would be insufficient. Rather, the lung bud replicates in a pattern very much like that of an upside-down tree. The original midline part of the bud condenses to form the trachea, which bifurcates downward into air tubes that separately feed the right and left chest cavities. These air tubes are now called the primary **bronchi**—a right **primary bronchus,** and a left **primary bronchus** (Fig. 4.4). The right bronchus and the left bronchus are not equal in size and shape. The left bronchus must accommodate the ultimate settling of the heart in the center-left chest cavity, so it branches off at a different angle. The right bronchus divides into three **secondary bronchi,** whereas the left bronchus, with a smaller cavity in which to grow, divides into only two.

This pattern of dividing continues almost infinitely. The primary bronchi divide into secondary bronchi, which divide into **tertiary bronchi,** and so on. At each new division, the caliber of the bronchus narrows, and its elasticity increases. Eventually,

FIGURE 4.3   **The coelom is divided into separate sacs.**

The lungs and heart initially grow against a single closed sac. In this cross-sectional series, follow the pleuropericardial folds as they grow inward from the body wall and divide that sac into three separate sacs (**A–C**). Given the bend in the sac at this time, the process is difficult to capture in a single view. The pleuropericardial folds meet in the midline and fuse to form a solid barrier between the lungs and their sacs and the heart and its sac (**B**). In the adult, this physical tissue is called the fibrous pericardium. (From Sadler TW. Langman's Essential Medical Embryology. Baltimore: Lippincott Williams & Wilkins, 2006. Figure 3.7.)

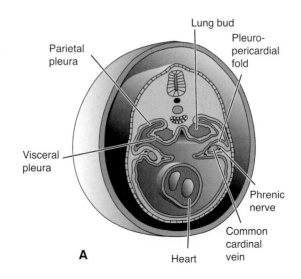

A

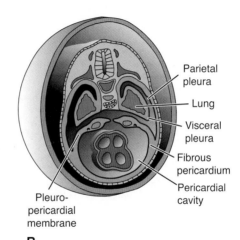

B

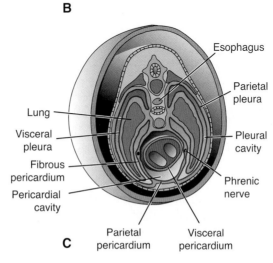

C

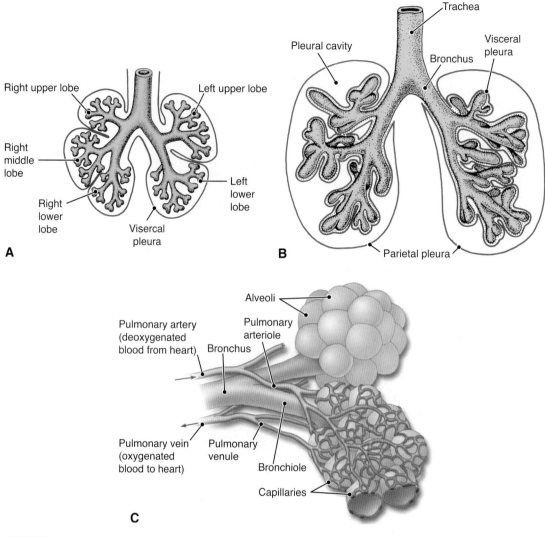

Right upper lobe

Left upper lobe

Right middle lobe

Right lower lobe

Left lower lobe

Visercal pleura

A

Trachea

Pleural cavity

Visceral pleura

Bronchus

Parietal pleura

B

Alveoli

Pulmonary artery (deoxygenated blood from heart)

Pulmonary arteriole

Bronchus

Pulmonary vein (oxygenated blood to heart)

Pulmonary venule

Bronchiole

Capillaries

C

FIGURE 4.4   **Maturation of the lungs.**

As the bronchi grow distally, they form ever smaller tubular units. Each secondary bronchus consti-tutes a named lobe of the lung (**A**). As the secondary bronchi divide into bronchioles and then into alveoli, they continue to push against the compliant pleura (**B**). Ultimately, a functional air sac forms at the end of each alveolus (**C**). (From Sadler TW. Langman's Medical Embryology, 9th Edition Image Bank. Baltimore: Lippincott Williams & Wilkins, 2004; from McArdle WD, Katch FI, Katch VL. Essen-tials of Exercise Physiology, 2nd Edition. Baltimore: Lippincott Williams and Wilkins, 2000.)

the network is as branched as it can be in the space provided, and the bronchial "twigs" end as endodermal "shoots" or "bubbles" called **alveolar sacs**. The combined surface areas of the many terminal sacs greatly exceed the simple surface area of the inner lining of the chest cavity. The functional lung is, thus, a tubular framework of bronchi (Fig. 4.4) that ends in an almost infinite multitude of absorbent sacs. Oxygen is absorbed into the surface of the sac and is transpired into the bloodstream by diffusion into rich pulmonary capillary beds. Waste gases accumulate and are expired in antici-pation of the next breath. After birth, the system continues to grow via branching of more and more alveoli. Thus, good air quality and physical activity during youth are necessary for full respiratory health during adulthood.

The lung develops sequentially, in the sense that the terminal sac of the lung is the last part to mature. The "trunk" (trachea) and "large branches" (bronchi) form first. This differentiation pathway is notable, because the fetus must have functional terminal sacs to survive outside the womb. These functional sacs also must be able to line themselves with a protective fluid called **surfactant**, which protects the young air sac from collapse under the pressure of the new air–water (blood) interface. In some sense, the total weight of the newborn is irrelevant—viability depends on how ready the lungs are to deal with the pressure (both literally and figuratively) of breathing. Lung development has been described as proceeding in four somewhat overlapping stages:

- **Pseudoglandular period** (weeks 5–17 of gestation): The lung architecture is too immature for respiration. Even if air could be introduced through the developing bronchi, it could not be absorbed, because terminal sacs have not formed.
- **Canalicular period** (weeks 16–25 of gestation): The bronchial tubes canalize (open fully), and the lung tissue is vascularized. Primitive alveoli form at the end of this period. Therefore, respiration is possible, but the sacs lack a surfactant to protect their surface tension against collapse. A fetus born at the end of this period may survive, but the chances are low, and the risk of lifelong complications is heightened.
- **Terminal sac period** (week 24 to birth): Terminal sacs (alveoli) proliferate during this period. Importantly, cells that produce pulmonary surfactant also begin to form. Adequate production of surfactant is key to the survival of infants born during this period.
- **Alveolar period** (late fetal period to ~8 years of age): Mature alveoli begin to replace terminal sacs and continue to do so for several years. Children exposed to harmful breathing environments during this time are at risk for failure to develop full lung capacity or function. (See Clinical Anatomy Box 4.1.)

CLINICAL ANATOMY OF THE ADULT LUNG

The mature lung passively inflates and deflates as you exploit the pressure differential between the atmosphere and the pleural sac. Because difficulty breathing is such a major clinical crisis and the lung functions regionally as much as globally, be aware of the relational anatomy of the lung to the pleural sac and the body wall all around the chest cavity (Fig. 4.5). The lobes of the lung, for example, border each other in predictable places (Fig. 4.6). The **fissures** that mark the space between the lobes pass deep to obvious places on the chest wall. The **horizontal fissure** between the **upper lobe** and **middle lobe** of the right lung is found deep to the line of the fourth rib. The **oblique fissure** between the **middle lobe** and **lower lobe** crosses the midclavicular line between the fifth and sixth ribs. These landmarks determine, for example, where to position the stethoscope to be comfortably within the bounds of just the upper lobe, or just the lower lobe, of a particular lung (Fig. 4.7).

The pleural sac extends beyond the limit of the lungs around the periphery of the chest cavity. This excess presents an opportunity to sample, without damaging the lung, the fluid that accumulates in the sac. Indeed, the regions of the sac are named for the areas that they line—**visceral pleura** for the part of the pleural sac adjacent to the lung surface, and **parietal pleura** for the part adjacent to everything else. The parietal pleura is further divided into **costal pleura** (against the ribs), **diaphragmatic pleura** (against the diaphragm), **mediastinal pleura** (against the mediastinum, or

FIGURE 4.5   **Named sections of the parietal pleura.**

The parietal pleura is further described by the name of the connective tissue against which it is pressed, such as costal for the ribs and diaphragmatic for the diaphragm. For the lungs to inflate most efficiently, the sac must fully line the thoracic cavity. The space between the parietal pleura and the inner chest wall is only a potential space. (From Moore KL, Dalley AF. Clinically Oriented Anatomy, 5th Edition. Baltimore: Lippincott Williams & Wilkins, 2006. Figure 1.23, p.113.)

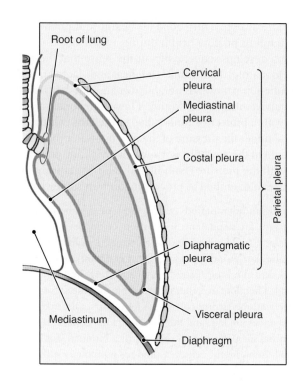

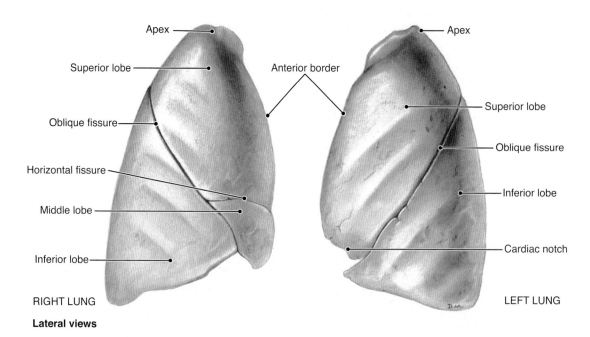

RIGHT LUNG

LEFT LUNG

Lateral views

FIGURE 4.6   **Lateral views of the adult lungs.**

Knowledge of the fissures between lungs facilitates a respiratory examination. Pneumonias and other fluid accumulations can be restricted to individual lung lobes and, thus, can be detected by appreciating a "line of dullness" or rubbing when the chest wall is tapped or the lungs are auscultated. (From Agur A, Dalley AF. Grant's Atlas of Anatomy, 11th Edition. Baltimore: Lippincott Williams & Wilkins, 2005. Figure 1.27A, p.122.)

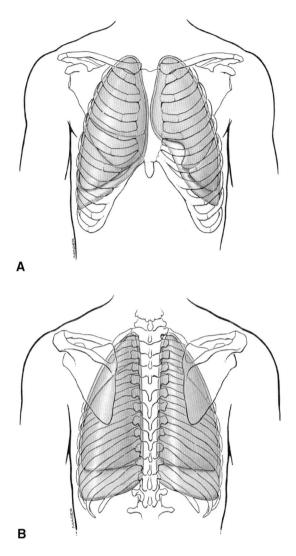

A

B

FIGURE 4.7 **Lung examination landmarks.**

The borders between lung lobes in a normal, seated patient generally correspond to the locations shown here. (**A**) Anterior view showing horizontal fissure of right lung behind the fourth rib, oblique fissure in the fifth intercostal space in the midclavicular line, and fissure of the left lung in the fifth intercostal space in the midclavicular line. (**B**) Posterior view showing inferior border of both lungs at the eighth rib in the midaxillary line and the tenth rib inferior to the scapula. The pleural sac reflections are lower (tenth rib in the midaxillary line and twelfth rib inferior to the scapula). (From Agur A, Dalley AF. Grant's Atlas of Anatomy, 11th Edition. Baltimore: Lippincott Williams & Wilkins, 2005.)

middle place, between the lungs), and **cervical pleura** (above the rib line in the soft well at the base of the neck) (Fig. 4.5).

The pleural sac droops below the limit of the lung in the deep **costodiaphragmatic recess** down the side of the chest wall. Gravity will bring excess pleural fluid into this recess when the patient stands. This location between the ninth and tenth ribs in the **midaxillary line** is practical for sampling pleural fluid (**thoracocentesis**) without risk to the lung (Fig. 4.8).

Unwanted air, blood, or other fluids can enter the pleural sac and fill it, which can make breathing difficult. The sac acts something like the air bag in a car. If the bag deploys, it pushes against you and makes it very difficult for you to push your face forward into the steering wheel. Likewise, a pressurized pleural sac (from the influx of air or fluid) prevents the delicate air sacs of the lung from inflating, thus making breathing difficult and potentially leading to a "collapsed" lung (Fig. 4.9). Excess air in the sac is a **pneumothorax**; excess blood in the sac is a **hemothorax**.

The delicate lining of the air sacs in the lung can deteriorate from chronic irritation, such as from the effects of smoking. If the lining breaks down, air will still enter the

FIGURE 4.8   The lung is at risk when pleural fluid is sampled.

Pleural fluid or other exudates will accumulate in the recesses at the inferior margins of the pleural sac. Thus, they can be sampled by needle aspiration (thoracocentesis) with lessened risk of injuring the lung tissue. (From Cohen BJ, Wood DL. Memmler's The Human Body in Health and Disease, 10th Edition. Baltimore: Lippincott Williams & Wilkins, 2004.)

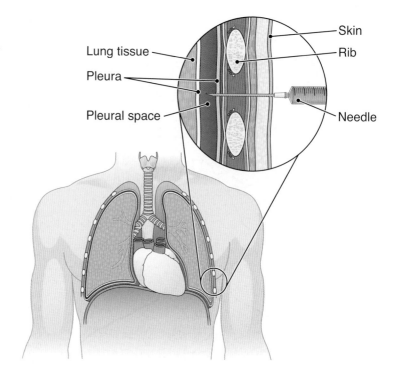

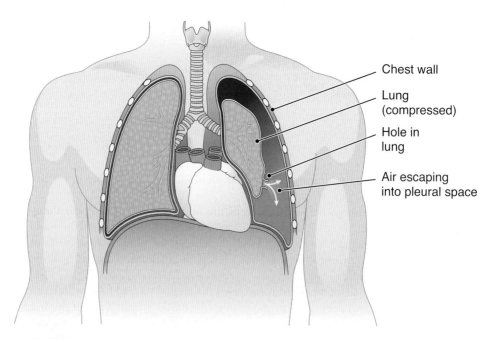

FIGURE 4.9   Positive pleural pressure "collapses" the lung.

Just as with the pericardial sac and the heart, pressure that builds up in the pleural sac (e.g., from air or blood) will overpower the ability of the air sacs to inflate against the pleural sac, resulting in a collapsed lung. (From Cohen BJ, Wood DL. Memmler's The Human Body in Health and Disease, 10th Edition. Baltimore: Lippincott Williams & Wilkins, 2004.)

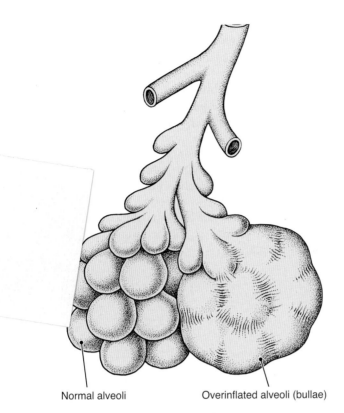

FIGURE 4.10   Emphysema.

The surface of a healthy lung is replete with tightly clustered air sacs. An emphysemic bronchiole does not function well, because the sacs have become slack or completely degraded. Inspired air fills the space but cannot be expired easily. (From Werner R, Benjamin, BE. A Massage Therapist's Guide to Pathology, 2nd Edition Baltimore: Lippincott Williams & Wilkins, 2002.)

Normal alveoli   Overinflated alveoli (bullae)

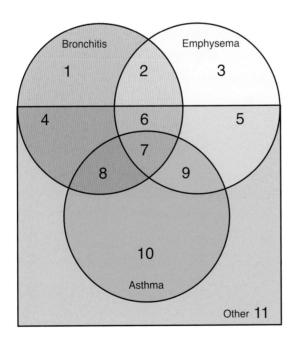

FIGURE 4.11   Major families of respiratory stress.

Most people who have difficulty breathing suffer from bronchitis, emphysema, asthma, or some combination of these. As shown schematically, a patient can experience one, two, or all three of these conditions at once. The box perimeter indicates patients with some form of airway obstruction (11). Patients with two or more of these conditions are more common than patients with only one. (From Snider GL, ed. Clinical Pulmonary Medicine. Boston: Little, Brown and Company, 1981 p. 249.)

relevant bronchiole, much like blowing into a skinny balloon with a hole at the far end, but the air will just escape into the space between the air sac and the pleural sac, or into flaccid air sacs. Localized erosion of functional lung tissue is called **emphysema** (Fig. 4.10).

Difficulty breathing can arise from an obstruction, such as asthma or bronchitis, that makes it difficult to get air through the respiratory tree. It also can also arise from compression, such as pleural effusion, or from incompetence, such as emphysema. A patient may suffer from more than one of these conditions at a time and/or for an extended period of time (Fig. 4.11). A significant component of primary care medicine concerns helping elderly patients with a history of smoking through a complex of respiratory conditions known as **chronic obstructive pulmonary disease (COPD)**. COPD involves one or more of the obstructive, compressive, or incompetency conditions of respiration. Studying the developmental anatomy of the respiratory tube and the relationship it maintains with the pleural sac will help you to anticipate the reasons why people have difficulty breathing.

5

Urinary and Reproductive Systems

INTRODUCTION

The body must eliminate what it cannot absorb, and it must deliver or receive sex cells to reproduce. These bodily functions are intimate to our sense of well-being, so complications of these functions distress patients greatly. We already have previewed how the hindgut forms and how it begins to interface with the outside world. In this chapter, we complete the picture of how the end of the tube grows, and we examine a region of the mesoderm between the paraxial column and the lateral plate column (recall Fig. 1.12).

The urinary system maintains vital fluid balances and chemistry. As with the respiratory system, the gross anatomy of the organ (the kidney) and the tubing is unremarkable compared to its critical clinical significance. Also, as with the respiratory system, mastery of how the structures appear radiographically is a goal of studying the anatomy.

Sexual reproduction in animals is believed to be a derivation of an original design in which species were self-reproducing—that is, of a design that did not involve "male" and "female" individuals. To derive the anatomy of sexual reproduction, "maleness" and "femaleness" result from co-opting the same tissue zones, but selectively and to opposing degrees. The three basic tissue types grow toward a goal of projection or invagination, which enables the coupling between individuals that is necessary to execute reproductive behaviors.

DEVELOPMENT OF THE KIDNEY AND URETER

Recall that mesoderm first condenses into three zones—paraxial, intermediate, and lateral plate (see Fig. 1.12). Paraxial mesoderm forms the axial skeleton and supporting musculature of the body. The lateral plate mesoderm helps to form the body wall that folds around and makes a trunk of the body. The mesoderm clump between the paraxial and lateral plate clusters, the **intermediate mesoderm,** is implicated in the growth of the urinary and reproductive systems.

In real space, the wedge of intermediate mesoderm lies beside the primitive aorta, just ventral to the somite columns that are becoming the vertebral bodies. The wedge bulges against the otherwise smooth continuity of the peritoneal membrane layer of cells, so it is referred to as the **urogenital ridge.** From the very beginning of formation, the ridge has a dedicated **nephrogenic cord** of cells for the urinary system and a **gonadal ridge,** or a **genital ridge,** for the reproductive system (Fig. 5.1). They cooperate because of the convenience of an exit portal that is provided by the former and the intriguing consequences of sex differentiation in the latter.

Even though it cannot do so directly to the outside world, the developing fetus must eliminate waste fluid. For this purpose, an internal system of drainage tubes develops

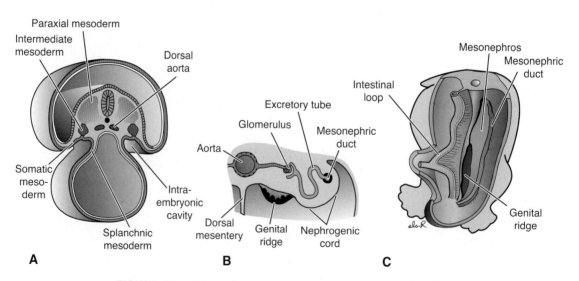

FIGURE 5.1　Intermediate mesoderm.

The intermediate mesoderm is adjacent to the peritoneum throughout lateral folding of the embryo (**A**). It develops into adjacent genital and nephric cell colonies (**B**). The proximity of these colonies to the peritoneum explains how their adult derivatives relate to the abdominal cavity and to each other (**C**). (From Sadler TW. Langman's Medical Embryology, 10th Edition. Baltimore: Lippincott Williams & Wilkins, 2006. Figure 15.1A, p. 230; Figure 15.17A,B, p. 240.)

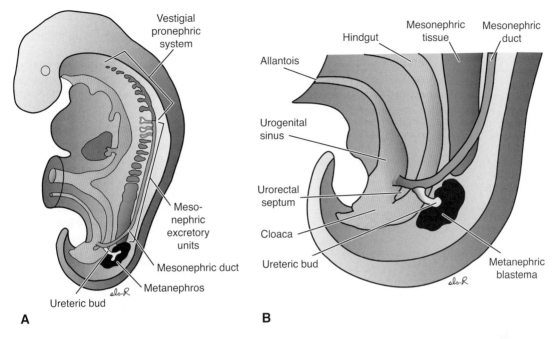

FIGURE 5.2   **Early fluid drainage in the embryo.**

The mesonephric duct runs the length of the embryonic body and terminates in the back wall of the gut tube, very close to the base of the allantois (**A**). The transverse tubules that drain fluid from the embryonic blood vessels will disintegrate over time, leaving just the longitudinal mesonephric duct behind (**B**). The future kidney buds off of the base of the mesonephric duct. The ureteric bud will develop into a kidney at its top end and a ureter connecting the kidney to the back of the future bladder. (From Sadler TW. Langman's Medical Embryology, 10th Edition. Baltimore: Lippincott Williams & Wilkins, 2006. Figure 15.2, p. 230; Figure 15.4, p. 231.)

early (and is eventually replaced by a permanent organ and duct). The temporary system forms within the nephrogenic cord as a series of drainage ducts (**glomeruli**) that connect in a lattice-like fashion to form an exit tube, or **mesonephric duct** (see Fig. 5.1B). The duct must go somewhere, and this is where the endodermal gut tube enters the picture. Remember that the urorectal septum of mesoderm bisected the cloacal end of the gut tube and separated it into a natural end to the gut tube (rectum) and a severed remnant with one end presenting to the outside world and the other end connected to the allantois. This severed remnant is well positioned for drainage to the outside world if only something would connect to it (Fig. 5.2).

The severed remnant is a blind pouch of endoderm, formally called the **urogenital sinus**. The sinus will communicate with the outside world through what used to be the upper half of the cloaca. This will become the **urinary** and **genital** orifices of the body, and it now is clear how those portals came to be "in front of," or anterior to, the anal portal. If, however, internal to this portal the urogenital sinus is a blind pouch, then it has nothing to excrete. The **mesonephric duct** will take advantage of this opportunity and connect the body's fluid-filtering system to an exitway, but only temporarily (see Fig. 5.2). Soon after connection, the sinus induces the permanent urinary system organs to form.

The mesonephric duct forms while the embryonic body is still differentiating. This duct is a dynamic latticework of draining tubes, with some forming in the lower part of the body at the same time that older, more superior ones are disintegrating.

While the latticework and original function of the duct system disappear, the duct itself persists on each side parallel to the vertebral column. It loses its waste fluid-filtering purpose but is available to be co-opted by the reproductive system.

Focus now on the bottom of the mesonephric duct, where it ports into the back of the urogenital sinus. As soon as this relationship is forged, the mesonephric duct grows an aggressive "bud," or **diverticulum**, from the junction point (see Fig. 5.2). This bid is called the **ureteric bud**, or the **metanephric blastema**. The term "ureteric bud" affirms that the ureter derives from this; the term "metanephric blastema" implies that this is a revised nephros, or **kidney**, system. It replaces the defunct mesonephric system.

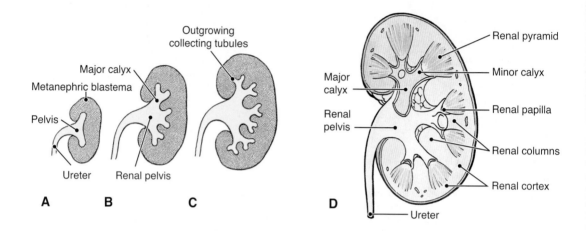

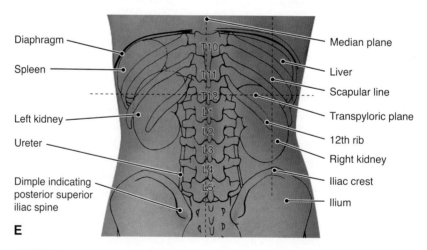

FIGURE 5.3   **Kidney development.**

The kidneys mature as an aggregate of collecting tubules (**A–C**). Longitudinal section of an adult kidney (**D**) demonstrates the confluence of drainage channels from the periphery to the ureter. The kidneys ascend (**E**) along the back of the abdominal wall until they come to rest just below the diaphragm (and below the liver on the right side). This means that the ureter must snake its way down the back of the abdominal wall and over the pelvic brim before it can port into the back of the bladder. (From Sadler TW. Langman's Medical Embryology, 9th Edition. Baltimore: Lippincott Williams & Wilkins, 2004. Figure 14.5. p. 325; from Moore KL, Agur AMR. Essential Clinical Anatomy, 2nd Edition. Baltimore: Lippincott Williams & Wilkins, 2002. Figures 3.34, p. 182 and p. 186.)

The origin of the ureteric bud is the complicated part. Once it has appeared, further growth of the ureter and kidney is largely just expansion of the tube (the future **ureter**) and its ear-shaped cap called the **metanephric blastema** (the future **kidney**) (Fig. 5.3). The developing kidney establishes a major vascular connection to the aorta as it becomes the central organ of urea filtration. As it expands, the mesonephric duct persists, but it no longer is connected to regional capillary beds by lattice-like glomeruli. Its upper end is open, and its lower end drains into the back of the **urogenital sinus**.

If the kidneys were located in the pelvis, this would be the end of the story regarding urinary system development. The kidneys are found more superior, however, overlapping with the lowest ribs and lining the posterior body wall at the same level as the duodenum and pancreas (see Fig. 5.3E). They must get there from their beginnings deep in the pelvic cavity, but the means by which they "ascend" are not clear. There is no functional reason for the kidneys to be located where they are in the adult. In part, they probably just drift into the available lumbar gutter as the fetus elongates and the herniated midgut returns to the abdominal cavity. The ureter is now quite elongated, and it remains a slender, smooth muscle tube connecting the kidney to the back of the urogenital sinus. It travels superficial to some structures (common iliac vessels) and deep to others (gonadal vessels) to reach the urogenital sinus, which remains in the pelvis (Fig. 5.4).

The gross anatomy of the adult kidney is appreciated best in a coronal section (see Fig. 5.4B). The organ matures as five relatively independent clusters of functioning tubules, each with its own dedicated branch of the renal artery. A cortex, which is heavily invested in fascia (renal capsule), houses pyramidal colonies of tubules that drain

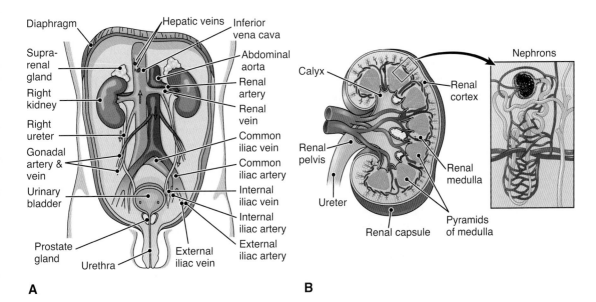

A   **B**

FIGURE 5.4   **The kidney and ureters in situ.**

The kidneys rest against the body wall in the lower thoracic and upper lumbar region of the vertebral column (**A**). Note that the ureter passes deep to the gonadal vessels en route to the bladder. Through compact, efficient, and pyramidal nephron communities (**B**), they rapidly filter the blood supply provided by and drained into the large renal vessels. (From Cohen BJ, Wood DL. Memmler's The Human Body in Health and Disease, 10th Edition. Baltimore: Lippincott Williams & Wilkins, 2004.)

toward the hilum of the kidney into dedicated calyces at the top of the ureter. Like a stream-and-river system, minor calyces merge into major calyces, which collectively form the renal pelvis, or delta. The conformation of calyces makes the inception of the ureter resemble a multitude of trumpets.

The ureter narrows considerably once it has received the output of the kidney. This narrowing complicates the transport of calcifications that can arise within the renal network (renal calculi, or kidney stones). Sharp edges of kidney stones may snag the inner lining of the ureter and become trapped, leading to smooth muscle spasming of the ureter, visceral pain, and partial restriction of urine drainage.

The right and left kidney "ascend" to different vertebral levels because of the physical barrier of the liver on the right side. Although both kidneys overlap the margins of the twelfth rib and the first lumbar vertebra, the right kidney is slightly more inferior, as seen in a frontal view, than is the left kidney. Both kidneys come to lie adjacent to the suprarenal glands, which, as their name implies, are found perched atop and alongside the superior pole of each kidney (see Fig. 5.4A). The two structures are related spatially but are mostly independent functionally.

DEVELOPMENT OF THE BLADDER AND URETHRA

The proximal part of the urinary system processes body fluid and transports it to a storage organ that develops from the urogenital sinus. The storage organ (the **urinary bladder**) matures in the same manner in both males and females, but its distal continuation to the outside world (the **urethra**) modifies differently according to sex.

Whereas the mesonephric duct and the ureteric bud both developed from intermediate mesoderm, the urogenital sinus is an endodermal structure. As with other endodermal derivatives of the gut tube, it is enveloped by a layer of mesoderm that has contractile properties (smooth muscle). In the adult state, this smooth muscle wrap of the bladder is called the **detrusor muscle**.

The urogenital sinus has three distinct parts: vesical, pelvic, and phallic (Fig. 5.5). At the top end, the **allantois**, that finger-like blind pouch now imprisoned at the base of the umbilical cord, balloons out as the **vesical** region to form the **urinary bladder**. It expands because the mesonephric duct and its associated ureteric bud invade the wall of the sinus (Fig. 5.5D–G). The tip of the allantois, however, stays tucked into the tight opening of the umbilical cord. It normally withers in place until it is just a fibrous band of tissue tethering the bladder wall to the inside of the abdominal wall (the **urachus**). If the allantois does not wither, however, then urine accumulating in the bladder can leak through the patency into a cyst near the umbilicus or even dribble out of the umbilical knot (a **urachal cyst**, or **fistula**) (Fig. 5.6.).

The **pelvic** part of the urogenital sinus is unremarkable. It simply connects the swelled bladder to the skin barrier, where the urinary orifice will be. In the mature state, this narrowed part of the sinus will be called the **pelvic urethra** and the **membranous urethra**. It is most notable clinically because in males it elaborates to form the secretory structures of the **prostate gland**. Prostatitis and prostate tumors, thus, impinge on the urethra, resulting in the major symptom of **impaired micturition** (difficulty voiding urine).

The **phallic** part of the urogenital sinus is quite remarkable. It has the same original configuration in all embryos, but it is radically altered in the presence of a Y chromosome (i.e., in males). The embryonic phallus is simply a bulge in the body wall just above where the gut tube exits the body (see Fig. 5.5C). In fact, the underside of

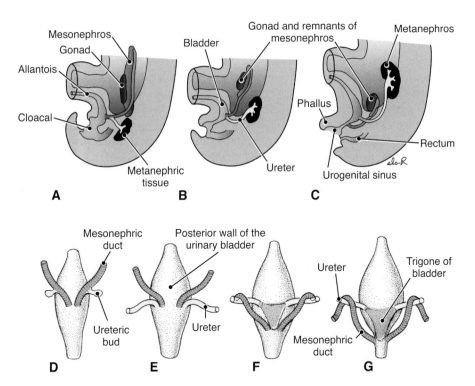

FIGURE 5.5 **The bladder develops from the base of the allantois.**

The back wall of the urogenital sinus is connected to the mesonephric duct (**A**). As the ureter and kidney grow, the root of the mesonephric duct burrows into the wall of the sinus (**B** and **C**). Eventually, enough of the duct sinks into the bladder wall so that the connection of the ureter and the mesonephric duct is lost, as seen in dorsal views of the developing bladder (**D–G**). (From Sadler TW. Langman's Medical Embryology, 10th Edition. Baltimore: Lippincott Williams & Wilkins, 2006. Figure 15.10, p. 236; Figure 15.14, p. 238.)

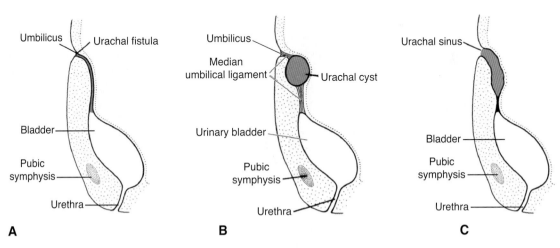

FIGURE 5.6 **Urachal cysts and fistulas.**

The withered allantois does not always resorb itself into a fibrous cord (the urachus, or median umbilical ligament) between the bladder and umbilicus. If the urachus remains patent, fluid can weep out of the umbilicus through a fistula (**A**) or can be trapped as a cyst (**B**). The urachus also may form a sinus connection to the outside but not to the bladder (**C**). (From Sadler TW. Langman's Essential Medical Embryology, 10th Edition. Baltimore: Lippincott Williams & Wilkins, 2006. Figure 7.6C–E p. 77).

the phallus is formed by the upper portion of the cloacal membrane. When the urorectal septum separates the cloacal membrane into an anal orifice and a urogenital orifice, the urogenital orifice is the part that remains along the underside of the phallus.

The **phallus** transforms differently in males than in females. In females, the phallus does not elaborate, so even though it is relatively large in the fetus, it is relatively small in the mature state. The relationship of the urogenital orifice to the phallus barely changes in females, as displayed in an external view of fetal development (Fig. 5.7). Indeed, the external structure of the mature female phallic region is a minimal modification of the fetal design. The phallic part of the urogenital sinus has very little "length," so the **urethra** in females is a short shunt from the bladder to the outside world.

In males, the phallus elongates and takes the phallic portion of the urogenital sinus with it. This means that the underside of the phallus is grooved by a long, slit-like orifice, which at this stage may be called the **urethral groove** (Fig. 5.8). In the mature state, this groove closes over and gets "swallowed up" within the phallus, where it is called the **penile urethra**. Despite being closed up inside the phallus, it must still get to the outside world, and this is a very interesting part of genital development (see below).

In summary, the body develops a filter for collecting fluid waste and uses a remnant of the gut tube as a route for this fluid to leave the body. The filter begins as a simple "sink and tube" design called the **mesonephros** (collecting tubules connected by a mesonephric duct). This temporary filter ultimately is replaced by its own bud, the **metanephros**. The metanephros expands to form a single filtering organ (the kidney), which is connected to the gut tube remnant by its own root (the ureteric bud, which is the future ureter). This filter empties fluid waste into the gut tube remnant, which

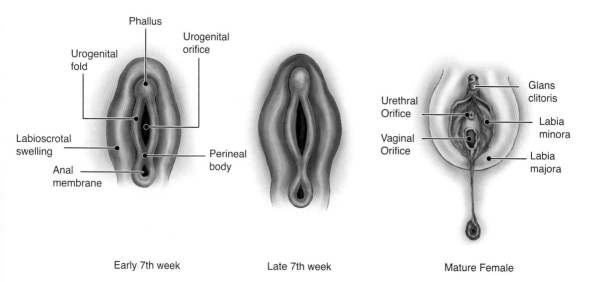

Phallus

Urogenital
orifice

Urogenital
fold

Labioscrotal
swelling

Anal
membrane

Perineal
body

Urethral
Orifice

Vaginal
Orifice

Glans
clitoris

Labia
minora

Labia
majora

Early 7th week   Late 7th week   Mature Female

FIGURE 5.7   **The urogenital sinus meets the outside world.**

As the perineal region matures from a sex-indifferent stage to a sex-specific genital design, the original design of a urogenital sinus "below" a phallus barely changes. These tissues, shown here in external view, will become the genitalia in both sexes. (Adapted from Larsen WJ. Human Embryology. New York: Churchill-Livingstone, 1993. Figure 10.18, p. 257.)

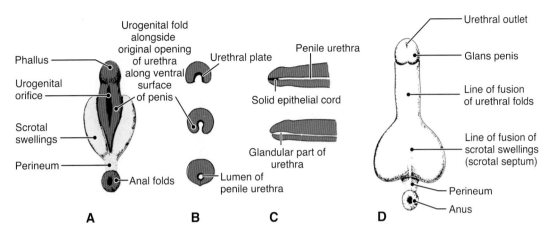

FIGURE 5.8   Male development alters the urogenital opening.

Although male genitalia look quite different from female genitalia, they derive from the same source tissue. The phallus elongates (**A**), taking the groove on its underside with it (**B**). The adult phallus, however, delivers urine and semen through an opening in its tip, so the underside exposure must be resorbed, which occurs through migration of the tissue on either side. This leaves a urethra embedded in the "shaft" of the phallus, but no escape to the outside world (**C**). A pit in the tip of the phallus bores its way inward until it links up with the end of the urethra, resulting in the postnatal configuration (**D**). (From Sadler TW. Langman's Medical Embryology, 10th Edition. Baltimore: Lippincott Williams & Wilkins, 2006. Figure 15.33a–d, p. 249.)

by now has an expanded top end (the bladder) and a narrowed, tubular bottom end (the urethra). The outer opening of the urethra is the adult derivative of the urogenital membrane half of the original cloacal membrane. Its configuration differs between males and females.

REPRODUCTIVE SYSTEM

The anatomy of the reproductive system obviously differs between males and females, but how and why? The "why" part involves genetic coding for the production of hormones that influence how cell colonies differentiate. The "how" part is the story of what happens to the discarded **mesonephric duct**.

The relevant cells are in the **intermediate mesoderm** (Fig. 5.9). One border of the mesoderm column is called the **genital ridge**, or the **gonadal ridge,** because germ cells cluster within it. The **gonad** will become the **testis** in the male and the **ovary** in the female, but they both arise in the back of the abdominal area within this gonadal ridge. Close to this ridge is the mesonephric duct, which runs vertically (longitudinally) down from the ridge and empties, as noted above, into the bladder. The important event to notice is how the **peritoneal lining** of the intermediate mesoderm "seeps in," or gets drawn into, the mesoderm column itself (Fig. 5.10). It is as if the mesonephric duct wanted a partner, so it drew in the border of its own territory into a second, parallel tube. This incorporated sleeve, or tube, logically is called the **paramesonephric duct**.

These two ducts factor heavily in the differentiation of male from female, which is logical given that there are two different adult pathways (male and female) and two

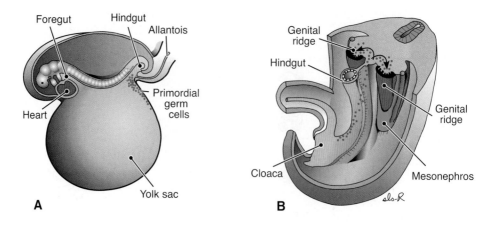

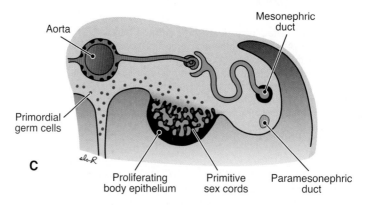

FIGURE 5.9   **Future sperm and egg cells gather in the genital ridge.**

Gametes arise in the gut tube endoderm (**A**) and migrate through the dorsal mesentery (**B**) to receptive primitive sex cords that are proliferating in the genital ridge (**C**). (From Sadler TW. Langman's Medical Embryology, 10th Edition. Baltimore: Lippincott Williams & Wilkins, 2006. Figure 15.18a,b, p. 240; Figure 15.19, p. 249.)

FIGURE 5.10   **Formation of the paramesonephric duct.**

As the gametes migrate into the gonadal ridge, the mesonephric duct system induces the peritoneal lining of the body wall to buckle inward (see left side). The resulting paramesonephric duct is, in fact, a sleeve of the peritoneal cavity with open upper and lower ends (see right side). (Adapted from Moore KL, Persaud TVN. The Developing Human, 5th Edition. Philadelphia: W.B. Saunders, 1988. Figure 13-20, p. 281.)

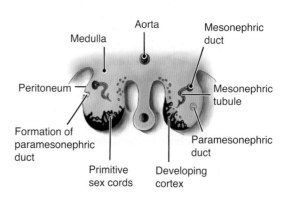

different "usable" ducts (mesonephric and paramesonephric). We now describe how the gonadal ridge uses one, but not the other, depending on the sex identity of the germ cells.

Female Reproductive Anatomy

Female identity results from an XX configuration of the twenty-third chromosome and subsequent formation of primordial germ cells in the yolk sac. These germ cells migrate toward the gonadal ridge. As they collect along the gonadal ridge, the ridge cells harbor them closely. Females develop a finite number of primary egg cells, or oocytes. They must be guarded closely and released sparingly (typically one per month for ~30–35 years). This may be why early in development the ridge cells form a capsule around the germ cells that prevents the germ cells from establishing a relationship with the nearby tubules of the mesonephric duct (Fig. 5.11). Remember that the tubules disintegrate as the kidney and ureter mature, so with no ability to drain egg cells from the female gonad, the mesonephric tubules are resorbed. In the absence of anything draining into the mesonephric duct at its top end, the duct also dissolves.

The **paramesonephric duct** remains as the most likely escape route for egg cells that the female gonad periodically releases. Physically, however, it is not related to the developing **ovary**, so at best, it can be a kind of "sink" for collecting the expelled egg (Fig. 5.12). This is one major challenge. The other major challenge is what to do with the egg once it has been collected by the open end of the paramesonephric duct. To meet this challenge, the paramesonephric duct distorts into a holding chamber called the **uterus** (Fig. 5.13). This is no small feat.

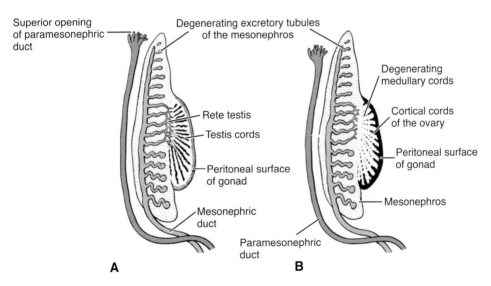

A   **B**

FIGURE 5.11   **Sexual differentiation in the genital ridge.**

The developing male reproductive tissue maintains a connection to the mesonephric duct system and a loose proximity to the peritoneal membrane (**A**). There is no function for the paramesonephric duct in males. By contrast, gametes in the developing female gonad are sequestered by strong cortical cords (**B**). In the absence of close contact with the gonad, the mesonephric duct degenerates, and the paramesonephric duct persists. (From Sadler TW. Langman's Medical Embryology, 9th Edition Image Bank. Baltimore: Lippincott Williams & Wilkins, 2004.)

FIGURE 5.12   **Formation of the ovary.**

The genital ridge forms a gonad in both males and females. The female gonad (ovary) is pressed against the peritoneal lining and remains virtually encapsulated by it. The mesonephric duct disintegrates (**A**), removing any possible connection of the ovary to the urinary tract. The paramesonephric duct has stepped up in its place, even developing an expanded opening with finger-like projections (**B**). (From Sadler TW. Langman's Medical Embryology, 10th Edition. Baltimore: Lippincott Williams & Wilkins, 2006. Figure 15.24, p. 243.)

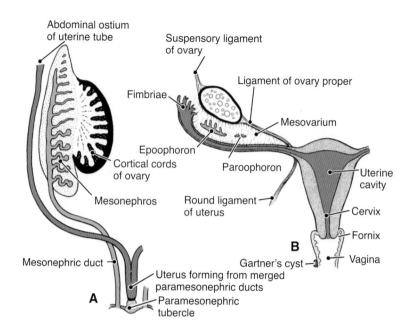

When the paramesonephric ducts first formed, they were just invaginations of the edge of a column of cells. **The top end was open to the peritoneal cavity and so was the bottom end**. If you were swimming about in the peritoneal cavity you could enter the top end of the duct and emerge, through the bottom end of the chute, in the very same peritoneal cavity. Likewise, if an egg cell is expressed through the peritoneal membrane by the ovary and gets drawn into the top end of the paramesonephric duct,

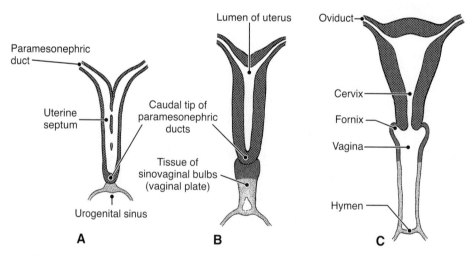

FIGURE 5.13   **Paramesonephric ducts merge to form a uterus.**

The paramesonephric ducts from each side merge into themselves at their bottoms and erode their walls to form a single chamber, the future uterus, as seen in schematic frontal view (**A**). The merger still abuts the back wall of the bladder (shown here as the urogenital sinus), but eventually, the duct draws up the back wall (**B**) and evacuates it to form a canal at the bottom end of the uterus (**C**). Importantly, as seen in the far right (**C**), this canal is still closed to the outside world because it never did break down the back wall of the bladder. (From Sadler TW. Langman's Medical Embryology, 9th Edition Image Bank. Baltimore: Lippincott Williams & Wilkins, 2004.)

it would end up back in the peritoneal cavity at the bottom of the abdomen—unless the bottoms of the right and left paramesonephric ducts sealed themselves together and swelled into a holding chamber, which is precisely what happens (see Fig. 5.13).

The uterus thus forms in the midline of the body, with two **uterine tubes** (**Fallopian tubes**, **oviducts**, or **salpinges**) reaching up on either side toward the encapsulated ovary. The merger of the paramesonephric ducts at their bottom ends, however, creates a closed loop. The uterus must reach the outside world so that two important things can happen: First, the germinating cell from a male can reach the egg, and second, the resulting conceptus can be birthed. Toward this goal, the paramesonephric duct, which is now the uterus, does what the mesonephric duct also did—it ports into the back of the urogenital sinus.

Unlike the mesonephric duct, which actually pokes into the sinus and opens a hole, the uterine union of the paramesonephric ducts only neighbors against the surface of the sinus (Fig. 5.14). After all, the bottom ends of the ducts already have sealed together into the uterine chamber; at best, it can abut the sinus wall with its own wall. When the wall of the uterine chamber impacts the wall of the sinus, the uterine wall induces the sinus wall to stretch out, and eventually, a cavity forms within the wall of the sinus itself. This is the early stage of the **vaginal cavity**. The top of the cavity, which is formed by the original impact of the uterine wall and the sinus wall, erodes, but the bottom of the cavity remains an intact wall. This will be important later.

At this point, therefore, the uterine cavity is on the verge of breaching the urogenital sinus cavity (the future bladder). Rather than commingle the pathway for fluid waste and germ cell transport, however, the uterovaginal cavity establishes its own advent to the outside world. Using its intact lower wall as a guide, the uterovaginal cavity pivots and drives its lower wall directly toward the urogenital orifice underneath the phallus (see Fig. 5.14C). It effectively extends itself into a canal parallel to the bladder and its urethra. This, of course, is the typical adult female configuration, in which the vaginal orifice is located "behind," or inferior to, the urethra and

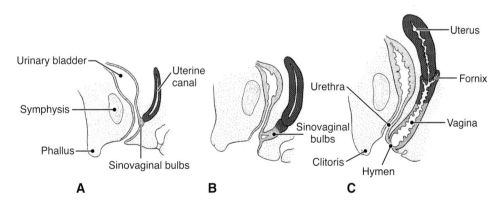

FIGURE 5.14   The uterus induces a vaginal canal.

As seen in lateral view, the uterus draws the bladder wall posteriorly (**A** and **B**), all the while evacuating the tissue into a canal that is open to the uterus. It never breaks through the back wall of the bladder, however (**C**). Rather, it pushes the back wall of the bladder downward and forward until it is directly presented to the outside world just below the true path of the urethra. Eventually, this wall, known as the hymen, will break down and allow the sex cell access to the outside world, and vice versa. (From Sadler TW. Langman's Medical Embryology, 9th Edition Image Bank. Baltimore: Lippincott Williams & Wilkins, 2004.)

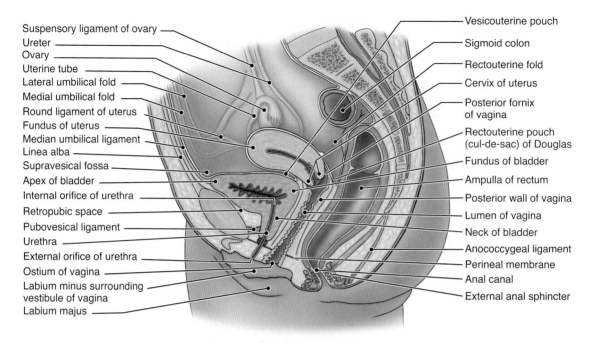

Suspensory ligament of ovary
Ureter
Ovary
Uterine tube
Lateral umbilical fold
Medial umbilical fold
Round ligament of uterus
Fundus of uterus
Median umbilical ligament
Linea alba
Supravesical fossa
Apex of bladder
Internal orifice of urethra
Retropubic space
Pubovesical ligament
Urethra
External orifice of urethra
Ostium of vagina
Labium minus surrounding
vestibule of vagina
Labium majus

Vesicouterine pouch
Sigmoid colon
Rectouterine fold
Cervix of uterus
Posterior fornix
of vagina
Rectouterine pouch
(cul-de-sac) of Douglas
Fundus of bladder
Ampulla of rectum
Posterior wall of vagina
Lumen of vagina
Neck of bladder
Anococcygeal ligament
Perineal membrane
Anal canal
External anal sphincter

FIGURE 5.15   **Sagittal view of the female pelvis.**

The peritoneal sac drapes over the ovary, reproductive organs, and rectum. The thick body of the uterus transitions to the vagina through a cervix. An archway, or fornix, at the upper end of the vaginal canal surrounds the cervix and brushes into contact with the peritoneum posteriorly. (From Moore KL, Dalley AF. Clinically Oriented Anatomy, 5th Edition. Baltimore: Lippincott Williams & Wilkins, 2006.)

the vaginal canal and uterus are located directly behind the bladder in the midline (Fig. 5.15).

During this entire process, the lower wall of the vaginal canal remains intact, effectively shutting off the female reproductive system from the outside world. For some time after birth, this wall (the **hymen**) persists. It disintegrates at a variable point in time before onset of the first **mensis**, or reproductive cycle.

As the kidneys are ascending to their mature location, the gonads descend away from their original location. In the female, the **ovary** remains tightly "shrink-wrapped" by the peritoneal lining against which it grew. The ovary migrates inferiorly to the edge of the **pelvic brim** (the inner "rim" of the pelvic skeleton), guided by a cord of tissue called the **gubernaculum**. For reasons that still are not clear, the gubernaculum in the female is "weaker" than the gubernaculum in the male—to the extent that in the female, it fails to "pull" the gonad very far at all. The ovary migrates approximately halfway around the abdominal wall before coming to rest in the pelvic cavity just below the pelvic brim. The gubernaculum persists, but as a loose, fibrofatty band of tissue called the **round ligament** (Fig. 5.16).

The uterine tubes remain physically apart from the ovary, with the tubes being separated from it by the layer of peritoneum that coats the ovary capsule. During **ovulation**, when the ovary releases an egg, the egg itself pierces the peritoneal lining on the ovary and, for the briefest of moments, enters the peritoneal cavity. Very nearby is the wide opening of the top of the uterine tube (formerly the paramesonephric duct), and the egg typically is "sucked into," or flows into, the opening and travels down the tube into the uterine chamber. This is the one and only natural occurrence of peritoneal sac rupture.

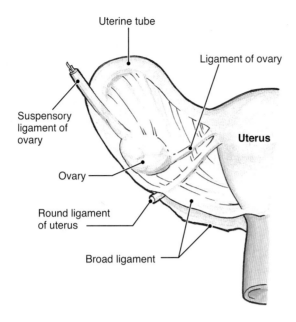

Uterine tube

Ligament of ovary

Suspensory
ligament of
ovary

Uterus

Ovary

Round ligament
of uterus

Broad ligament

FIGURE 5.16   Schematic position of the adult ovary.

This frontal view is intended to show that the female gonad also migrates, just not as far as the male gonad. As it migrates, the ovary pushes against the peritoneal lining until it is completely "shrink-wrapped" by peritoneum. It also drags its blood supply with it, so the ovarian artery and vein slip through the only corridor between the peritoneal reflection (called the suspensory ligament of the ovary). The drape of peritoneum over the uterine tube and uterus is the broad ligament, the wrinkles of which (ligament of the ovary and round ligament) are fibrous remnants of the tether between the gonad and the abdominal wall. Ovulation is the process by which the ovary "expels" an egg by bursting it through the peritoneal lining and into the peritoneal cavity, thus the "pitting" in the surface of the ovary that is seen over time and the painful sensation experienced by some women at ovulation. The egg cell then "falls" into the paramesonephric duct. (From Moore KL, Agur AMR. Essential Clinical Anatomy, 2nd Edition. Baltimore: Lippincott Williams & Wilkins, 2002. Figure 4.20A, p. 244.)

The complicated part of the female reproductive system is now complete. The shapes of the external surfaces of the system barely differ from those of the early fetal stage (Fig. 5.17). The female external genitalia are a **maturation** of the basic plan. The male genitalia, by contrast, **transform** the basic plan. This basic plan consists of the genital tubercle, or phallus; the folds of skin that form around it; and the **urogenital orifice** that runs under it. Two skinfolds are important to realize. The outer one is a swelling of the ectoderm and underlying fascia (loose mesoderm) of the abdominal wall called the **labioscrotal swelling**. In females, this fat-filled, pendulous pouch presses against the one from the other side as an effective, if passive, closure of the **vestibule** containing the openings to the urinary and reproductive systems.

Medial to these labioscrotal swellings are less pudgy folds of ectoderm that closely parallel the vestibule; they run the length of the original urethral groove, or urogenital orifice, along the underside of the phallus. These are called the **urogenital folds**. They have no fatty layer underneath them, but they do house a spongy body of tissue that can store a large amount of blood—it has the capacity to become turgid with fluid pressure. In females, this spongy body is called the **bulb of the vestibule**. In the mature female, the labioscrotal swellings become the **labia majora**, and the urogenital folds become the **labia minora**, both of which attend the vestibule that holds the now-separated openings to the **urethra** and the **vaginal canal** (see Fig. 5.17).

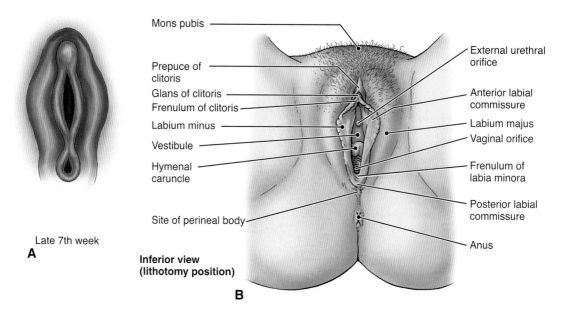

Mons pubis

Prepuce of
clitoris

Glans of clitoris

Frenulum of clitoris

Labium minus

Vestibule

Hymenal
caruncle

Site of perineal body

External urethral
orifice

Anterior labial
commissure

Labium majus

Vaginal orifice

Frenulum of
labia minora

Posterior labial
commissure

Anus

Late 7th week
A

**Inferior view
(lithotomy position)**

B

FIGURE 5.17   **Fetal and adult female external genitalia.**

In females, the little-modified phallus houses the erectile tissues of the clitoris. The urogenital folds
on either side of the orifice (**A**) remain a small flap of tissue (labium minus) that closes passively over
the urethral and vaginal openings (collectively called a vestibule) (**B**). The initial labioscrotal swelling
fails to receive a gonad but, instead, maintains an underlayer of fatty tissue and becomes the labium
majus, which provides a more buffered passive closure to the vestibule. (From Moore KL, Dalley AF.
Clinically Oriented Anatomy, 5th Edition. Baltimore: Lippincott Williams & Wilkins, 2006.)

As mentioned above, the phallus in the female does not proliferate. In the mature
state, it remains a bulb of ectoderm at the top of the vestibule. Like the labia minora,
this part of the phallus houses a rich vascular bed that can swell with blood (the **corpus
cavernosum**). The tip of this bed, the midline culmination of the genital tubercle, is
the **clitoris** in the mature female.

Male Reproductive Anatomy

The transformation to maleness starts from the same basic design of mesonephric and
paramesonephric ducts (see Fig. 5.11). As the germ cells accumulate along the gonadal
ridge, however, no firm capsule encloses them. Males produce an almost infinite number of sex cells throughout their adult lives, so the imperative is not to harbor them
closely but to release them. An avenue for this release is conveniently in place in the form
of the original collecting tubules of the mesonephric duct (Fig. 5.18). Thus, in the presence of male sex cells, the mesonephric duct remains intact as the most convenient portal for their transmission, because it is linked to a large number of tubules. The duct
persists as the **ductus deferens**, connected to the gonad via the mature tubules, now
called the **rete testis**. This induced preservation signals the death of the paramesonephric duct, which begins to degenerate at the same time.

In keeping with the theme of minimization of male internal reproductive anatomy,
the released sex cells simply co-opt the **urinary pathway** to reach the outside world. The
mesonephric duct does not have to manufacture a new facility for handling the released

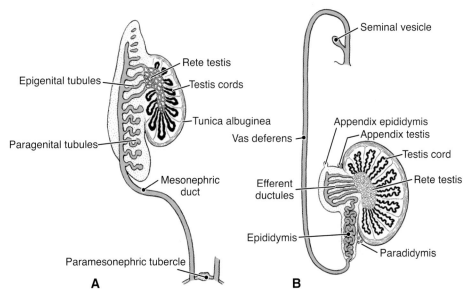

FIGURE 5.18   **Formation of the testis.**

In the male, the urogenital ridge contributes basic structure to the testis, which does not adhere tightly to the adjacent peritoneal lining. Rather, the sex cells condense into a medulla that is close enough to the original collecting tubules of the mesonephric duct system to use them as conduits (**A**). With more liberty to migrate, the testis descends, taking the duct with it (**B**). (From Sadler TW. Langman's Medical Embryology, 10th Edition. Baltimore: Lippincott Williams & Wilkins, 2006.)

sex cells, because it already is ported into the back of where the bladder becomes the prostate. The real energy of development during the male transformation is spent in two other ways—first, getting the gonad to descend to the very bottom of the trunk so that it can suspend away from the body, and second, growing a genital extension of the urethral groove.

Core body temperature is too hot for sperm cells housed in the gonad to survive. The gonad needs to free itself of this temperature trap, but how? The remarkable process of male gonadal descent "bubbles out" the bottom of the abdominal wall into a sac that is so thin the gonad it holds enjoys the cooling effect of being "outside" the body cavity and as "exposed" to the elements as the nose or the fingertips. This, of course, makes that part of the abdominal wall vulnerable to other internal pressures. Many of these manifest as **hernias**; thus, studying the anatomy of the abdominal wall must include an emphasis on the **inguinal canal** and the opening forged by the descending gonad.

As noted above, the gonads develop in the back of the abdominal region in the fetus. As noted below, the mesoderm of the abdominal wall forms a three-layered sandwich of muscles. The gonad develops in the space between the innermost layer of this sandwich and the **peritoneal membrane** (Fig. 5.19). In males as well as females, a gubernaculum of fibrofatty tissue will direct the gonad around the abdominal wall. In males, however, the gubernaculum "tows" the gonad all the way around to the front of the abdominal wall. As it does so, it induces the wall to pouch outward such that the **labioscrotal swelling** becomes a true **scrotal sac**. In keeping with conservative embryologic patterning, all tissue layers between the gonad and the skin follow the pouch—the **transversalis fascia**, the **internal abdominal oblique**, the **external abdominal oblique**, the **superficial fascia**, and the **skin** (Fig. 5.20). The innermost wall muscle (the **transversus**

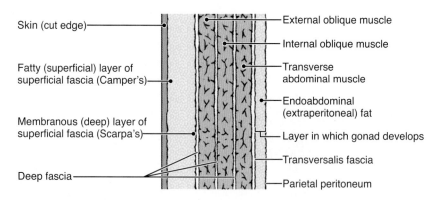

FIGURE 5.19   **The gonadal position relative to the abdominal wall.**

The gonad develops in the loose tissue between the peritoneum and the body wall musculature. As the male gonad descends, it travels around the body wall but never "breaks through" or punctures a layer anterior to it. It simply pushes that layer ahead of itself and into the scrotal sac. (From Moore KL, Dalley AF. Clinically Oriented Anatomy, 5th Edition. Baltimore: Lippincott Williams & Wilkins, 2006. Figure 2.4, p. 197.)

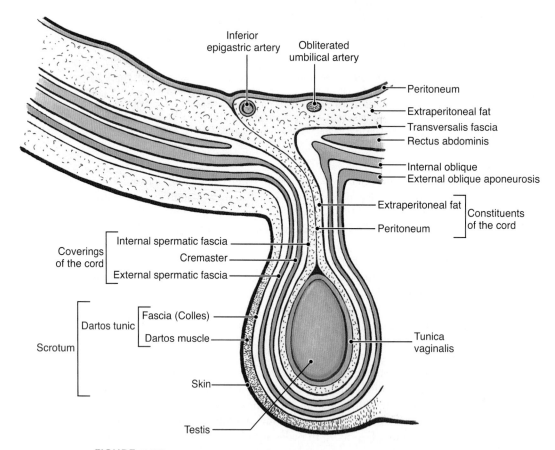

FIGURE 5.20   **The testis descends into the labioscrotal swelling.**

In this cross-section of the abdominal wall and scrotum, the gonad has migrated around the abdominal wall, staying in its home space between the peritoneum and the body wall musculature. At the very front of the wall, the gonad pouches outward, taking all forward layers with it, into the scrotum, which is the male derivative of the labioscrotal swelling. Thus, an inherent weakness exists in the inguinal region of the anterior abdominal wall where these layers stretch out to conform to the scrotal sac. (From Agur A, Dalley AF. Grant's Atlas of Anatomy, 11th Edition. Baltimore: Lippincott Williams & Wilkins, 2005.)

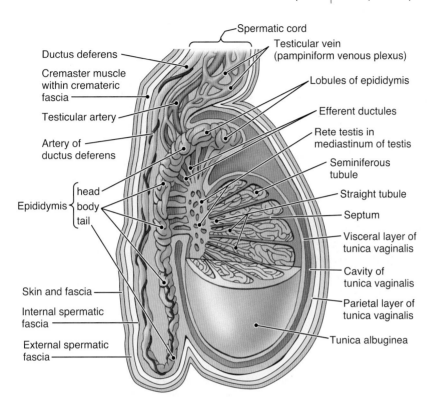

Spermatic cord

Testicular vein
(pampiniform venous plexus)

Ductus deferens

Cremaster muscle
within cremateric
fascia

Lobules of epididymis

Testicular artery

Efferent ductules

Artery of
ductus deferens

Rete testis in
mediastinum of testis

Seminiferous
tubule

Epididymis { head / body / tail

Straight tubule

Septum

Visceral layer of
tunica vaginalis

Skin and fascia

Cavity of
tunica vaginalis

Internal spermatic
fascia

Parietal layer of
tunica vaginalis

External spermatic
fascia

Tunica albuginea

FIGURE 5.21   **Tissue layers around the descended testis.**

The testis is wrapped by the layers of the abdominal wall that followed it into the scrotal sac. These layers also wrap the blood vessels and duct that run from the testis back into the body cavity. Together, this complex is called the spermatic cord. Note that during its migration, the testis "pinched off" a slip of the peritoneum that had drooped into the labioscrotal swelling before the arrival of the testis. This becomes the closed sac (tunica vaginalis) against the gonad, much like the pleural, pericardial, and peritoneal sacs. Like those, the tunica vaginalis can swell with excess fluid and disrupt function of the organ.

abdominis) does not extend inferiorly enough to be in the path of the inguinal canal, so it does not participate in the formation of the **spermatic cord**. Once pouched away from the abdominal wall, these tissue layers are called the **internal spermatic fascia**, the **cremaster muscle**, the **external spermatic fascia**, the **dartos muscle**, and the **skin**, respectively (Fig. 5.20).

The testis must still be connected to the inside world of the body, so a neurovascular bundle and a sperm duct still connect to it and travel between it and the body cavity through the inguinal canal. The **testicular artery** of the bundle remains a direct branch off of the abdominal aorta, which means that it runs a rather winding course down and around the body wall to keep track of the migrated gonad (Fig. 5.21). The **ductus deferens**, which is a remnant of the mesonephric duct, connects the **testis** to the **bladder** as originally designed, so it curls into the pelvic cavity immediately on leaving the inguinal canal at the **deep inguinal ring**.

The point at which the scrotal sac first pouches away from the abdominal wall represents a significant weakening of the wall, because each tissue layer "bubbles out" and stretches considerably. This point of the abdominal wall is called the **superficial inguinal ring**, and it is the location of inguinal **hernias** when excessive internal pressure

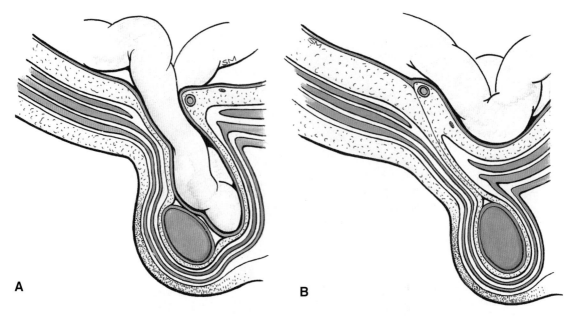

A

B

FIGURE 5.22   **The gut tube can herniate into the path of the testis.**

Inguinal hernias breach the weakness of the abdominal wall around the path of the testis. Indirect inguinal hernias (**A**) result when a section of intestine follows the same route as the testis, pushing the peritoneum into the bulge that it created during migration. Indirect hernias parallel the spermatic cord and can distend the scrotum. Direct inguinal hernias (**B**) result when abdominal pressure exceeds the strength of the abdominal wall medial to the superficial inguinal ring and the path of the inferior epigastric artery. They are caused by intense pressure, such as when lifting a heavy weight improperly, and form a bulge of the abdominal wall, typically above the root of the scrotal sac. (From Agur A, Dalley AF. Grant's Atlas of Anatomy, 11th Edition. Baltimore: Lippincott Williams & Wilkins, 2005.)

forces the gut tube either through the inguinal canal (**indirect hernia**) or through the remaining muscular wall of the abdomen between the superficial inguinal ring and the midline (**direct hernia**) (Fig. 5.22).

If the gubernaculum successfully draws the testis into the scrotal sac, the gubernaculum then reduces to nothing more than a miniscule ligament that binds the testis to the bottom of the sac. Success is not guaranteed, however, and the testis may get trapped along the way and take up to a year after birth to descend completely. The condition of incomplete testis descent is called **cryptorchidism**. (See Clinical Anatomy Box 5.1.)

Remember that unlike the developing ovary, the maturing male gonad allies more closely with the collecting tubules than with the peritoneum that lines the gonadal ridge. The **medulla** of the **testis** becomes a production factory for male sex cells, and it remains interfingered with the mesonephric tubules. The other tubules of the mesonephric duct degenerate as part of the planned transfer of urinary function to the metanephros. The mesonephric duct, however, remains (and is now the **ductus deferens**, or **vas deferens**), and the junction of it and the metanephros with the bladder becomes a point of interest.

In the mature state, the ureter and the ductus deferens enter the back of the bladder in different places, but in the fetal state, they are two branches of a single trunk that is "rooted" into the back of the urogenital sinus (Fig. 5.23). This trunk progressively burrows into the back of the sinus (now the bladder) such that it melds into the wall of the bladder itself in the shape of a triangle, or **trigone**. This burrowing absorbs the full

CLINICAL ANATOMY

Box 5.1

CRYPTORCHIDISM

The birth of a child is one of the most exciting, but also distressing, moments of life. When parents first see their baby, they naturally want everything to look "normal." Development, however, can be interrupted, perturbed, or even just slightly out of sync. One of the most valuable roles you can play as a health care professional is to explain a newborn baby's condition to worried parents. For example, parents expecting a boy may be distressed at the sight of a scrotal area that looks asymmetric or "flat." This may be a result of **cryptorchidism**, a condition in which the gonad has not descended completely into the scrotal sac.

In approximately 3% of newborn males, a testis or testes remain undescended at birth. Normally, the tardy gonad will descend during the first three months after birth. If the gonad remains sequestered, however, it may fail to mature properly, which can lead to infertility, renal problems, and testicular tumors.

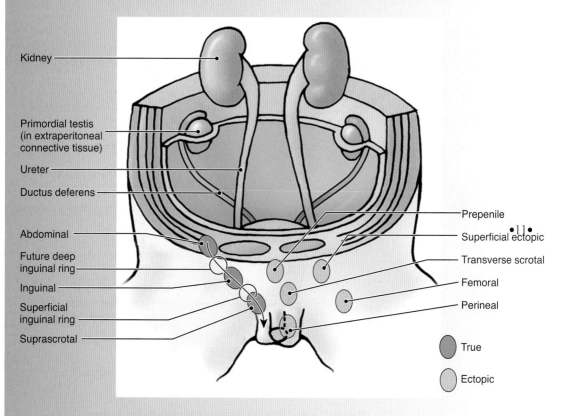

Kidney

Primordial testis (in extraperitoneal connective tissue)

Ureter

Ductus deferens

Abdominal

Future deep inguinal ring

Inguinal

Superficial inguinal ring

Suprascrotal

Prepenile

Superficial ectopic

Transverse scrotal

Femoral

Perineal

True

Ectopic

Cryptorchidism.

extent of the shared tube between the mesonephric and metanephric ducts, and in the end, each tube empties into the bladder in a different place. This difference is affected by the descent of the gonad, which causes the mesonephric duct (ductus deferens) to bend around the perimeter of the bladder. This detailed moment of development is important because it explains two things about adult male anatomy—first, why the ductus deferens appears to drape **over** the ureter, and second, why the ductus deferens empties into the prostate below the bladder (rather than the back of the bladder, where the process began) (see Fig. 5.23). This prostatic position of the sperm duct enables a basic separation of collected urine (in the bladder, trapped by a sphincter) and semen, which enters the urethra below the bladder.

To preserve the integrity of the sex cells in the common channel of the urethra, accessory organs of reproduction form near the base of the bladder. One is the **seminal vesicle**, which is a pouch of the bottom of the mesonephric duct itself, much like the original ureteric bud. The other is the **prostate gland**, which is a ballooning of the lining of the urethra itself, packaged within a coat of mesoderm (Fig. 5.23). Anatomically, the prostate gland surrounds the initial part of the urethra. The ductus deferens receives the output of the seminal vesicle, at which point the duct is called the **ejaculatory duct**. This duct is embedded in the substance of the prostate, so the point at which male sex cells first enter the urinary system is in the **prostatic urethra** (Fig. 5.24). Because the

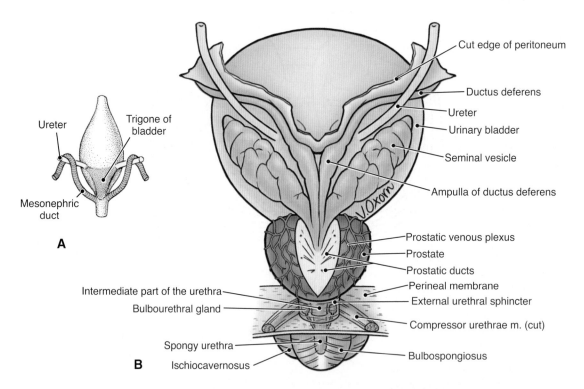

FIGURE 5.23   Male fetal and adult internal urinary and reproductive anatomy.

The mesonephric duct burrows so far into the back wall of the bladder that it forms a "trigone" zone (**A**). Once the reproductive duct is independent of the ureter, there is relatively little change into the adult state, as seen posteriorly (**B**). A prostate gland proliferates from the interface of the mesonephric duct and the urethra, and a seminal gland buds off of the reproductive duct. These glands provide critical fluids and media for the sperm cells produced in the testis. m. = muscle (From Moore KL, Agur AMR. Essential Clinical Anatomy, 2nd Edition. Baltimore: Lippincott Williams & Wilkins, 2002. Figure 4.13, p. 281.)

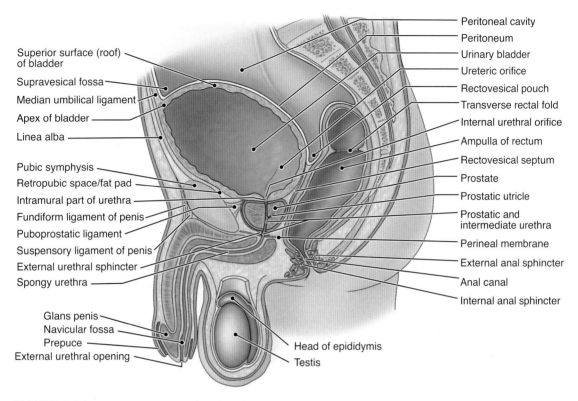

Superior surface (roof) of bladder
Supravesical fossa
Median umbilical ligament
Apex of bladder
Linea alba
Pubic symphysis
Retropubic space/fat pad
Intramural part of urethra
Fundiform ligament of penis
Puboprostatic ligament
Suspensory ligament of penis
External urethral sphincter
Spongy urethra
Glans penis
Navicular fossa
Prepuce
External urethral opening
Head of epididymis
Testis
Peritoneal cavity
Peritoneum
Urinary bladder
Ureteric orifice
Rectovesical pouch
Transverse rectal fold
Internal urethral orifice
Ampulla of rectum
Rectovesical septum
Prostate
Prostatic utricle
Prostatic and intermediate urethra
Perineal membrane
External anal sphincter
Anal canal
Internal anal sphincter

FIGURE 5.24   **Sagittal section of the male pelvis.**

The peritoneum drapes over the relatively simple topology of the bladder and rectum. The prostate gland, which is subject to hyperplasia with advancing age, can be palpated via the rectum. (From Moore KL, Dalley AF. Clinically Oriented Anatomy, 5th Edition. Baltimore: Lippincott Williams & Wilkins, 2006. Figure 3.17A, p. 397.)

urethra is wholly enclosed in the prostate gland, enlargement of the prostate because of prostatitis or prostate cancer can constrict the flow of urine. The frequent urge to urinate followed by diminished flow is a primary symptom of prostate disease.

Male and female reproductive anatomy logically is complementary. Female internal anatomy is elaborate, but the external anatomy is little modified. Male internal anatomy is especially minimal, but external anatomy is greatly modified. Male anatomy seizes on the opportunity to use the phallus as an extender of the urethra. The original tissues available to be incorporated are the same as those for the female—the **genital tubercle**, the **labioscrotal swelling**, and the **urogenital folds** bordering the urethral groove (see Figs. 5.7 and 5.8). In males, the genital tubercle drives the forward development of the reproductive system.

As described earlier, the underside of the tubercle is grooved by the urethra, which is the exit point for excretion of urine and ejaculation of sex cells. As the tubercle elongates in males, it draws the groove out along with it. The vascular bed of the tubercle is described as cavernous because it can retain a large volume of blood. We identify this major portion of the developing **penis** as the **corpus cavernosum**, or **cavernous body**, and this portion is homologous to the body of the clitoris (Fig. 5.25). The urogenital folds also extend along the length of the penis because as in the female, they border the urethral orifice. At the "top," or forward, end of the urethral groove, the urogenital folds

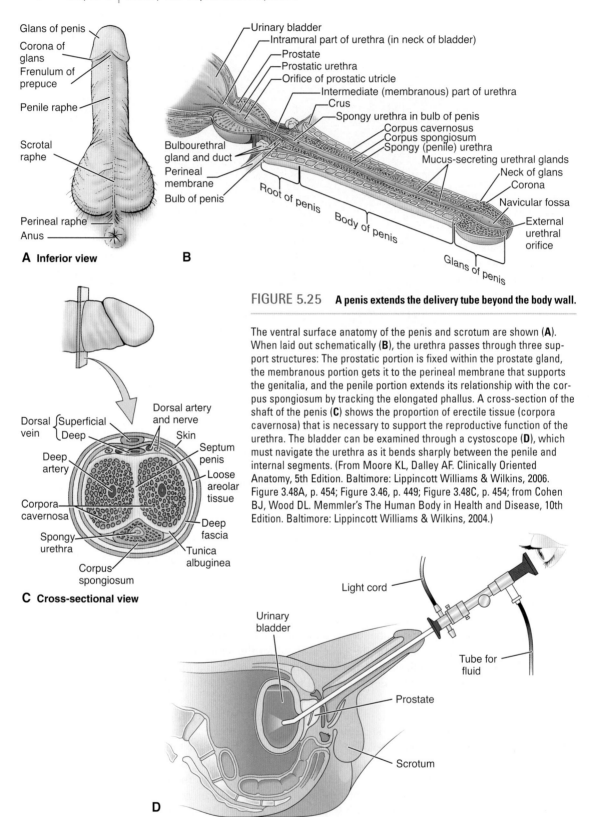

A Inferior view

Glans of penis
Corona of glans
Frenulum of prepuce
Penile raphe
Scrotal raphe
Perineal raphe
Anus

B

Urinary bladder
Intramural part of urethra (in neck of bladder)
Prostate
Prostatic urethra
Orifice of prostatic utricle
Intermediate (membranous) part of urethra
Crus
Spongy urethra in bulb of penis
Corpus cavernosus
Corpus spongiosum
Spongy (penile) urethra
Mucus-secreting urethral glands
Neck of glans
Corona
Navicular fossa
External urethral orifice

Bulbourethral gland and duct
Perineal membrane
Bulb of penis

Root of penis
Body of penis
Glans of penis

C Cross-sectional view

Dorsal vein { Superficial, Deep }
Deep artery
Corpora cavernosa
Spongy urethra
Corpus spongiosum

Dorsal artery and nerve
Skin
Septum penis
Loose areolar tissue
Deep fascia
Tunica albuginea

FIGURE 5.25   A penis extends the delivery tube beyond the body wall.

The ventral surface anatomy of the penis and scrotum are shown (**A**). When laid out schematically (**B**), the urethra passes through three support structures: The prostatic portion is fixed within the prostate gland, the membranous portion gets it to the perineal membrane that supports the genitalia, and the penile portion extends its relationship with the corpus spongiosum by tracking the elongated phallus. A cross-section of the shaft of the penis (**C**) shows the proportion of erectile tissue (corpora cavernosa) that is necessary to support the reproductive function of the urethra. The bladder can be examined through a cystoscope (**D**), which must navigate the urethra as it bends sharply between the penile and internal segments. (From Moore KL, Dalley AF. Clinically Oriented Anatomy, 5th Edition. Baltimore: Lippincott Williams & Wilkins, 2006. Figure 3.48A, p. 454; Figure 3.46, p. 449; Figure 3.48C, p. 454; from Cohen BJ, Wood DL. Memmler's The Human Body in Health and Disease, 10th Edition. Baltimore: Lippincott Williams & Wilkins, 2004.)

Light cord
Urinary bladder
Tube for fluid
Prostate
Scrotum

D

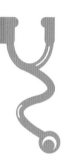

CLINICAL ANATOMY

Box 5.2

HYPOSPADIAS

I f the spongy body of the penis fails to fuse over the urethral groove, the newborn's urethra will open along the "underpart," or ventral part, of the shaft instead of at the tip of the head. Called **hypospadias**, this condition can range from a minor transposition of the urethral orifice to a major, slit-like opening in the shaft. The baby can still urinate, just not from where you might expect it. Indeed, many cases of hypospadias are clinically benign or go undetected and untreated until adolescence, when boys take a deeper interest in their own bodies. By knowing the way in which the penis develops, you can help to explain the treatment options for this simple, but strange-looking, condition to the parents.

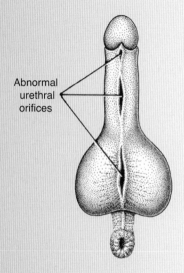

Abnormal urethral orifices

Hypospadias. (From Sadler TW. Langman's Medical Embryology, 10th Edition. Baltimore: Lippincott Williams & Wilkins, 2006. Figure 15.35A, p. 250.)

come together to form a natural boundary to the groove. This boundary cap mushrooms into a kind of "head" to the penis. In the mature state, the urogenital fold in the male is called the **corpus spongiosum**, or **spongy body**, and its top end is called the **glans penis**.

The anatomic configuration now has the basic shape of a mature penis, but the long opening of the urethra looks very strange along the underside of the penile shaft. In normal development, the urogenital folds will zip together and close over this exposure. This solves the problem along the penile shaft, but it creates another problem—the urethra now has no opening to the outside world. To solve this problem, the "top," or forward, end of the spongy body, now the glans penis, cavitates, or bores a hole into itself (see Fig. 5.8). The glans penis thus develops a pit that tunnels inward until it reaches the enclosed urethra. Failure of this process to complete leads to a relatively common clinical anomaly of the male reproductive system called **hypospadias**. (See Clinical Anatomy Box 5.2.)

6

Nervous System

INTRODUCTION

An adult head and neck develops to meet the needs of the top ends of the nervous system and the absorbing systems (digestion and respiration). From its position lying along the dorsal or posterior border of the vertebral bodies, the neural tube expands at its top. This expansion must be covered by ectoderm. In humans, it is so big that it curls, or forces down into flexion, the anatomy in front of the vertebral bodies. This anatomy is the top of the gut tube, and the result is an adult head in which the brain sits atop a plank of bone connected to the vertebral bodies, and the "face" hangs below that same perch (Fig. 6.1).

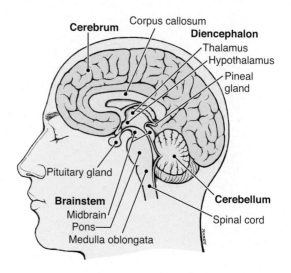

FIGURE 6.1   Schematic profile of the head, with a sagittal view of the brain.

The head is part brain and part face. (From Stedman's Medical Dictionary, 27th Edition. Baltimore: Lippincott Williams & Wilkins, 2006.)

DEVELOPMENT AND ORGANIZATION OF THE HEAD AND NECK

The face is comprised of ectoderm and mesoderm tissue that grows as a security gate for the absorbing endoderm. An entryway to the respiratory system must form (the **nose**), and a processing station for the digestive system must form (the **oral cavity**). Through and around this anatomy, the central nervous system must reach out to the outside world with endings that are sensitive to special waves—light waves (**vision**), sound waves (**hearing**), chemical waves (**smell** and **taste**), and fluid waves (**balance**). Some of these require cooperation with the face (smell and taste); others just squeeze out to the sides (hearing) or on top (vision) of it.

Finally, an artifact of the mammalian biological past must be resolved. When the embryo folds from a disk into a "body," the cervical region ectoderm and mesoderm fold around to complete the tube design, but ribs do not extend from the transverse processes of the vertebrae. Instead, a relatively "loose" cylinder of connective tissue (the neck) develops between the trunk cavity and the tops of the neural and gut tubes. This is the branchial or gill region in water-breathing animals and the pharyngeal/laryngeal region in air-breathing animals (Fig. 6.2). Mammalian embryos transform a neck with the rudiments of a water-breathing anatomy into a supple neck lacking any bumps, grooves, or dimples.

The essential adaptation of water-breathing organisms is to develop a series of arches around the arc from the anterior part of the trunk back to the vertebrae. Figure 6.2 captures a sense of how the arch framework looks. The idea is to provide a permeable membrane of exchange between the circulatory system of the animal and the water in which that animal lives. The branchial arches each contain a complete bone–muscle–nerve–blood vessel unit, and the gaps between the arches allow water to flow against tissue layers that could exchange gas with it (the **gills**). From this basis, the adult human head and neck develop with the same dedicated bone––muscle–nerve–artery units in each pharyngeal arch.

The advent of terrestrial life and the opportunity to absorb oxygen from the atmosphere resulted in lungs developing from the gut tube. The lungs are very effective, but they do not derive from or work with the gill arches. The terrestrial body form has no room or reason for a gill system that is exposed to the outside world. The arch system transformed in reptiles and mammals by closing in on itself, so the neck region in

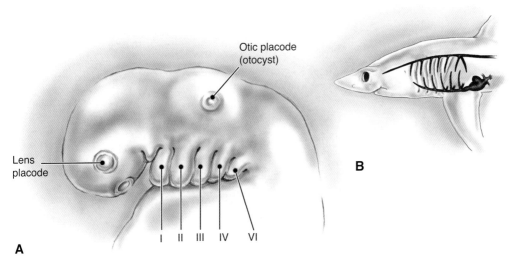

Lens
placode

A

B

FIGURE 6.2   **Pharyngeal arches derive from an ancient life in the hydrosphere.**

The pharyngeal arches of the human embryo (**A**) are homologous to the structures that become gill slits in fish (**B**). Patterns of face, throat, and neck anatomy are best understood by tracking the fates of these arches.

these animals is effectively closed to the outside world. How the arches transform explains why cranial nerves serve some muscles but not others and why the aortic arch gives off the subclavian and carotid arteries in the way that it does.

In gross anatomy, it is important to use embryology to understand adult structure. It is less important to comprehend the step-by-step account of how the head and neck develop. In this section, note how the recently folded embryo transforms its arches and grows a face underneath its brain. Many specific details will be excluded in favor of mastering the general plan.

The Pharyngeal Arches

During the fourth and fifth week of development, the presumptive neck region of the embryo develops a series of arches that are best appreciated in a coronal section (Fig. 6.3). The arch design is simple, and every surface is important. The arch itself consists of a core of **mesenchyme** from lateral plate and paraxial mesoderm. Within the arch is a clump of **neural crest cells**, a dedicated **artery**, and a dedicated **nerve**. The outside surface of the arch is ectoderm, and the inside surface is effectively the **pharyngeal** region of the endoderm.

The arches are not truly separated from one another as the gills of fishes are. Rather, a thin layer of ectoderm lies over the outside of the arches from superior to inferior, and the pharyngeal endoderm lays over the inside for the same distance. In between the arches, the ectoderm and the endoderm come together, giving the neck a series of **clefts** between the arches as seen from the outside and a series of **pouches** between the arches as seen from the inside. Some arches, clefts, and pouches remain as distinct anatomies in the body, such as the core of the lower jaw and the auditory tube.

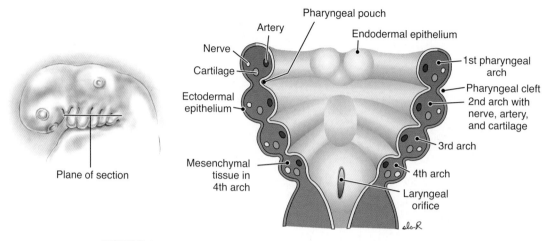

FIGURE 6.3   **A coronal slice through the pharyngeal arches.**

This anterior view shows the cut surfaces and inner lining of the pharyngeal arches. All surfaces are relevant to development of the face and neck. Each arch has a dedicated nerve, artery, and cartilage. Between each arch is an external cleft and an internal pouch. (From Sadler TW. Langman's Medical Embryology, 10th Edition. Baltimore: Lippincott Williams & Wilkins, 2006. Figure 16.6A, p. 260.)

Try to visualize that above the arches, the endodermal tube ends like the end of a garden hose, in which the nozzle near the top is ribbed (the arches) and the hose ends just above it. Perched in back and bending the end of the hose forward is a giant **neural tube** that sends feelers, such as the future eye and the future ear, toward the surface. As the arches transform, they will "swallow up" the end of the gut tube and pack in muscles and bones both around it and between it and the outside world. In time, they effectively become the **face** that protects the endoderm, especially in terms of the **maxilla** and **mandible**.

The embryo develops six pharyngeal arches over the course of two to three weeks. They are numbered from the top down, but for ancient biological regions the fifth pharyngeal arch either fails to generate or degenerates very shortly after forming. So, there are effectively five total arches, but they are numbered 1, 2, 3, 4, and 6. The story of arch transformation at this point proceeds arch by arch, cleft by cleft, and pouch by pouch.

First pharyngeal arch

The mesenchyme of the first pharyngeal arch becomes the maxilla, the zygomatic bone, part of the temporal bone, and the mandible. In some animals, the lower jaw consists of three interacting bones. In humans, one of these bones, the mandible, has become dominant. The other two bones develop as remnants from a section of the first arch cartilage called **Meckel's cartilage**. They are shriveled up at the back end of the first arch or at the back end of the mandible, and they are the **malleus** and the **incus** bones of the ear (Fig. 6.4).

The dedicated nerve of the first arch is cranial nerve V, the **trigeminal nerve**. Muscles that act on the first arch bone derivatives are likely to be innervated by this nerve (e.g., the muscles of mastication). One muscle, the tensor tympani, acts on the malleus, so its innervation from cranial nerve V makes sense. Some muscles that act on the mandible, such as the mylohyoid and the anterior digastric, also are innervated by cranial nerve V. The rules of these "arch nerves" are not absolute, but the pattern does explain much of the motor dedication of cranial nerves V, VII, IX, and X.

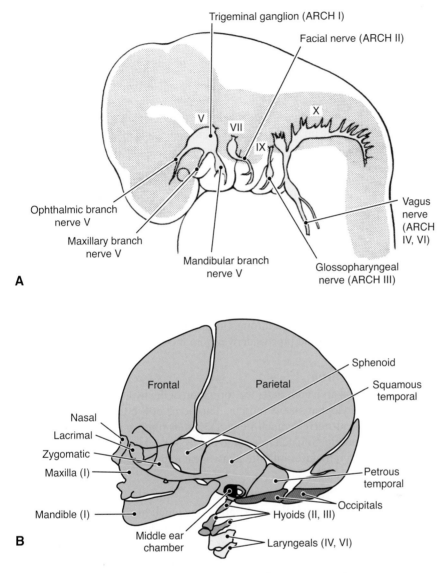

FIGURE 6.4   **Dedicated nerves and cartilage fates of the pharyngeal arches.**

Muscles that act across the bones that derive from each arch are likely to be motored by the nerves that are dedicated to that arch (**A**). The auditory ossicles (**B**) ultimately are sequestered in a middle ear chamber deep to skin that stretches tight enough to be sensitive to sound waves. (From Sadler TW. Langman's Medical Embryology, 10th Edition. Baltimore: Lippincott Williams & Wilkins, 2006. Figure 16.7, p. 261.)

Cranial nerve V is predominantly a sensory nerve (see below). It is the principal sensory nerve to the skin of the face. Because the first pharyngeal arch matures into the bony framework of the face, it is no surprise that the overlying skin is serviced by the same dedicated cranial nerve. The first arch will morph into a facial structure that guards the entrance to the gut tube. This would be simple except for the fact that at the same time it is developing, the gut tube is budding off a respiratory system. It, too, must reach the outside world, so the elaboration of the face is a little more complicated than just wrapping some lips around a membrane. That means that it deserves a section of its own, because many clinical problems and birth defects are associated with the formation of the face. The geometry and migration of the tissue changes will make more sense after the "endings," or fates, of each of the arches and the clefts and the pouches are itemized.

Second pharyngeal arch

The second pharyngeal arch is sometimes called the **hyoid arch**. The cartilage of this arch gives rise to the stapes bone of the ear, the styloid process of the temporal bone, the stylohyoid ligament, and the lesser horn and upper body of the hyoid bone. In the adult, these structures lie on a kind of arc both around and up the neck toward the mastoid process behind the ear (see Fig. 6.4). This arc follows below the derivatives of the first arch, which makes perfect sense.

The fact that cranial nerve VII, the **facial nerve**, is the dedicated cranial nerve of this arch also makes some sense, because it comes after the nerve of the first arch (cranial nerve V). The muscles innervated by the **facial nerve** (posterior digastric, stylohyoid, and stapedius) operate on the bones of the second pharyngeal arch. The facial nerve also provides motor innervation to the muscles in the skin of the face that enable expression. These **muscles of facial expression** do not fit the pharyngeal arch model as closely as the other motor targets of the facial nerve do, because the muscles of facial expression range all over the head and neck. They arise initially in the neck, however, and then migrate over the head, taking fibers of cranial nerve VII with them. The fibers of the facial nerve responsible for this leave the skull through the stylomastoid foramen, which makes perfect sense, because the styloid process derives from the second arch.

Third pharyngeal arch

The third pharyngeal arch completes the formation of the hyoid bone and leads to only one muscle—the stylopharyngeus muscle. The nerve of the third pharyngeal arch is the **glossopharyngeal nerve** (cranial nerve IX), so its only voluntary motor fibers are dedicated to this muscle. Situated inferior to the second, or hyoid, pharyngeal arch, the third pharyngeal arch matures into the pharyngeal region of the throat.

Fourth and sixth pharyngeal arches

The fourth and sixth pharyngeal arches derive very much in concert with one another. Remember that the fifth pharyngeal arch is a vestige of development in simpler vertebrates and is absent in human development. The cartilage components of the fourth and sixth pharyngeal arches fuse to form the cartilaginous framework of the **larynx**. The muscles that grow from the mesenchyme in these arches include the cricothyroid muscle, the elevator of the soft palate, and the pharyngeal constrictors. These muscles are innervated by the superior laryngeal branch of the **vagus nerve**, which is the dedicated nerve of the fourth pharyngeal arch.

All the other intrinsic muscles of the larynx are innervated by a different branch of the vagus nerve, the **recurrent laryngeal nerve**. This fiber bundle of cranial nerve X is considered to be the dedicated nerve of the sixth pharyngeal arch. Cranial nerve X also delivers parasympathetic innervation to a great part of the body. Its role in the head is focused on the pharynx and larynx, which is the region of the throat derived from the pharyngeal arches, for which it is the dedicated cranial nerve.

The Pharyngeal Pouches

The endoderm pouches also transform. Return to Figure. 6.3, and imagine how the endoderm that lines the inner surface of the pharyngeal arches remains continuous and unbroken. The "throat," however, is not perfectly smooth from the back of the mouth down the gut tube, because the sequence of arches and pouches does not smooth over completely. Some of the pouches remain pouches, and some transform into glands of the throat.

The first pharyngeal pouch, which is between the first and second pharyngeal arches, remains the most pouch-like, hardly changing from the embryonic to the adult state. Remember that the first pharyngeal arch is becoming the connective tissue of the face and that the second pharyngeal arch is sweeping along underneath it, back to the side of the head and what is now the developing ear region. The first pharyngeal pouch remains in the space between the changes in the first and second pharyngeal arches and forms the **auditory tube**, or **eustachian tube**, in the adult.

The auditory tube is a pouch that is lined with endoderm at the very back, top, and sides of the oral cavity (Fig. 6.5). It leads to a dead end that is nothing more than the original lining of ectoderm between the first and second pharyngeal arches. In the adult body, this intact juncture of endoderm and ectoderm between the fates of the first and second pharyngeal arches is the **tympanic membrane**, or **eardrum**. Its ectodermal side is exposed to the outside world and is so thin that changes in sound waves make it vibrate.

The second pharyngeal pouch, which is between the second and third pharyngeal arches, disappears almost completely. The little bit of mesoderm between it and the second pharyngeal cleft migrates up as the first pharyngeal arch matures and, eventually, becomes the palatine tonsil. This is a swelling of lymphoid tissue (derived from mesoderm) that is particularly sensitive to immunologic pressures in the oral cavity. The second pharyngeal pouch remains as a small crypt in the lining of the oral cavity that houses the bump that is the palatine tonsil (Fig. 6.6). The appearance of this region is a key part of any oral examination.

The third pharyngeal pouch actually expands and comes to look like a bulb. The third and fourth pharyngeal arches close together around it, however, effectively trapping the pouch as a blind endodermal sac in the connective tissue of the neck. The pouch then migrates inferiorly to settle very near the bottom of the neck and the top of the chest cavity in a fascial space just deep to the sternum. It now has the properties of a gland and is called the **thymus gland**. It is an important regulator of the immune system shortly after birth. The third pharyngeal pouch also encapsulates a small gland called the **inferior parathyroid gland**, which travels with the thymus down the neck and comes to lie just beside the thyroid gland (hence its name) (see Fig. 6.5).

The fact that the connective tissue above and below this pouch merges behind it is the first signal that the lining of the rest of the "throat" will be smooth. Indeed, from approximately the level of the tonsils down, only the respiratory system interrupts the smooth lining of the gut tube endoderm.

The fourth pharyngeal pouch mimics the third pharyngeal pouch. It collapses on itself, assuring the smooth lining of the inside of the pharynx. It also encapsulates the **superior parathyroid gland**, which comes to lie above and to the side of the thyroid gland, and it gives rise to the final internal body of the derived pouches, the **ultimobranchial body**. This body of cells assists the thyroid gland's ability to provide important calcium regulation.

The **thyroid gland** is the largest endocrine gland of the body. It develops from clumps of endoderm cells that become enmeshed in cords of mesoderm in the midline ventral wall of the early pharynx. The thyroid gland is the first endocrine gland to develop, at approximately 24 days after conception, at the junction where the first and second pharyngeal arches are forming the tongue bud (see below). Eventually, it migrates downward and comes to rest just inferior to the big thyroid cartilages of the larynx. The gland is easy to locate, because it is easy to see and palpate the projecting

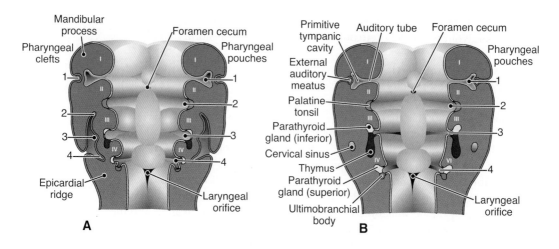

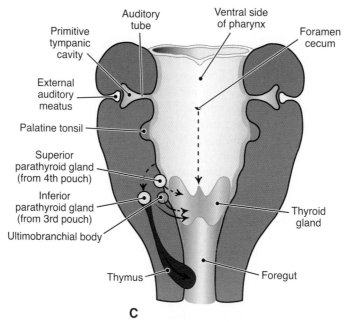

FIGURE 6.5   **Coronal views of pharyngeal arch transformations.**

The first pouch hardly changes (**A**). It remains as a thin barrier between outside and inside—the tympanic membrane of the ear. On the inner side is the auditory tube, which is open to the throat, and on the outer side is the ear canal. The remaining clefts smooth over as a result of expansion and descent of the second arch, leaving the possibility of a trapped cyst or fistula in the connective tissue of the neck (**B**). The second pouch harbors a condensation of lymphatic tissue—the future tonsil (**C**). Parathyroid glands and critical immunologic tissue (the thymus gland) develop from involutions of the third and fourth pouches. From the midline of the ventral pharynx, the thyroid gland originates from the lining of the foramen cecum and descends external to the gut tube (**C**). (Adapted from Sadler TW. Langman's Medical Embryology, 10th Edition. Baltimore: Lippincott Williams & Wilkins, 2006. Figure 16.10A,B, p. 263; Figure 16.11, p. 264.)

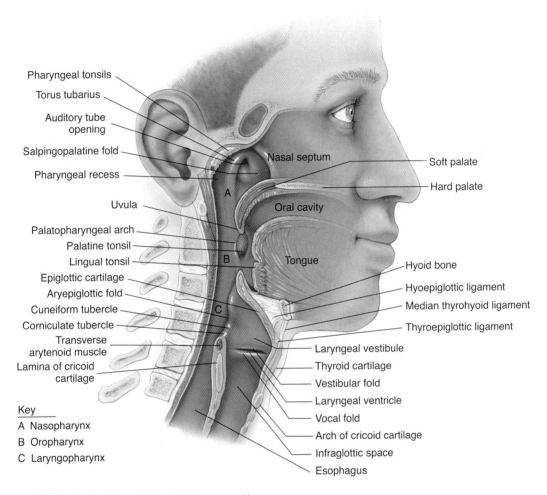

FIGURE 6.6   Sagittal view of the adult pharynx and larynx.

The opening of the auditory (eustachian) tube and the tonsillar crypt are obvious derivatives of the pouch system. A complex face fronts the pharynx and develops from dramatic growth of the first arch. (Anatomical Chart Company, copyright 2007.)

thyroid cartilages superior to it. **A goiter** is an enlargement of the thyroid gland that usually results from a lack of iodine in a local water supply (Fig. 6.7).

The Pharyngeal Clefts

Just as the inner lining of the arch system transforms, so does the outer lining, the pharyngeal clefts. Obviously, the end result of changes in the embryologic neck is that the ectoderm smooths out instead of remaining arched. The pharyngeal clefts complement the pouches in several ways. The first pharyngeal cleft remains more or less intact (as did the first pharyngeal pouch), and the second, third, and fourth pharyngeal clefts collapse on themselves (as did the third and fourth pharyngeal pouches, in a manner of speaking).

The first pharyngeal cleft is the most interesting one, because it persists almost undisturbed as the first pharyngeal arch above it migrates aggressively into the future

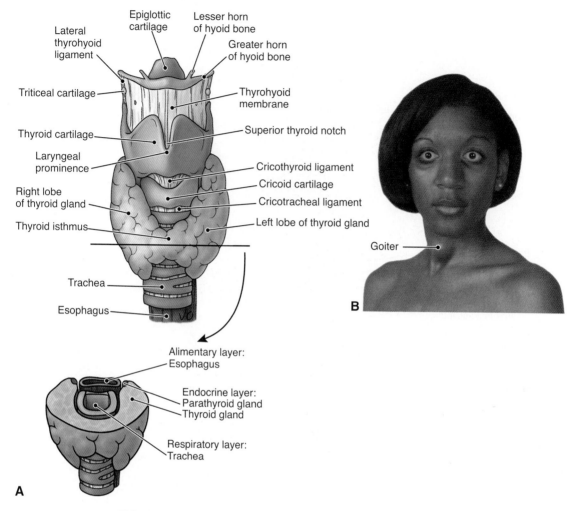

FIGURE 6.7   **An inflamed thyroid gland is a goiter.**

Anterior view of the thyroid gland inferior to the prominent thyroid cartilage is shown (**A**). Inflamma-
tion of the thyroid gland (goiter) presents as a progressive swelling near to and usually including the
midline of the neck below the palpable thyroid cartilage (**B**). (From Moore KL, Agur AMR. Essential
Clinical Anatomy, 2nd Edition. Baltimore: Lippincott Williams & Wilkins, 2002. Figure 9.12, p. 619; from
Moore KL, Dalley AF. Clinically Oriented Anatomy, 5th Edition. Baltimore: Lippincott Williams &
Wilkins, 2006. Figure B8.8, p. 1086.)

face. Remember that the first pharyngeal pouch persists as the auditory tube. Only a
thin membrane of ectoderm and endoderm, the **tympanic membrane** in the adult,
separates the auditory tube from the outside world (see Fig. 6.5).

As the first pharyngeal arch expands and migrates, the core of the arch, which
becomes the mandible, dominates the lower and anterior part of the arch. Its other two
bony components, the malleus and incus, are left behind as **ossicles** (literally, "tiny
bones") and pushed back to the rear of the arch. The rear of the arch is near the developing cervical vertebrae or, effectively, the side of the head. The second pharyngeal
arch contours to the first, and its bony derivatives likewise are retracted to the far side
of the head (the styloid process and the stapes ear ossicle).

This expansion of the front part of the arches at the expense of the back part of the arches reduces the cleft between the first and second pharyngeal arches to something like a finger hole in a glove, an external pouch that is exactly opposite its internal pouch (now the auditory tube). This external pouch ends as the ectodermal surface of the tympanic membrane, and the tubular pouch itself is now called the **ear canal**.

The end result is that the head now has a built-in surface that is so thin it vibrates when sound waves change. All it needs is an extension of the brain (cranial nerve VIII) to take advantage of this capability. The ectoderm around the first cleft elaborates into a wave-collecting dish (the **ear**), and the remnant bones of the first and second pharyngeal arches (malleus, incus, and stapes) become puppets of the vibrating tympanic membrane, transmitting vibrations to cranial nerve endings housed in a sturdy growth of bone that surrounds the middle and inner ear canal.

The second, third, and fourth pharyngeal clefts "undimple" as the neck elongates, and the second pharyngeal arch droops down over the lower two (see Fig. 6.5). One muscle of facial expression ranges inferiorly in the superficial fascia from the mandible to the clavicle. This muscle is the platysma muscle, and it may run the length of the neck as a result of the second pharyngeal arch drooping down over the exteriors of the third, fourth, and sixth pharyngeal arches.

Development of the Face

A major process of head and neck development is the transformation of the arch around the top of the endoderm into the face. The first pharyngeal arch becomes everything from mucous membranes to sinus-evacuated bones to the elaborate hardening of ectoderm into **teeth**. The important topography of what you see when you ask the patient to say "Ahhh" is the story of how the rim around the endoderm becomes a forward guardhouse, hanging from a shelf below the brain.

Above the vertebral column, the embryonic occipital somites and neural crest cells combine to form a shelf of bone underlying the neural tube. The bone plank, or shelf, is composed of the singular midline bones in the head: occipital, sphenoid, and ethmoid. They extend as if they were additional vertebral bodies, but they also bend forward (because the neural tube resting above them is so big and flexed) (Fig. 6.8).

The forward and downward flexion of the brain reorients the opening of the gut tube. It now points more or less forward, like the end of a periscope, and it carries the first pharyngeal arch with it. Remember that the first pharyngeal arch develops into the face bones and the mandible, so the logical position is for the top half of the arch to become the face bones and the bottom half to become the mandible and ear ossicles. This is exactly what happens.

The portion of the first pharyngeal arch that leads to the face bones is called the **maxillary process**, and the part that leads to the mandible is called the **mandibular process** (Fig. 6.9). As the arch system bends forward in response to the growing brain, the oropharyngeal membrane resembles the opening of a giant mouth. The borders of the stomodeum, or the mouth opening, are five distinct swellings. The "bottom" of the opening is the solid ventral wall, or floor, of the pharyngeal arches. The "sides" of the opening are the first arch processes, the mandibular below and maxillary above. The "top" of the opening is the ectoderm and dermis covering the very top of the neural tube, the budding frontonasal prominence.

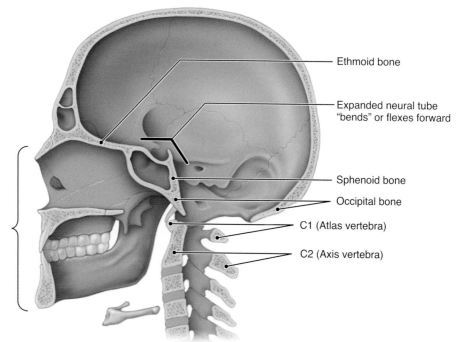

FIGURE 6.8   **A shelf of bone bears the brain and hangs the face.**

The expanded neural tube rests on a midline basicranial plank (occipital, sphenoid, and ethmoid bones) that, in turn, is the mounting for the facial skeleton and tissue at the top of the gut tube.

From this "sock-puppet" beginning, the two sides of the oral cavity will fuse in the midline (Fig. 6.10). For approximately six weeks after the first month of development, the five facial swellings will swell even more to present a forward "mouth" and "nose." The frontonasal prominence descends a swollen knob of tissue in the midline called the **intermaxillary process**. Two nasal pits invaginate the ectoderm at the bottom of this knob, dividing the hump on each side into a **medial nasal process** and a **lateral nasal process**. This leaves a groove between the sides of the nasal process and the maxillary swelling. This groove persists in the body as the **nasolacrimal duct** that draws excess tears into the nasal cavity.

The intermaxillary process spills down to hang below the two pits and, thus, forms the philtrum, or the "Angel's kiss," of the upper lip. It fuses with the maxillary swellings on each side to complete closure of the upper lip. Failure to meet in the middle results in two of the most common congenital anomalies of the head, **cleft lip** and **cleft palate**. (See Clin. Anat. Box 6.1.)

The exterior of the face is now coming together. The first pharyngeal arch effectively splits into two bony cores that are connected by a skin flap (the **cheek**). The upper core swells out and forward to become the maxilla and other bones. The lower core matures into a single mandible, which is as forward as the maxilla. In between the maxillary cores is a swollen nasal prominence, which still must become an open passage back to the pharynx that is separate from the oral passage. The barrier between the oral and nasal passages is already in place as the **palate**, which forms from the primary and secondary plates of the maxilla. The nasal passages develop because the nasal pits keep pitting inward. They pit so much, in fact, that they fuse

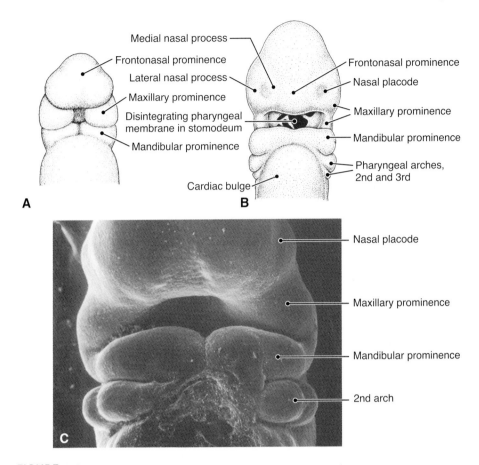

FIGURE 6.9   **The face grows from five positions.**

The first pharyngeal arch on each side proliferates a mandibular and maxillary swelling at the top of the gut tube. Meanwhile, neural crest cells and undifferentiated mesenchyme condense superior to the neural tube (**A** and **B**). These five prominences rotate toward each other to create a face; resolution of the clefts between adjacent prominences results in continuity from forehead to chin. Scanning electron micrograph of an embryo at a similar stage of growth is shown (**C**). (From Sadler TW. Langman's Medical Embryology, 10th Edition. Baltimore: Lippincott Williams & Wilkins, 2006. Figure 16.5a–c, p. 260.)

into each other to form a single big nasal sac with a tenuous membrane between it and the oral cavity below (Fig. 6.11). This tenuous membrane cannot hold everywhere, and indeed, it ruptures to form a **choana** between the back part of the nasal sac and the top of the pharynx.

The palates

The intermaxillary segment of the nasal process grows a hardened shelf in a backward direction to keep the evacuating nasal passage separate from the oral cavity. This is the **primary palate**, but it is not enough. The maxillary processes chime in with their own shelf contribution, on either side and largely behind the primary palate. These palatine shelves merge with each other in the midline and with the primary palate up front to form the composite **secondary palate**. The magnificent potential of mesoderm to range from elastic to rigid shows in the final step: The front part of the secondary palate

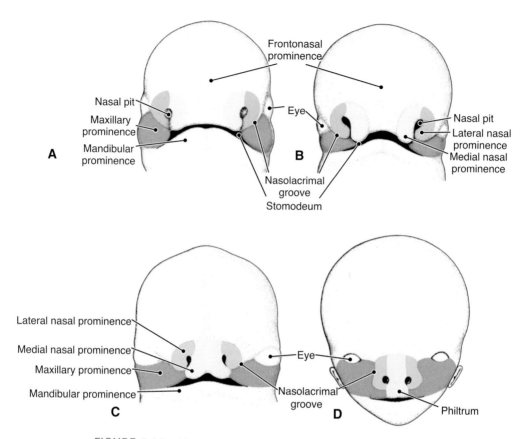

FIGURE 6.10   **The face comes together when the five swellings rotate together.**

The lower jaw solidifies early, but the upper jaw, lip, and nose merge over a period of weeks. The middle of the upper lip is formed by continuation of the frontonasal prominence (**A, B**). The maxillary and mandibular swellings merge enough to reduce the breadth of the mouth (**C**). The pharyngeal arch and mesenchymal swellings rotate in concert with expansion of the brain and rotation of the orbits toward stereoscopy (**D**). (From Sadler TW. Langman's Medical Embryology, 10th Edition. Baltimore: Lippincott Williams & Wilkins, 2006. Figure 16.22A,B, p. 263; Figure 16.23A,B, p. 264.)

fully hardens into bone, while the back part of the secondary palate remains cartilaginous and muscular—the **soft palate** at the back of the roof of the mouth.

A vertical growth of bone down from the top of the nasal prominence in the middle of the sac fuses with the secondary palate to form a thin but sturdy midline **nasal septum**. Within the nasal passages, curly scrolls of bone and thick membranes over them develop in a tiered pattern. This provides a great deal more surface area for treating inhaled air before it enters the unprotected respiratory system. Two other modified surfaces (the **teeth** and the **tongue**) deal with what is put in the mouth before it is swallowed.

The teeth

The teeth are specializations of the connective tissue surface lining of the first pharyngeal arch (Fig. 6.12). The care and treatment of teeth constitute an entirely separate medical field (dentistry). The human dental battery includes front teeth (**incisors**) for nipping small bits of food off of larger ones; staging teeth (**canines** and "bicuspids,"

CLINICAL ANATOMY

Box 6.1

CLEFT LIP AND CLEFT PALATE

Any adult structure that results from two halves coming together (A) can fail to form if the two halves do not meet properly. In the face, this risk is compounded by the fact that the front of the palate forms from a different tissue source than the back of the palate does. For this reason, a person can be born with a cleft lip on one side (B), indicating a forward gap between the premaxillary segment and the lip; a cleft lip that also involves the primary palate (C); clefting on both sides (D), because the intermaxillary segment grows independently of the adjacent swellings; clefting of only the secondary palate (E); or radical clefting of both primary and secondary growth areas (F). Clefts can be detected with ultrasound as early as the fifth month of gestation. Clefting of some kind occurs in approximately 1 in 700 live births. Among these, 20% are an isolated cleft lip, 50% are a cleft lip and cleft palate, and 30% are an isolated cleft palate. For reasons that have yet to be understood fully, a cleft lip with cleft palate occurs more frequently in males than in females, but isolated cleft palates (1 in 2,000 live births) occur more frequently in females than in males. These conditions can be corrected surgically, but long-term medical management is necessary to reduce adverse effects on speaking and swallowing.

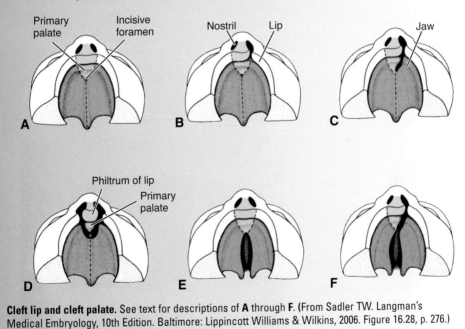

Cleft lip and cleft palate. See text for descriptions of **A** through **F**. (From Sadler TW. Langman's Medical Embryology, 10th Edition. Baltimore: Lippincott Williams & Wilkins, 2006. Figure 16.28, p. 276.)

or **premolars**) for holding and positioning the bits of food; and powerful crushers (**molars**) for reducing everything to a pulp before swallowing. Because the teeth develop in sockets of the bones of the first pharyngeal arch, it is logical and correct to assume that their sensory innervation comes from **cranial nerve V**. Likewise, general sensory innervation to all the modified ectoderm that lines the oral and nasal cavities is the province of the same nerve.

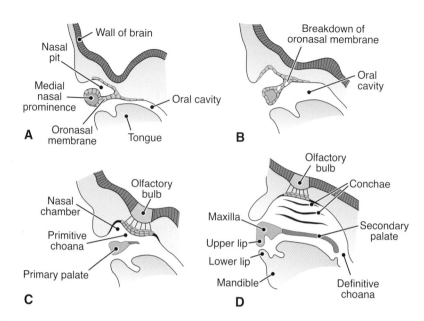

FIGURE 6.11   The nasal passage must bore its way into the pharynx.

The external surface of the frontonasal prominence includes a nasal pit, but there is no initial connection between this indentation and the gut tube (**A**). Rather, the incipient nasal passage connects to the throat when the intervening membrane erodes (**B**). This connection is further modified when the secondary palate expands (**C** and **D**). (From Sadler TW. Langman's Medical Embryology, 10th Edition. Baltimore: Lippincott Williams & Wilkins, 2006. Figure 16.32a–d, p. 280.)

FIGURE 6.12   The dental battery.

A substantial amount of mandibular and maxillary bone is devoted to housing the teeth. From front to back, the battery includes two incisors, one canine, two premolars and three molars. Note that the roots of the upper teeth intimately border the bottom of the maxillary sinus, which invites abscess and spread of infection following traumatic tooth extraction.

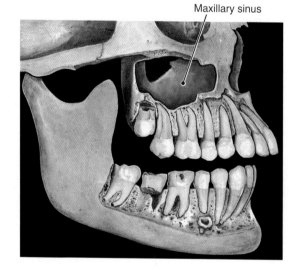

The tongue

The **tongue** provides what the teeth do not: mobility, taste, and expression. Tongue development is one of the best examples of how embryology explains the gross anatomy of the adult. The tongue receives innervation from **cranial nerves V, VII, and IX**, and this is best explained by studying how the tongue develops.

The tongue begins as a swelling of mesenchyme in the ventral floor of the pharyngeal arch system (Fig. 6.13). This swelling overlaps the territories of the first, second, and third pharyngeal arches, which explains how the cranial nerves become involved. Growth of the tongue "zones" is not equal, however, in the sense that the contribution of the first pharyngeal arch to the tongue is quite large (approximately two-thirds of the total tongue). Thus, general sensory coverage of the anterior two-thirds of the tongue is delivered by **cranial nerve V**.

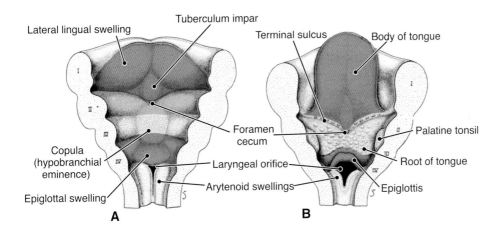

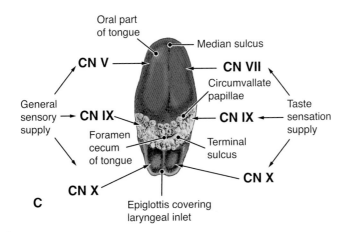

FIGURE 6.13   **The tongue is a raised surface of the mouth that is embedded with muscles.**

The ventral midline of pharynx swells along all of the pharyngeal arches (**A**). Aggressive swelling of the first arch and migration of the third arch (**B**) result in the elevated surface of a tongue. The back of the tongue also is elaborated from the floor of the pharynx as an epiglottis, which passively closes off the larynx during swallowing. General innervation of the tongue surface comes from the cranial nerves dedicated to the arches from which it derives (**C**); the special sense cells of the second arch migrate into the anterior two-thirds of the tongue, which explains why taste from there is carried back to the brain by cranial nerve (CN) VII. (From Sadler TW. Langman's Medical Embryology, 10th Edition. Baltimore: Lippincott Williams & Wilkins, 2006. Figure 16.17, p. 269.)

The second pharyngeal arch component to the tongue swelling is almost completely overrun by the third pharyngeal arch component. The only remnants are the **taste buds** of the anterior two-thirds of the tongue, which are served by **cranial nerve VII**. The swelling under the floor of the third pharyngeal arch expands to be the posterior one-third of the tongue, taste buds and all. **Cranial nerve IX** therefore provides both **general sensory** and **taste sensory** innervation to this part of the tongue; it begins as the row of bumps (**vallate papillae**) that signals the back, or base, of the tongue.

The very back root of the tongue arises from a swelling in the fourth pharyngeal arch, but this swelling mostly becomes the epiglottis, which closes like a toilet seat over the opening to the larynx. Therefore, some sensory and taste fibers at the very back root of the tongue and along the surface of the epiglottis may lead back to **cranial nerve X**.

The tongue is more than just an internal swelling on the floor of the pharyngeal arch system, however. It has a strong core of intrinsic muscles that make up its "flesh" and several extrinsic muscles that connect its "body" to surrounding bones, such as the mandible and hyoid. For the most part, these muscles migrate into the tongue swelling from regular somites near the occipital bone, and they carry cranial nerve XII (the **hypoglossal nerve**) with them for motor support.

The base of the tongue is therefore an outgrowth of the front of the throat, just above where the respiratory system tops out and joins the pharynx. The body of the tongue lies up and forward (projects superior and anterior) from its root, parallel to the arc of the mandible. Stretching from one side of the bottom of the mandible down to the hyoid bone and up to the other side of the mandible is a kind of trampoline, or diaphragm, muscle called the **mylohyoid**. This muscle is effectively the floor of the mouth, and the tongue flops around on it instead of on the loose skin under the chin.

The wet-lined skin of the inner cheek is continuous with the wet-lined endoderm at the very back of the oral cavity. The endoderm begins where the sensory distribution of cranial nerve V ends, because the bottom of the first pharyngeal arch rims the very top of the endodermal tube. The "face" is an elaborate extension of connective tissue beyond the endoderm, the purpose of which is to encounter and treat the sources of energy that must be absorbed. The same elaboration does not apply to the bottom of the gut tube, where endoderm meets ectoderm in a less-celebrated junction just inside the anal orifice. This lower junction is a transition of elimination, from unprotected to protected surfaces, and of substances that have been processed completely before reaching the ectoderm–endoderm transition.

Development of the Head and Central Nervous System

The neural tube swells above the final occipital somite. The large, developing human brain flexes over the front edge of the occipital bone produced by those somites, and it would droop into the back of the nose and mouth were it not for an extra shelf of bone that "extends" the occipital bone forward and underneath the weighty brain. This extra shelf is called the **basicranium**, and its cell source is actually a cluster of neural crest cells—that is, pinched off parts of the neural tube with dynamic potential for inducing tissues. The sphenoid bone that fuses to the occipital bone at the basisphenoid synchondrosis, and the ethmoid bone between the sphenoid bone and the very top of the nasal cavity, constitute this "plank" on which the brain rests (see Fig. 6.8).

That leaves nothing much around the sides and top of the neural tube from which to grow a bony cover. The "flat" bones of the cranium, including parts of the **temporal bone**, **parietal bones**, and the **frontal bone**, form **intramembranously** from the mesenchyme of the connective tissue membrane covering the neural tube. The dermis essentially lays down a hard basement layer over the swelling brain that it covers.

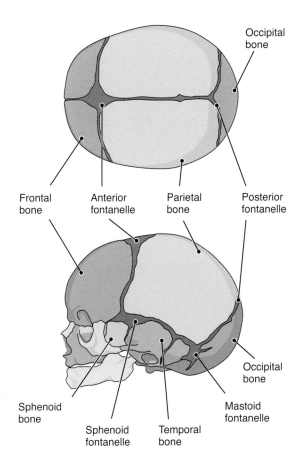

Occipital bone

Frontal bone

Anterior fontanelle

Parietal bone

Posterior fontanelle

Sphenoid bone

Sphenoid fontanelle

Temporal bone

Mastoid fontanelle

Occipital bone

FIGURE 6.14   "Soft spots" in **the skull allow the brain to keep growing.**

The neurocranial bones (frontal, parietal, temporal, and occipital) grow mainly through intramembranous ossification. Persistence of membranes between the bones (fontanelles) allows continued brain growth after birth. (From Cohen BJ, Wood DL. Memmler's The Human Body in Health and Disease, 10th Edition. Baltimore: Lippincott Williams & Wilkins, 2004.)

This process takes several years, because the brain continues to grow for 8 to 10 years after birth. **Fontanelles**, or "soft spots," can be felt in babies between the hardened centers of the cranial vault bones and their expanding perimeters (Fig. 6.14).

The brain reaches the outside world to exercise special capacities to sense chemical waves (smell and taste), sound waves (hearing), and light waves (vision). Each of these special sense pathways governs bone formation at the interface of the nerve with the outside world. Olfactory nerve endings are embedded in a cribriform plate of the ethmoid bone. Auditory nerve endings are housed in a chamber of the temporal bone, far removed from the sound waves that impact the skin (tympanic membrane) but exposed in elongation along a tubular pathway (the cochlea; see below) where sound is channeled by the ear ossicles. The sense of vision occupies a position below the swollen brain but above the face. The brain extends itself in the form of an optic nerve (cranial nerve II) underneath the frontal bone. The maxillary prominence has formed a ready shelf below this trajectory in the form of the maxilla and zygomatic bones, and the beginnings of a protective bony cone are in place.

During later growth, the zygomatic bone reaches up along the sides to articulate with the edge of the frontal bone, and the midline bones (sphenoid and ethmoid) complete the shell medially. The end result is a protective, bony cone called the **orbit** that is unusual in the animal world. Protected on all sides by some type of bony sheet, the optic nerve rests in the cone and induces the surface ectoderm to form a **lens**. (Ectoderm, thus, can develop over time into membranes as delicate as the **tympanic membrane**, as derived as the **cornea**, and as hard as the **tooth enamel**.)

Development of the head and neck is a very complicated topic because it involves multiple systems, biological complexity, and a large region for which the whole is greater than the sum of its parts. Even anatomists need extra time to command the transformations of head and neck development. Use a sense of what must occur at the top of the neural and endodermal tubes to anticipate where structures are located and what they are called.

THE NERVOUS SYSTEM

Definition

The nervous system includes the areas where "decisions" are made by the body in response to sensations, the structures that detect the sensations, and the structures that deliver the responses to the sensations. The decision areas are the **spinal cord** and the **brain**, which are termed the **central nervous system**. The nerves that emanate from them, which contain fibers that are used to import or export the necessary signals, constitute the **peripheral nervous system** (Fig. 6.15).

FIGURE 6.15   Schematic anatomy of the central nervous system.

The central nervous system receives, associates, and transmits impulses that route through 12 pairs of cranial nerves, 31 pairs of spinal nerves, and associated sympathetic and parasympathetic fibers. Note that the spinal cord is connected to nerves at all vertebral levels but does not extend beyond the second or third lumbar vertebra. (From Moore KL, Dalley AF. Clinically Oriented Anatomy, 5th Edition. Baltimore: Lippincott Williams & Wilkins, 2006. Figure I.28, p. 49.)

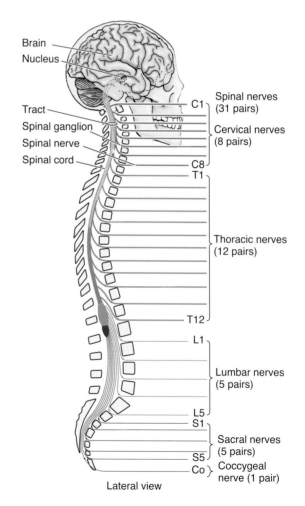

Lateral view

Gross Anatomy of the Central Nervous System

This section presents only the gross anatomic features of the brain and spinal cord, and it refers the physiology, function, and clinical aspects to courses in neuroscience. Begin by returning to the neurulation process of the third week of development (see Figs. 1.14 and 1.15). As the head end of the neural tube matures, it dilates in size, making it look quite different than the rest of the tube inferior to it. The end result is a "swollen" brain at the top end and its spinal cord "tail." The dilation prevents the somites of the mesoderm from forming a bony arch around it, which is one reason why the bones that cover the brain form by intramembranous instead of endochondral ossification. Intramembranous bone grows in response to the tissue underneath it, which explains why brain growth normally is not restricted by its bony covering.

Although the brain and spinal cord appear to be solid structures, they begin as a tube and forever have a canal at their center. The very small canal of the spinal cord expands with the brain to form elaborate **ventricles** of space. **Cerebrospinal fluid,** which is so important for maintaining neural tissue, bathes the central nervous system, and in so doing, it collects in the central canal and ventricular network of the spinal cord and brain (Fig. 6.16).

The **spinal cord** maintains a simple design. Cells with similar functions cluster into long columns, and the columns congregate together in the same region of the cord. This gives the gray matter of the cord a characteristic "butterfly" or H-shaped appearance in cross-section (Fig. 6.17). The **posterior horn** of the gray matter contains axons that carry **sensory** information to the spinal cord; this is also called the **dorsal horn.** By contrast, the **ventral horn** contains axons that carry **motor** impulses **away** from the spinal cord. In between these two "arms" of the H-shape is an **intermediate column,** and within it is the **intermediolateral gray horn,** which contains **sympathetic fibers** of the autonomic nerves (see below). These fibers are found between the T1-L2 spinal nerves in the cord.

All around this butterfly design of gray matter is the **white matter,** which contains fibers that help one level of the spinal cord communicate with other levels and with the brain. The basic design of gray matter and white matter is preserved as the tube expands to become the brain.

Recall that during neurulation, some cells become pinched off as the neural plate closes into a neural tube. These are the **neural crest cells.** Some of them develop into layers of cells that blanket the central nervous system. Collectively, these cells are called the **meninges** and include the **dura mater,** the **arachnoid mater,** and the **pia mater.** In addition to protecting the spinal cord and brain, they create a space for the flow of cerebrospinal fluid.

The dura mater is grossly tangible, and the arachnoid matter is (as its name implies) "spidery," or web-like. The pia mater is "intimate" to the surface of the brain and spinal cord, like a sheer shrink-wrap. The arachnoid mater webs out between the pia mater and the dura mater. Wisps of it are visible in the cadaver when the dura mater is slit open. The dura ("tough") mater is the outermost coating, and it also is the thickest. It covers the brain, but it also expands a few channels, or sinuses, within itself so that venous drainage of the brain can circulate around the inside of the skull. These channels are called the **dural venous sinuses,** and they converge toward the back of the head and drain down into the jugular foramen to become the **jugular vein.** The clinical terms **subdural hematoma** and **epidural hematoma** refer to a dangerous

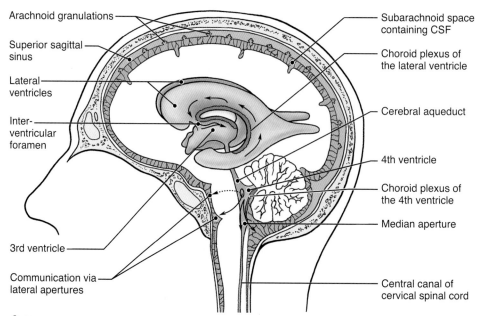

A Median section with ventricles viewed from the left

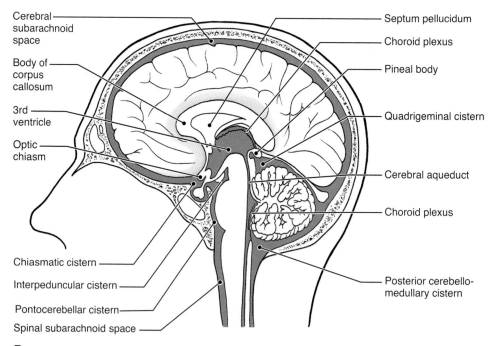

B Medial view, right half of hemisected brain

FIGURE 6.16   **Flow of cerebrospinal fluid.**

Nutrient fluid circulates through and around the central nervous system within the central canal of the spinal cord, which elaborates into a ventricular network in the brain (**A**). Cerebrospinal fluid (CSF) keeps the central nervous system tissue bathed by circulating around it in the subarachnoid space (**B**). Pools of cerebrospinal fluid collect in natural anatomic cisterns and inferior to the end of the spinal cord. (From Moore KL, Agur AMR. Essential Clinical Anatomy, 2nd Edition. Baltimore: Lippincott Williams & Wilkins, 2002. Figure 8.13, p. 526.)

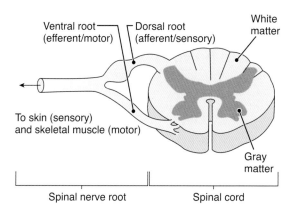

Ventral root (efferent/motor)

Dorsal root (afferent/sensory)

White matter

To skin (sensory) and skeletal muscle (motor)

Gray matter

Spinal nerve root   Spinal cord

FIGURE 6.17   **Simple cross-section of the spinal cord and spinal nerve roots.**

(Bickley, LS and Szilagyi, P. Bates' Guide to Physical Exam and History Taking. Philadelphia; Lippincott, Williams and Wilkins, 2003. Figure 60-10.)

bleeding deep to the dura mater or between it and the skull, respectively. (See Clinical Anatomy Box 6.2.)

As mentioned above, the spinal cord is connected to the rest of the ectoderm (and to the mesoderm, for that matter) by what are called **nerves**. These are part of the peripheral nervous system described below. The nerves do not just stick out of the spinal cord randomly. They conform to segments that correspond to each individual bony vertebra, all the way down to the coccyx vertebra. During fetal growth, however, something unusual happens. The body of the fetus grows more than its central nervous system does.

Shortly after the neural tube forms, the tube is as long as the growing vertebral column. Soon, however, the vertebral column increases in length, and the neural tube stays in place. The "deficit" is seen entirely in the lower region of the vertebral column. The spinal cord ends at approximately the level of the third lumbar vertebra in the adult body. It stays connected to the coccyx vertebrae by a thin filament of pia mater called the **filum terminale**, or terminal thread. The bottom of the cord is called the **conus medullaris**.

The discrepancy between the end of the cord and the end of the vertebral column means that the nerves leaving the spinal cord in the original lower lumbar or sacral regions now can only exit the vertebral canal by hanging down from the cord until they reach the level of the appropriate intervertebral foramen. This gives the end of the cord and the flowing nerve fibers the appearance of a horse's tail, the classical term for which is **cauda equina**. In some ways, this is a useful discrepancy, because below the end of the cord, the cerebrospinal fluid accumulates like a pool. For various clinical reasons, you may need to sample the cerebrospinal fluid, and this is a good place to introduce the needle (because you will not hit the spinal cord itself) (Fig. 6.18).

At the other end of the cord, the transition is from the spinal cord to the brain. Traditionally, this is marked by the bony rim of the **foramen magnum** in the occipital bone. Above this level, the gray matter and the white matter take on several expansive shapes and wriggles. Developmentally, this part of the tube dilates into three segments: a **forebrain**, a **midbrain**, and a **hindbrain**. The hindbrain develops into the **medulla oblongata** and the **pons** (at its top end). The hindbrain also grows a large bulb called the **cerebellum** on its dorsal surface. The midbrain together with the hindbrain is called the **brainstem**, which is the home to several vital bodily functions. The neural tube continues forward as the forebrain into a variety of interactive structures, including the **thalamus**, the **hypothalamus**, and the **cerebrum**. The cerebrum is so big in

Box 6.2

MENINGES AND HEMATOMAS

Throughout the central nervous system, three tissue layers coat the brain, spinal cord, and varying extents of the nerves that connect to them (A). As its name implies, the dura mater is resistant. Brain tissue, however, is not. When blood accumulates in the meningeal spaces, the only tissue that is displaced is brain tissue. Hematomas are very serious conditions, because depression and/or ischemia of neural tissue can have permanent effects in a very short period of time. An epidural hematoma (B) results from a tear in the arteries that serve the dura mater, principally the middle meningeal artery. This can result from a hard impact to the cranium, with or without fracture of the bone itself. Blood accumulates between the dura and the cranium, and the swelling quickly depresses the brain matter. Neural effects follow quickly and do not subside. A more insidious injury is a subarachnoid hemorrhage (C), in which an artery that feeds the brain tears and blood spills into the sinuous subarachnoid space. This can result from an ischemic attack, or stroke, in one of the vessels or from concussion, whiplash, or shaking types of injury to the head. In this case, neural deficits result from the loss of blood to intended tissues as well as from the depression of neural tissue caused by pooling blood. In this condition, symptoms may take longer to appear, so extended monitoring of the injury is essential.

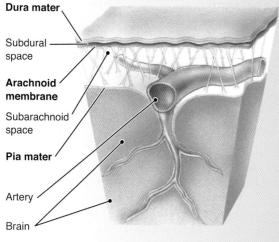

Dura mater
Subdural space
Arachnoid membrane
Subarachnoid space
Pia mater
Artery
Brain

A

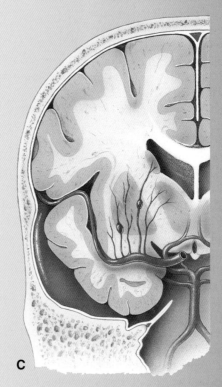

C

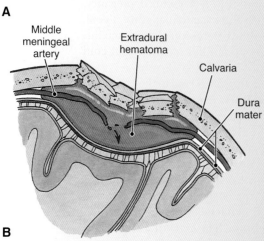

Middle meningeal artery
Extradural hematoma
Calvaria
Dura mater

B

Meninges and hematomas. See text for descriptions of **A** through **C**. (From Bear MF, Connors BW, Parasido MA. Neuroscience—Exploring the Brain, 2nd Edition. Philadelphia: Lippincott Williams & Wilkins. 2001; from Moore KL, Agur AMR. Essential Clinical Anatomy, 2nd Edition. Baltimore: Lippincott Williams & Wilkins, 2002; Anatomical Chart Company, 2002.)

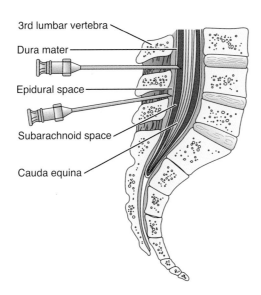

3rd lumbar vertebra

Dura mater

Epidural space

Subarachnoid space

Cauda equina

FIGURE 6.18   **Lumbar puncture and epidural anesthesia.**

Because the spinal cord ends before the neural canal of the vertebral column constricts, a substantial amount of cerebrospinal fluid can accumulate in the lower lumbar regions of the subarachnoid space. Needles can be introduced in the space between L3 and L4 to sample cerebrospinal fluid (a "spinal tap" or lumbar puncture) without risk to the spinal cord itself. Likewise, anaesthetic can be introduced to the epidural space at the same levels. (From Taylor C, Lillis CA, LeMone P. Fundamentals of Nursing, 2nd Edition. Philadelphia: JB Lippincott, 1993.)

humans that it must contort to fit into its bony house; thus, the cerebrum forms **lobes**, **sulci**, and **gyri** (Fig. 6.19).

Gross Anatomy of the Peripheral Nervous System

Parts of the system

For the nervous system, anatomists use terms that relate to what signal the nerve provides, what part of the body the nerve serves, and whether the nerve is under conscious control. There are other ways to classify the nervous system, however, so gravitate to the classification scheme that helps you to learn the system most efficiently.

Basic terms

The word *nerve* is familiar. Its familiarity breeds confusion, however, because it can refer to many different things. For gross anatomy, a nerve implies a collection of nerve cells, regardless of their function. Some nerves conduct purely sensory information, some purely motor information, and some both types of information (a "mixed" nerve). A nerve in gross anatomy is visible to the naked eye, and it is named in general (e.g., "a **cutaneous nerve**") if it is not the exclusive provider of a function (e.g., you have millions of cutaneous nerves detecting sensation in the skin) and in specific (e.g., "the **median nerve**") if it is a discrete bundle with an exclusive function. Often, specifically named nerves are found in the same location of everybody's body with little variation, which is another hallmark of providing a specific name to a structure in gross anatomy. **Injuries to nerves with specific names tend to have major ramifications, whereas injuries to nerves with general names tend to have less significant consequences**. Nerves can be very short or nearly the length of an entire limb. If a nerve has a specific name, the name typically says more about the location of the nerve in the body than it says about the function of the nerve. The **femoral nerve**, for example, is in the thigh, but its name does not indicate whether it is a sensory, motor, or mixed nerve.

Nerve bundles contain fibers that transmit an impulse either toward the central nervous system or from the central nervous system toward a target organ (or cell) in the

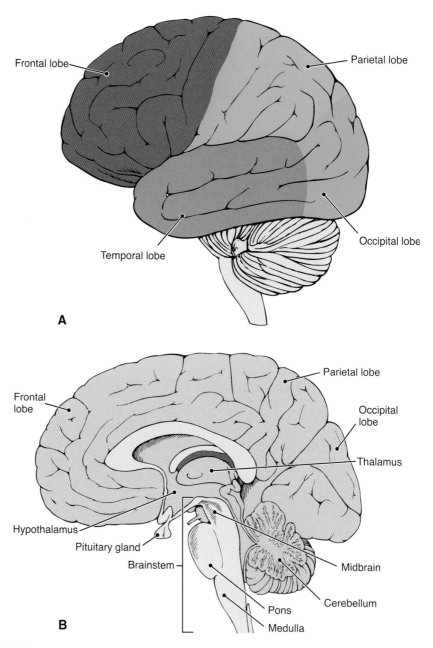

FIGURE 6.19   **External (A) and sagittal (B) profiles of the brain.**

(Bickley, LS and Szilagyi, P. Bates' Guide to Physical Exam and History Taking. Philadelphia; Lippincott, Williams and Wilkins, 2003. Figure 60-2; Figure 60-3.)

body. Some nerve bundles contain fibers of both types. A fiber that delivers an impulse to the central nervous system is called a **sensory fiber**; more formally, it is called an **afferent fiber** (from the classical language term meaning "to bear toward"). A fiber that delivers an impulse from the central nervous system to a body tissue is called a **motor fiber**; more formally, it is called an **efferent fiber** (from the classical language term meaning "to bear away"). For both types of fibers, injuries close to the central nervous system (i.e., near the skull or the vertebral column) are more serious than injuries near the tissues being served, because as nerves converge toward the spinal cord or brain, they tend to merge into larger and larger bundles.

When nerves of separate origin in the central nervous system criss-cross each other and exchange fibers, they form what is called a **plexus**. Two major plexuses (or plexi) serve the limbs: a **brachial plexus** of nerves in the upper limb and a **lumbosacral plexus** of nerves in the lower limb. Plexuses also are found where nerves come together to serve a major organ, such as the heart (the **cardiac plexus**).

Nerves can be classified according to their two basic destinations: the structural or somatic tissues (muscles, bones, and skin) and the "organ" or visceral tissues (glands, heart, digestive tube, etc). Each type of tissue needs a detection (sensory) and a reaction (motor) capability. Innervation of the organ tissues often is a simple matter of powering them on or purposefully shutting them down, either to meet a challenge (sympathetic) or to stay calm between challenges (parasympathetic). A basic scheme for the nerves, then, may look like this:

Somatic
   Sensory
   Motor

Visceral
   Sensory
   Motor
      Sympathetic
      Parasympathetic

Grouping 1: To excite or relax?

The nervous system detects conditions in two worlds: the world outside of the body (the environment), and the world of the body, which seeks to stay in a certain state of equilibrium, or **homeostasis**, in the face of changing environmental conditions. Nerve fibers that serve the skin and "framework" of the body for detecting and responding to the outside world are independent of nerve fibers that serve the smooth muscle organs, blood vessels, and glands of the body that maintain homeostasis. A nerve is called **somatic** if it serves skeletal muscle and the general sensory surfaces of the body, and a nerve is called **visceral** if it serves the organs, vessels, and glands. Both somatic and visceral nerves can include afferent and efferent fibers, so a basic means of describing the function of a named nerve is as follows:

- Somatic afferent
- Somatic efferent
- Visceral afferent
- Visceral efferent

A **somatic afferent nerve fiber** detects the basic sensory impressions: pain, pressure, touch, temperature, and proprioception from the parts of the body that make direct contact with the environment. A **somatic efferent nerve fiber** delivers an impulse for contraction to a fiber of skeletal, or striated, muscle. Somatic efferent nerve fibers can be thought of as the voluntary motor control network.

The involuntary activities of the body need some means of notifying the central nervous system of their state of being, and this is the domain of visceral afferent nerves. The digestive system organs, for example, can transmit signals of fullness. A **visceral efferent nerve fiber** transmits an impulse for contraction of involuntary muscle fibers, such as those of the smooth and cardiac tissue types. An example would be peristalsis of the digestive tract, or constriction of the smooth muscle walls of blood vessels. A visceral efferent nerve fiber also can feed an impulse to the glands of the body to increase or decrease their secretions.

Grouping 2: To excite or relax?

Within the group of visceral efferent nerves, separate fibers respond to urgent needs (as perceived in the brain) versus to keep the body in a rested state (equilibrium, or homeostasis). Involuntary reactions to urgent needs include, for example, blushing when embarrassed or widening the pupil when in dim light. Nerve fibers that control these classic "fight or flight" responses are called **sympathetic nerve fibers**, and those that restore the status quo or keep the body in a resting state are called **parasympathetic nerve fibers**.

The visceral efferent nerves are so important to health that they are classified in their own system—the **autonomic nervous system**, which is composed of sympathetic and parasympathetic divisions (Fig. 6.20). The **sympathetic system** begins as cell bodies in the spinal cord, between the first thoracic and the second or third lumbar spinal nerve regions. (For this reason, it sometimes is called a **thoracolumbar system**.) Sympathetic nerves can cause smooth muscle to contract (or inhibit it from contracting), trigger sweat glands to secrete, and inhibit other glands from secreting. Most extensively, sympathetic nerve impulses constrict the smooth muscle in the walls of arteries, so sympathetic fibers must cover the entire arterial circuit. For the most part, these nerves do not have specific names, but the specific level of the spinal cord where they originate is significant.

Once the sympathetic fibers leave the spinal cord they form a "necklace" or "chain," or a trunk, of fibers and cell bodies (**ganglia**) that lie immediately beside the vertebral column. (For this reason, the chain is sometimes called a **paravertebral chain**). This chain is studded with ganglia at each vertebral level from the thoracic to the coccygeal, and at the bottom of the vertebral column, it crosses over, just as a necklace would. At the superior end of the trunk, however, the left and right sides of the chain do not meet; rather, they independently follow a major artery (the carotid) through the neck and into the head. So, the chain is really not a literal necklace but, rather, is more like a giant U-shape. The cervical portion of the sympathetic chain typically includes three more ganglia (**inferior cervical ganglia, middle cervical ganglia**, and **superior cervical ganglia**).

Sympathetic fibers may exit the chain structure and join the somatic nerve fibers en route to distant parts of the body. They also may exit the chain structure and follow blood vessels toward the organs of the body. Before exiting the chain, the fibers may travel a considerable distance up or down the body within the chain (Fig. 6.21).

The original cell bodies of the parasympathetic nervous system are found in the **brain** and in the **sacral** spinal nerve region of the spinal cord (see Fig. 6.20), which sometimes is called the **craniosacral system**. Parasympathetic functions are subtle, because they maintain the "normal" activity of involuntary tissue. Parasympathetic nerve fibers do not act on the smooth muscles of arteries or on the sweat glands, so their distribution in the body is much more limited than the sympathetic distribution. Parasympathetic nerve fibers are very active in the head, lungs, heart, and digestive organs.

Parasympathetic nerve fibers do not coalesce into a chain or network once they depart from the central nervous system. Those of cranial origin travel in four of the twelve **cranial nerves** (cranial nerves III, VII, IX, and X), and those of sacral origin travel a short distance in a fishnet-like design of **pelvic splanchnic nerves** to their organ targets in the pelvis and lower digestive tract. All the parasympathetic innervation of the lungs, heart, and first two-thirds of the digestive tract travels in one cranial nerve, the **vagus nerve (cranial nerve X)**. The gross anatomy of major organ system homeostasis therefore is accounted for in the pathway of single nerve bundle.

The ganglia for the parasympathetic system tend to be microscopic in size. They also tend to be found close to or within the tissue being served. This is another reason why there is no equivalent parasympathetic "chain" or trunk where groups of cell bodies are located.

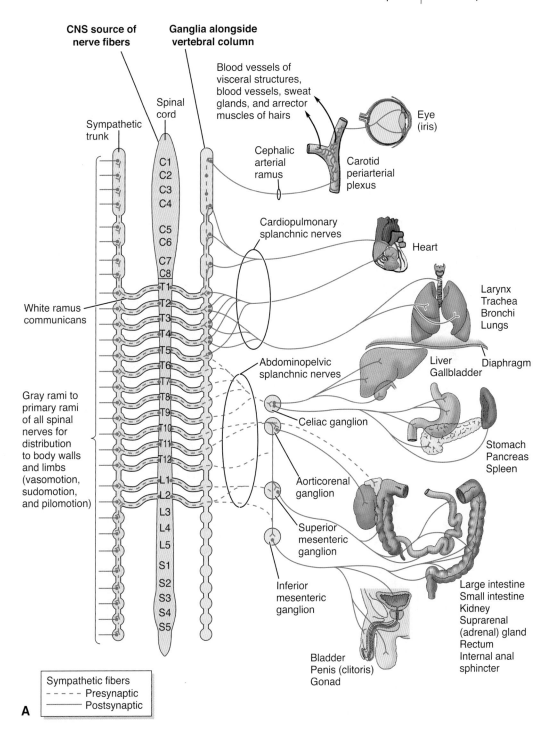

FIGURE 6.20   **The autonomic nervous system at a glance. (*continues*)**

Sympathetic nerve pathways and targets (**A**) as well as parasympathetic nerve pathways and targets (**B**) are shown. CN = cranial nerve; CNS = central nevous system; CSF = cerebrospinal fluid.

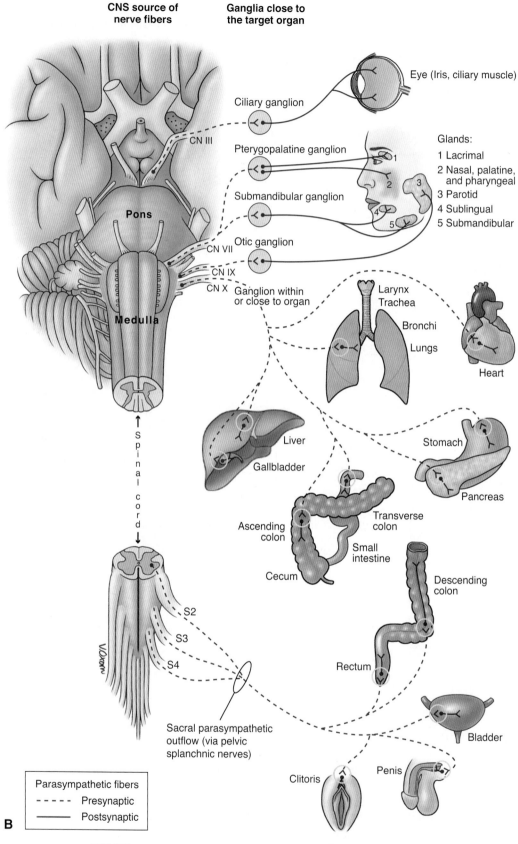

CNS source of nerve fibers

Ganglia close to the target organ

Eye (Iris, ciliary muscle)

Ciliary ganglion

CN III

Pterygopalatine ganglion

Glands:
1 Lacrimal
2 Nasal, palatine, and pharyngeal
3 Parotid
4 Sublingual
5 Submandibular

Submandibular ganglion

Pons

Otic ganglion

CN VII

CN IX

CN X

Medulla

Ganglion within or close to organ

Larynx
Trachea

Bronchi

Lungs

Heart

Spinal cord

Liver

Gallbladder

Stomach

Pancreas

Transverse colon

Ascending colon

Small intestine

Cecum

Descending colon

S2

S3

S4

Rectum

Bladder

Sacral parasympathetic outflow (via pelvic splanchnic nerves)

Clitoris

Penis

Parasympathetic fibers
- - - - Presynaptic
——— Postsynaptic

B

FIGURE 6.20 *(continued)* The autonomic nervous system at a glance.

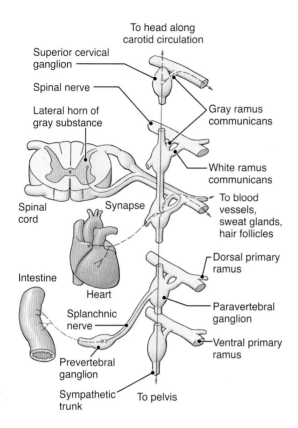

To head along
carotid circulation

Superior cervical
ganglion

Spinal nerve

Lateral horn of
gray substance

Gray ramus
communicans

White ramus
communicans

To blood
vessels,
sweat glands,
hair follicles

Spinal
cord

Synapse

Intestine

Dorsal primary
ramus

Heart

Splanchnic
nerve

Paravertebral
ganglion

Ventral primary
ramus

Prevertebral
ganglion

Sympathetic
trunk

To pelvis

FIGURE 6.21   Sympathetic nerve routes.

Sympathetic nerve impulses reach all parts of the body to constrict arteries, govern smooth muscle, and suppress or stimulate glandular secretions. All nerve fibers enter the chain of ganglia, but once there, they can go in a variety of directions depending on their purpose. Fibers going to peripheral targets throughout the body, such as arteries and sweat glands, get there most efficiently by returning to the spinal nerve and routing with it. Fibers going to thoracic and abdominal viscera pass through the chain and angle toward plexuses along the aorta. Fibers going to areas not served by spinal nerves, such as the head, ascend to the end of the chain (cervical ganglia), then typically jump to nearby blood vessels. (From Moore KL, Agur AMR. Essential Clinical Anatomy, 2nd Edition. Baltimore: Lippincott Williams & Wilkins, 2002. Figure 1.23, p. 44.)

Because the nerve connections in the autonomic nervous system are composed of two cell bodies (or neurons), there must be a synapse somewhere. This means that fibers can be described as either **presynaptic** or **postsynaptic**. This distinction is different from knowing which parts are **preganglionic**, meaning that they carry the impulse before the fiber reaches a ganglion, and which parts are **postganglionic**, meaning that they carry the impulse after the fiber has left a ganglion, because sympathetic fibers do not necessarily synapse in the first ganglion through which they travel.

Gross Anatomy of the Peripheral Nervous System

The spinal nerves

Remember that the body develops on a segmented plan. The somatic nerves that govern so much of sensation and movement all originate in the spinal cord, and they do so segmentally rather than like a random assortment of wires. Both sensory and motor impulses travel in the anatomic unit that we call a **spinal nerve**, and the nerve is further connected to the sympathetic chain of nerve fibers by tiny communicating fibers. Mastery of the spinal nerves should begin with studying a generic model for a typical spinal nerve (see Figs. 1.32–1.34).

Some of the dorsal and ventral rami are large enough, or significant enough, to be given a specific name. The **suboccipital nerve**, for example, is the specific name given to a bundle of fibers of the dorsal ramus of the first cervical spinal nerve (**C1 dorsal ramus**). It gives motor innervation to a set of muscles deep in the neck that help to stabilize the head on the vertebral column. In some cases, the rami of adjacent spinal nerves merge to form a **plexus** of fibers, the terminal branches of which also are given specific names. The **median nerve**, for example, is a major nerve of the forearm and hand, and it is a bundling of pieces of the ventral rami of C5, C6, C7, C8, and T1. Although the coverage of these nerve rami in the body is infinite, the number of nerve bundles significant enough to be given specific names is limited.

The 31 pairs of spinal nerves (eight cervical, twelve thoracic, five lumbar, five sacral, and one coccygeal) serve the entire body exclusive of the "head," which is broadly the domain of nerves that exit the brain rather than the spinal cord (see the discussion of cranial nerves below). The gross anatomy of the dorsal rami is relatively simple. Most of the action that is familiar to you occurs in the ventral rami.

Dorsal Rami

In general, the dorsal rami of all spinal nerves provide motor fibers to the "intrinsic" muscles of the back, or those muscles that derive from epimeric regions of the mesoderm somites. They also provide general sensory information from the skin that derives from the corresponding dermomyotomes (the skin that lies over the muscles in question). This is a relatively small area of muscle and skin; the dorsal rami generally are minor in size compared to their ventral counterparts. Only a few of them are given specific names in gross anatomy (Fig. 6.22).

- ■ **Suboccipital Nerve (C1):** The suboccipital nerve provides **motor** innervation to the muscles of the **suboccipital triangle** and to **semispinalis**.

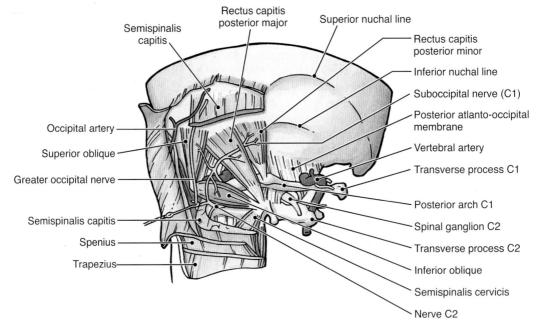

FIGURE 6.22   **Dorsal rami nerves in the deep neck.**

Musculature and skin of the vertebral column are served segmentally by unnamed dorsal rami of the spinal nerves. In the suboccipital region, the fibers of the first two cervical dorsal rami have more specific roles. The suboccipital nerve (C1) provides motor innervation to the suboccipital triangle muscles. The greater occipital nerve (C2) runs a lengthy course through this area before emerging to serve the skin over it. (From Moore KL, Agur AMR. Essential Clinical Anatomy, 2nd Edition. Baltimore: Lippincott Williams & Wilkins, 2002. Figure 5.12, p. 300.)

■ **Greater Occipital Nerve (C2):** The greater occipital nerve is the largest dorsal ramus. It provides **sensory** innervation to the posterior part of the scalp. It also networks extensively with neighboring sensory nerves.

■ **Third Occipital Nerve (C3):** The third occipital nerve is tiny dorsal ramus that provides **sensory** innervation to the lower scalp and the uppermost neck region in the back of the head.

Ventral Rami

Ventral rami provide the motor innervation to all the other muscles (i.e., those derived from the hypomeric regions of the mesoderm somites). They also provide general sensory innervation to all the rest of the skin. Because the limbs bud off of confined regions of the body wall, the few spinal nerves that correspond to those regions are quite large and interwoven. As a result, the spinal cord in these regions is "swollen"—that is, it has a wider diameter than in other regions. Sources vary on exactly which spinal nerve levels contribute to some of the larger nerves, and you will confirm that on the cadavers in the laboratory.

The first five cervical ventral rami serve the neck (Fig. 6.23). The motor fibers and the sensory fibers form discrete, separate nerve bundles once the ventral rami emerge. The **motor** fibers are referred to as the **ansa cervicalis**, because they form a loop, or **ansa**. The **sensory** fibers are just called the **cervical plexus** as a group, but four bundles of them get specific names. These bundles fill in the area between the part of the scalp covered by dorsal rami and the part of the face and head supplied by cranial nerve V (the trigeminal nerve):

Cervical Plexus (C1-C5)

■ **Lesser Occipital Nerve (C2-C3):** The lesser occipital nerve provides **sensory** innervation to the upper lateral part of the neck and around the mastoid process.

■ **Great Auricular Nerve (C2-C3):** The great auricular nerve provides **sensory** innervation to the auricle and the skin around the back of the jaw line.

■ **Transverse Cervical Nerve (C2-C3):** The transverse cervical nerve provides **sensory** innervation to the upper neck between the jaw line and the skin over sternocleidomastoid muscle.

■ **Supraclavicular Nerves (C3-C4):** The supraclavicular nerves are **sensory** to the neck from sternocleidomastoid muscle down to the line of the clavicle.

Ansa Cervicalis (C1-C3)   This elegant loop of nerves lies over the carotid sheath and sends **motor** fibers to the following muscles:

■ Geniohyoid (C1)
■ Thyrohyoid (C1)
■ Sternohyoid (C1-C3)
■ Sternothyroid (C1-C3)
■ Omohyoid (C1-C3)

Phrenic Nerve (C3-C5)   Remember that the adult **diaphragm** started out as a transverse septum of mesoderm at the very top end of the unfolded embryo. Its motor innervation thus derives from relatively high in the spinal cord and follows the muscle when it migrates into the trunk of the body (Fig. 6.24). **The phrenic nerve is the sole motor innervation to the diaphragm.** It also provides some sensory innervation to the central part of the diaphragm and some sensory innervation to the parietal pericardium, parietal pleura, and parietal peritoneum.

Two developmental concepts are relevant here. First, the adult diaphragm is formed, in part, by the body wall migrating inward to meet the original septum transversum; thus, the edges of the diaphragm draw their sensory innervation from the

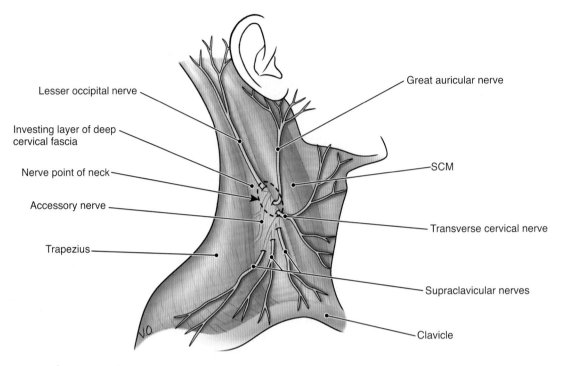

Lesser occipital nerve

Investing layer of deep
cervical fascia

Nerve point of neck

Accessory nerve

Trapezius

Great auricular nerve

SCM

Transverse cervical nerve

Supraclavicular nerves

Clavicle

A Cervical plexus

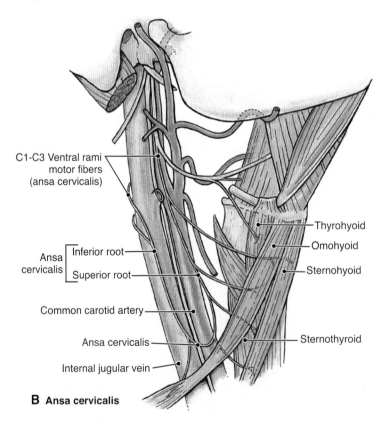

C1-C3 Ventral rami
motor fibers
(ansa cervicalis)

Ansa
cervicalis { Inferior root
Superior root

Common carotid artery

Ansa cervicalis

Internal jugular vein

Thyrohyoid

Omohyoid

Sternohyoid

Sternothyroid

B Ansa cervicalis

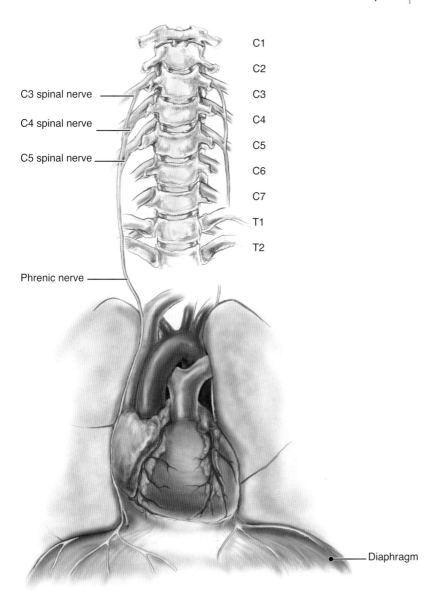

C1

C2

C3 spinal nerve ——   C3

C4 spinal nerve ——   C4

                       C5

C5 spinal nerve ——   C6

                       C7

                       T1

                       T2

Phrenic nerve ——

                                                        —— Diaphragm

FIGURE 6.24   **Phrenic nerve.**

The C3-C5 rami fibers originally served the septum transversum and adjacent mesoderm. In the adult, these tissues migrated and became the diaphragm and the pleural and pericardial sacs. Accordingly, the phrenic nerve provides motor innervation to the diaphragm and provides sensory innervation to the parietal pleura and fibrous pericardium along the way.

FIGURE 6.23   **The cervical plexus and ansa cervicalis spinal nerves.**

The first four cervical ventral rami split into separate sensory and motor fiber bundles. The sensory fibers constitute a cervical plexus (**A**) serving the side of the neck from the mandible to the clavicle. The motor fibers loop in front of the carotid artery and jugular vein as dedicated muscle bundle branches to the hyoid strap muscles (**B**). SCM = sternocleidomastoid. (From Moore KL, Agur AMR. Essential Clinical Anatomy, 2nd Edition. Baltimore: Lippincott Williams & Wilkins, 2002. Figure 9.4, p. 605; from Agur A, Dalley AF. Grant's Atlas of Anatomy, 11th Edition. Baltimore: Lippincott Williams & Wilkins, 2005. Figure 8.10A, p. 741.)

nearby **intercostal nerves** (thoracic ventral rami). Second, the sacs against which the major organs grow (the pleura, pericardium, and peritoneum) have sensory innervation on the surfaces that do not touch the organs. This sensory innervation comes from the nerves that are closest to them. The phrenic nerve just happens to run between the pleura and pericardium (and reaches out to both of them), and it terminates along the upper surface of the peritoneum (just below the diaphragm).

Brachial Plexus (C5-T1)   The **ventral rami from C5 through T1** are more or less completely dedicated to the **upper limb**, which buds off of the trunk in this region. The nerve bundle (the **brachial plexus**) is huge and complicated (Fig. 6.25). The plexus can be injured directly because it is exposed in the root of the neck and down into the armpit. The precise location of the injury determines how much motor and sensory innervation is lost, which in severe cases can lead to characteristic upper limb postures and movement deficits.

The motor fibers that come out of the plexus serve muscles of the upper limb. Some of these muscles are located in the back, as part of the complex that anchors the scapula to the axial skeleton. Anatomists designate four regions of the plexus from the ventral ramus outward to the named nerve. In order, these regions are **roots**, **trunks**, **divisions**, and **cords**. These designations are driven by visual appearance of the plexus and by a clever separation of the nerve bundles into those that serve muscles of flexion and those that serve muscles of extension.

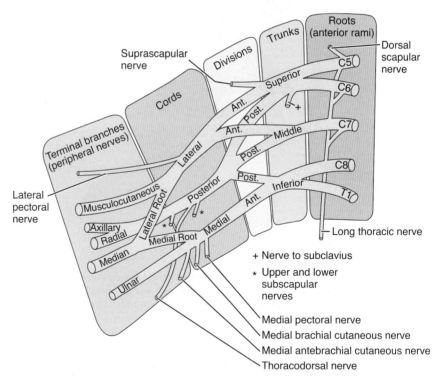

FIGURE 6.25   **Schematic design of the brachial plexus.**

The many named components of this intricate plexus all serve the muscles of the upper extremity. The division of each trunk into anterior (Ant.) and posterior (Post.) halves matches the opposition of the muscles of flexion (all served by anterior division nerves) and the muscles of extension (all served by posterior division nerves). (From Moore KL, Dalley AF. Clinically Oriented Anatomy, 5th Edition. Baltimore: Lippincott Williams & Wilkins, 2006. Figure 6.5, p. 776.)

Roots of the Plexus These are the five separate ventral nerve rami (C5-T1) as they appear just outside of the vertebral column. Two named nerve bundles come together directly from them:

- **Dorsal Scapular Nerve** (C5, sometimes C4): The dorsal scapular nerve provides motor innervation to the rhomboids.
- **Long Thoracic Nerve** (C5-C7): The long thoracic nerve provides motor innervation to the serratus anterior.

Trunks of the Plexus The five rami merge into three trunks:

- **Superior Trunk:** C5 and C6 roots.
- **Middle Trunk:** C7 root.
- **Inferior Trunk:** C8 and T1 roots

Two named nerves branch directly from the superior trunk:

- **Nerve to Subclavius:** The subclavius is a small muscle between the clavicle and rib cage.
- **Suprascapular Nerve** (C5-C6): The suprascapular nerve provides motor innervation to the supraspinatus and infraspinatus.

Divisions of the Plexus Each trunk divides into an **anterior division** and a **posterior division**. Fibers headed to muscles of flexion comprise the anterior division, and fibers headed to muscles of extension comprise the posterior division. The divisions coalesce to form **cords**.

Cords of the Plexus The cords are named based on their relationship to the large axillary artery, which travels in parallel toward the upper limb:

- **Lateral Cord:** The lateral cord is formed by the anterior divisions of the upper and middle trunks (C5-C7). It contributes to the musculocutaneous and median nerves.
- **Medial Cord:** The medial cord is formed by the anterior division of the inferior trunk (C8-T1). It contributes to the median, ulnar, and medial brachial cutaneous and medial antebrachial cutaneous nerves.
- **Posterior Cord:** The posterior cord is formed by the posterior divisions of all the trunks. It is the sole cord serving the muscles of extension. It contributes to the axillary and radial nerves.

Several named nerves branch directly from the cords:

- **Lateral Pectoral Nerve:** The lateral pectoral nerve branches from the lateral cord and provides motor to the pectoralis major.
- **Medial Pectoral Nerve:** The medial pectoral nerve branches from the medial cord and provides motor to the pectoralis major and the pectoralis minor.
- **Medial Brachial Cutaneous Nerve:** The medial brachial cutaneous nerve branches from the medial cord and is a large sensory nerve to the skin along the inside of the arm.
- **Medial Antebrachial Cutaneous Nerve:** The medial antebrachial cutaneous nerve branches from the medial cord and is a large sensory nerve to the skin along the inside of the forearm.
- **Upper Subscapular Nerve:** The upper subscapular nerve branches from the posterior cord and provides motor to the subscapularis.
- **Thoracodorsal Nerve:** The thoracodorsal nerve branches from the posterior cord and provides motor to the latissimus dorsi.
- **Lower Subscapular Nerve:** The lower subscapular nerve branches from the posterior cord and provides motor to the teres major.

The cords now become the **terminal nerves** of the plexus. These five nerves provide motor to the muscles within the arm, forearm, and hand. Continuing fibers also provide sensory information from corresponding skin zones:

- **Musculocutaneous Nerve:** The musculocutaneous nerve is derived from the lateral cord only. It provides motor to the flexors of the arm and forearm (biceps brachii, coracobrachialis, and brachialis). It continues into the forearm as the lateral cutaneous nerve of the forearm (Fig. 6.26).
- **Median Nerve:** The median nerve is derived from both the lateral cord and the medial cord. It provides motor to several muscles of flexion in the forearm and hand (see Fig. 6.26):
  - Pronator teres
  - Flexor carpi radialis

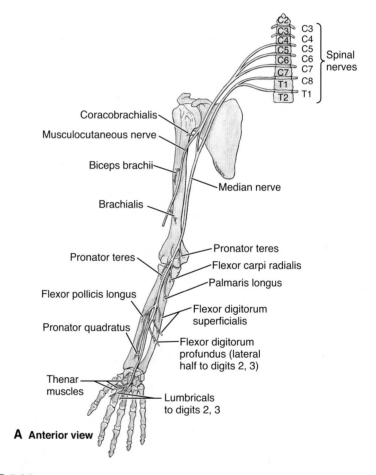

A Anterior view

FIGURE 6.26   **The median, ulnar, and radial nerves. (*continues*)**

Schematic views of the motor components of the median (**A**), ulnar (**B**), and radial (**C**) nerves, with the names of innervated muscles. The median nerve dominates the flexor muscles of the wrist and fingers and, especially, the thumb. The ulnar nerve serves flexor muscles on the medial side of the forearm and provides motor innervation to all intrinsic hand muscles except the thenar eminence thumb muscles. The radial nerve is the exclusive nerve of extension from triceps to the fingers. (From Moore KL, Dalley AF. Clinically Oriented Anatomy, 5th Edition. Baltimore: Lippincott Williams & Wilkins, 2006. Figures 6.30B,C,D, pp. 778–779.)

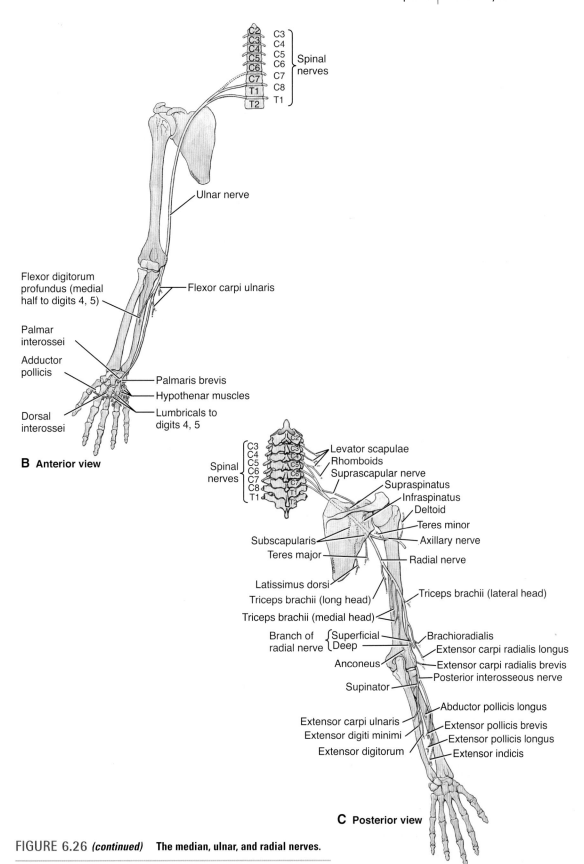

B Anterior view

C3 ⎫
C4 ⎪
C5 ⎪
C6 ⎬ Spinal nerves
C7 ⎪
C8 ⎪
T1 ⎭

Ulnar nerve

Flexor digitorum profundus (medial half to digits 4, 5)

Flexor carpi ulnaris

Palmar interossei

Adductor pollicis

Palmaris brevis

Hypothenar muscles

Dorsal interossei

Lumbricals to digits 4, 5

C3 ⎫
C4 ⎪
C5 ⎪
C6 ⎬ Spinal nerves
C7 ⎪
C8 ⎪
T1 ⎭

Levator scapulae
Rhomboids
Suprascapular nerve
Supraspinatus
Infraspinatus
Deltoid
Teres minor
Axillary nerve
Radial nerve

Subscapularis
Teres major

Latissimus dorsi
Triceps brachii (long head)
Triceps brachii (medial head)
Triceps brachii (lateral head)

Branch of radial nerve { Superficial / Deep }

Brachioradialis
Extensor carpi radialis longus
Anconeus
Extensor carpi radialis brevis
Posterior interosseous nerve
Supinator

Abductor pollicis longus
Extensor carpi ulnaris
Extensor pollicis brevis
Extensor digiti minimi
Extensor pollicis longus
Extensor digitorum
Extensor indicis

C Posterior view

FIGURE 6.26 *(continued)* The median, ulnar, and radial nerves.

- Palmaris longus
- Flexor digitorum profundus (half)
- Flexor digitorum superficialis
- Pronator quadratus
- Palmaris brevis
- Flexor pollicis longus
- Flexor pollicis brevis
- Abductor pollicis brevis
- Opponens pollicis
- First and second lumbrical

The median nerve also provides sensory innervation to the palm of the hand and to the palmar and dorsal aspects of the thumb and the first three fingers.

- **Ulnar Nerve:** The ulnar nerve is derived from the medial cord only. It provides motor to the rest of the muscles of flexion in the forearm and hand (see Fig. 6.26):
  - Flexor carpi ulnaris
  - Flexor digitorum profundus (half)
  - Flexor digiti minimi
  - Opponens digiti minimi
  - Abductor digiti minimi
  - Adductor pollicis
  - Dorsal interossei
  - Palmar interossei
  - Third and fourth lumbrical

  Refer to Figure 6.27 for a sense (no pun intended!) of the sensory distribution of the ulnar nerve.

- **Axillary Nerve:** The axillary nerve is derived from the posterior cord only—and generally from its uppermost rami (C5-C6) only. It provides motor to the deltoid and to teres minor muscles in the shoulder, and it continues onward to provide sensation to the skin over the lower part of the deltoid and the upper part of the triceps brachii (see Fig. 6.26).

- **Radial Nerve:** The radial nerve is derived from the posterior cord only and provides motor to every muscle of extension in the arm, forearm, and hand (see Fig. 6.26):
  - Triceps brachii
  - Anconeus
  - Supinator
  - Brachioradialis
  - Extensor carpi radialis brevis
  - Extensor carpi radialis longus
  - Extensor carpi ulnaris
  - Extensor digitorum
  - Extensor pollicis longus
  - Extensor pollicis brevis
  - Extensor indicis
  - Abductor pollicis longus

Given how the plexus is designed and positioned, injuries to the upper rami or the lower rami are more common than injuries to the middle rami. These injuries are classified as **upper plexus injuries** and **lower plexus injuries**. (See Clinical Anatomy Box 6.3.)

Thoracic Ventral Rami   The thoracic region of the adult body maintains the segmented nature of nerve distribution more than any other region of the body. As a result, the thoracic ventral rami perform almost identical functions. They provide

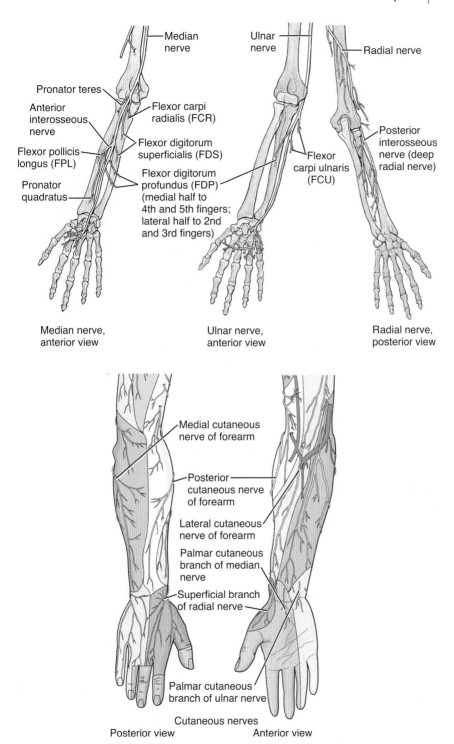

FIGURE 6.27   **Cutaneous distribution of the median, ulnar, and radial nerves.**

(From Moore KL, Dalley AF. Clinically Oriented Anatomy, 5th Edition. Baltimore: Lippincott Williams & Wilkins, 2006. Figure 6.10, p. 820.)

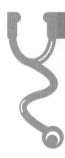

CLINICAL ANATOMY

Box 6.3

BRACHIAL PLEXUS INJURIES

Tension on the webbing between the neck and chest can shear the upper brachial plexus fibers (A–C), and tension on an outstretched arm can shear the lower brachial plexus fibers (D–F). Upper plexus injuries in adults result from trauma that wrenches the head forcibly to one side (A). Newborns also can suffer upper plexus injuries during childbirth if their heads are torqued too far as they are delivered (C). Results of upper plexus injuries will impact the muscles served by the C5 and C6 ventral rami contributions to the plexus. The arm tends to be medially rotated and fixed at the side because an impaired motor innervation to scapular retractors and humeral abductors (B).

Lower plexus injuries in adults can result from breaking a fall by grabbing something with an outstretched hand (D). Newborns also can suffer lower plexus injuries if their arms are stretched to facilitate delivery (E). Results of lower plexus injuries will affect muscles served by the C8 and T1 ventral rami contributions to the plexus. These muscles are mostly in the hand. Atrophy of the interosseous muscles, hyperextension of the metacarpophalangeal joints, and flexion of the interphalangeal joints puts the hand in a "clawed" position (F). Lower plexus injuries are much less common than upper plexus injuries.

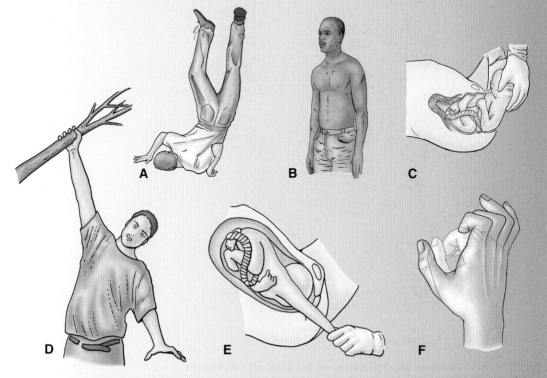

Brachial plexus injuries. See text for descriptions of **A** through **F**. (From Moore KL, Dalley AF. Clinically Oriented Anatomy, 5th Edition. Baltimore: Lippincott Williams & Wilkins, 2006. Figure B6.12, p. 780.)

motor innervation to the muscles of the body wall (intercostal and abdominal oblique muscles) and **sensory innervation to a swath of skin (a dermatome) over the "latitudinal" path of the ramus**. They also provide sensory innervation to the adjacent regions of the parietal pleura and parietal peritoneum.

The ventral rami run deep to the lower margin of the rib of the same thoracic level. A classic cross-sectional diagram in gross anatomy is the diagram of a segment of the trunk showing a typical thoracic ventral ramus and its cutaneous branches (Fig. 6.28).

Recall that the **sympathetic** part of the autonomic nervous system is headquartered in the **T1-L2** range of spinal nerve segments in the spinal cord. This means that a **white ramus communicans** is found as part of the thoracic spinal nerves. It represents the path for sympathetic fibers to exit the spinal cord, to travel through the ventral root of the spinal nerve, and ultimately, to leave the spinal nerve to connect to the sympathetic chain. This communicating fiber often seems to be emerging from the spinal nerve at the base of the ventral ramus. Recall also that sympathetic fibers leave the chain via a **gray ramus communicans** to route to the sweat glands and arterial smooth muscles. Gray rami communicantes are found from T1 to the lower limit of the spinal cord.

Lumbar Ventral Rami   The lumbar ventral rami serve the body wall in the same way as the thoracic ventral rami do. As the trunk nears its bottom, however, the lower limb buds away, much like the upper limb. The lower limb buds away from the region between the L2 and S3 spinal nerve levels of the central nervous system, so combinations

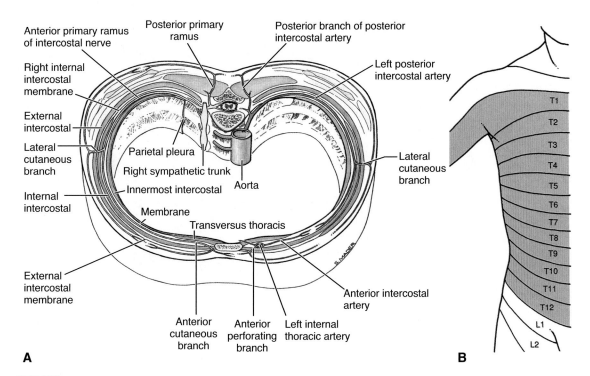

A   **B**

FIGURE 6.28   **A typical thoracic spinal nerve.**

The body wall is innervated segmentally by thoracic spinal nerve ventral rami. A transverse section of the thorax (**A**) shows how a typical nerve sends branches to the body wall musculature and to a band of skin (dermatome), both of which overlap with the branches of the succeeding spinal nerve (**B**). (From Moore KL, Agur AMR. Essential Clinical Anatomy, 2nd Edition. Baltimore: Lippincott Williams & Wilkins, 2002. Figure 2.9, p. 64; Figure 2.12B, p. 66.)

of ventral rami from these levels are devoted primarily to serve the lower limb. This bundle includes seven spinal nerves and numerous cross-overs (plexuses). The plexus is well protected against the back wall of the abdomen and pelvis, however, so in gross anatomy only the terminal nerves and the levels that compose them are emphasized.

The Lumbar Plexus   The lumbar plexus accounts for the various combinations of L1-L4 ventral rami, which are found just lateral to the vertebral column (Fig. 6.29). Nearby muscles, such as the piriformis and quadratus lumborum, get their motor innervation from unnamed ("muscular") direct branches of the plexus. Study the named terminal nerves and how they distribute:

- **Iliohypogastric (L1):** The iliohypogastric nerve runs in the sandwich of the abdominal wall muscles and provides sensory innervation to the skin of the upper hip and the inguinal region. Along with other lumbar ventral rami, it also provides motor innervation to the muscles of the abdominal wall.
- **Ilioinguinal (L1):** The ilioinguinal nerve parallels the iliohypogastric nerve, but it runs a slightly inferior course. It provides sensory innervation to the skin that pouches out to

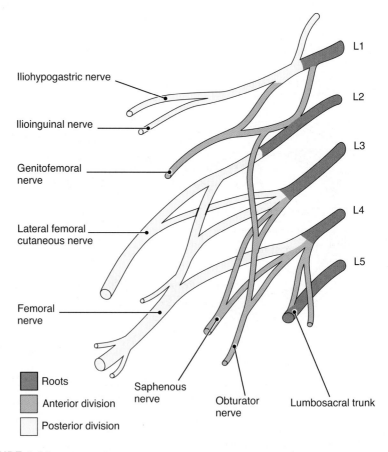

FIGURE 6.29   **The lumbar spinal nerves.**

The lumbar ventral rami continue the segmental distribution of the thoracic nerves, but in addition, they form a plexus to serve the lower extremity, which develops from the L2–S3 regions of the trunk. The saphenous nerve travels within the femoral nerve bundle. Part of the L4 and all of the L5 ventral rami descend to the pelvis to join a sacral plexus of nerves serving the lower limb. (From Premkumar K. The Massage Connection: Anatomy and Physiology. Baltimore: Lippincott Williams & Wilkins, 2004.)

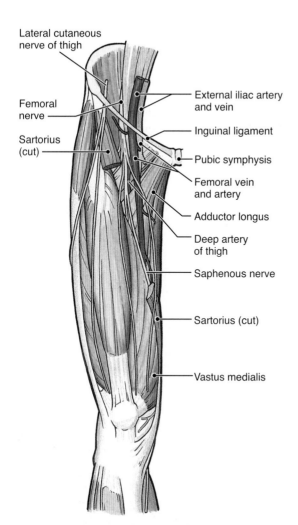

Lateral cutaneous
nerve of thigh

Femoral
nerve

Sartorius
(cut)

External iliac artery
and vein

Inguinal ligament

Pubic symphysis

Femoral vein
and artery

Adductor longus

Deep artery
of thigh

Saphenous nerve

Sartorius (cut)

Vastus medialis

FIGURE 6.30   **Lumbar plexus
nerves in the anterior thigh.**

The L2-L4 ventral rami combine to
form three large nerves serving
the anterior and medial thigh: the
lateral cutaneous, the femoral, and
the obturator (not shown). (From
Moore KL, Agur AMR. Essential
Clinical Anatomy, 2nd Edition.
Baltimore: Lippincott Williams &
Wilkins, 2002. Figure 6.11A, p. 339.)

become the scrotum in males and the labium majus in females. It also provides motor
to the abdominal wall muscles through which it passes to reach the inguinal and inner
thigh region.

■ **Lateral Femoral Cutaneous (L2-L3):** The lateral femoral cutaneous nerve pops out at
approximately the point of the anterior superior iliac spine of the pelvis bone. As the
name implies, the lateral femoral cutaneous nerve runs down the side of the thigh and
provides sensory innervation along the way (Fig. 6.30).

■ **Genitofemoral (L1-L2):** The name implies that the genitofemoral nerve has something
to do with the genitalia and something to do with the thigh. In the male, the genital
branch runs with the spermatic cord, where it provides motor innervation to the cremaster muscle. In the female, the genital branch runs with the homologous round ligament. In both sexes, this branch provides sensation to the skin of the scrotum or labium
majus. The femoral branch follows the femoral artery and vein under the inguinal ligament and provides sensation to a small patch of skin overlying them in a region called
the **femoral triangle**.

■ **Femoral (L2-L4):** The femoral nerve is the first of the major lower limb nerves (see Fig.
6.30). It enters the thigh just underneath the vulnerable inguinal ligament and rests virtually against the skin, below the crease where the thigh joins the trunk. Because of the
way the lower limb rotates during development to support an upright posture, the equivalent of the "armpit" in the lower extremity is exposed and faces forward (the femoral

triangle). In addition to the femoral nerve, the large femoral artery and femoral vein are vulnerable here as well (see above). Once in the thigh, the femoral nerve is the principal motor nerve of the quadriceps muscles and other anterior thigh muscles (sartorius, iliacus, and pectineus). Thus, it governs flexion of the hip and extension of the knee. It also provides skin sensation over a long swath of skin from the femoral triangle down to the inside arch of the foot. Some of these branches are quite large, so they are given specific names: anterior cutaneous nerve, medial cutaneous nerve, and saphenous nerve (for the one going past the knee joint into the leg and foot).

■ **Obturator (L2-L4):** The obturator nerve is formed from the same spinal nerve segments as the femoral nerve, but it is destined for the medial thigh (the adductor muscle group and inner thigh skin). The sensory component of the nerve commonly is absent.

■ **Lumbosacral Trunk (L4-L5):** The final named nerve of the lumbar plexus, the lumbosacral trunk nerve, is the union of the ventral rami of L4 and L5 into a nerve trunk that will participate in a large sacral plexus of spinal nerves serving the perineum and lower limb. As just noted above, the L4 ventral ramus also serves other nerves, but the L5 ramus is dedicated wholly to the lumbosacral trunk (Fig. 6.31). The trunk quickly joins forces with the sacral spinal nerves to form the robust "sciatic" nerve that serves the entire posterior part of the lower limb.

Sacral Plexus   The sacral plexus of L4-S4 gives rise to several named nerves, all but one of which (**nerve to piriformis**) immediately leaves the pelvis via the **greater sciatic foramen**. Some of these nerves are difficult to uncover during dissection of the cadaver. Others, such as the common fibular, tibial, and pudendal nerves, are much more apparent in the cadaver.

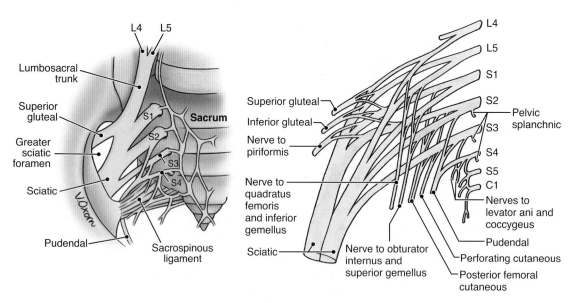

FIGURE 6.31   **The sacral plexus of spinal nerves.**

The ventral rami of L4–S3 form a plexus en route to the skin and muscles of the lower extremity. The S2-S5 and coccygeal ventral rami are dedicated also to the muscles and skin of the perineum. The most dominant nerve of this group is the pudendal nerve (S2-S4), which provides sensory innervation to the genital and anal skin, motor service to the voluntary sphincters of the bladder and anus, and motor innervation to the muscles that squeeze erectile tissue. (From Moore KL, Agur AMR. Essential Clinical Anatomy, 2nd Edition. Baltimore: Lippincott Williams & Wilkins, 2002. Figure 4.3, p. 220.)

The remaining named nerves must serve the lower limb and the anatomy at the "bottom of the trunk," which includes the critical anal and urogenital regions. These nerves are presented here in two groups: a sort of "local" group serving nearby pelvic and buttock structures and a "migrant" group serving the rest of the lower limb. The nerves of the local group are numerous but easy to remember because their names give them away. The nerves of the migrant group are only two in number but are devilish to remember because they do so many things.

Sacral Plexus Nerves in the Pelvis and Buttock The nerves of the sacral plexus in the pelvis and buttock are:

- **Nerve to Piriformis (S1-S2):** The motor fibers to the piriformis muscle arise from S1 and S2. They enter the muscle immediately, because the muscle originates around the S1 and S2 ventral foramina on the sacrum (see Fig. 6.31).
- **Nerve to Obturator Internus and Superior Gemellus (L5-S2):** This nerve bundle provides motor to the nearby obturator internus muscle and its upper assistant, the superior gemellus.
- **Nerve to Quadratus Femoris and Inferior Gemellus (L4-S1):** This nerve bundle provides motor to the nearby quadratus femoris and the lower assistant to the obturator internus, the inferior gemellus.
- **Superior Gluteal Nerve (L4-S1):** The gluteal muscles that form the mass of the buttock are served by two nerve bundles, one of which passes above the piriformis muscle on its way out of the pelvis and one of which passes below it. The superior gluteal nerve provides motor innervation to the **gluteus medius**, **gluteus minimus**, and **tensor fascia lata**.
- **Inferior Gluteal Nerve (L5-S2):** Because the bulk of the gluteus maximus actually is lower down in the buttock, it receives motor innervation from the inferior gluteal nerve.
- **Posterior Femoral Cutaneous Nerve (S1-S3):** The skin along the back of the thigh, beginning just below the buttock, is the domain of this sensory nerve. Other sensory nerves in the buttock are called the cluneal nerves and are either direct branches of the sacral spinal nerves or branches of the posterior femoral cutaneous bundle.
- **Pudendal Nerve (S1-S5):** The pudendal nerve arises from the S2-S4 ventral rami, with occasional contributions from S1 and S5. It is a remarkable nerve and provides **motor to most of the muscles of the perineum**, which is the region of the bottom of the pelvis and which includes a muscular diaphragm and all the muscles associated with the genitalia. It also provides sensory innervation to these key regions. Its anatomic course is elegant and complex, and its functions collectively were "shameful" to ancient anatomists, hence the name **pudendal**.
- **Nerve to Levator Ani (S3-S4):** Most of the pelvic diaphragm that slings the gut tube and the urogenital tract into place at the bottom of the pelvis is innervated by direct fibers of the pudendal nerve. This part is called the levator ani, and it includes the muscles that you consciously contract during a bowel movement or when straining to lift a weight. (The rest of the diaphragm is the coccygeus muscle, which gets a direct branch from the sacral plexus.)
- **Inferior Rectal Nerve (S2-S4):** Shortly after serving the levator ani and exiting the pelvic cavity, the pudendal nerve loops forward, underneath the pelvic diaphragm. It sends inferior rectal fibers toward the midline to grab the nearby external anal sphincter. Sensory fibers continue to the skin surface to serve the sensitive area around the anal orifice.
- **Perineal Nerve (S2-S4):** The remaining fibers of the pudendal nerve collectively are called the **perineal nerve**. They are destined to serve the skin from the anal orifice forward onto the genitalia and to serve the muscles of the urogenital region. The muscles served include the deep and superficial transverse perineus, external urethral sphincter, bulbospongiosus, and ischiocavernosus.

Damage to the first three of these nerves will affect hip rotation, but neither the muscles nor their nerves are particularly vulnerable. These three nerves are difficult to obtain during dissection.

Of the sensory fibers to the genitalia, the named ones to be studied are the dorsal nerve of the clitoris and the homologous dorsal nerve of the penis. These fibers run onto the "top" surface of the clitoris and penis (as you look down), just underneath the arch of the bony pubic symphysis.

Because the pudendal nerve runs so close to the ischial tuberosity, chronic pressure to this area can "numb" or suppress sensation throughout the perineum and genitalia. This is a possible temporary consequence of childbirth, and it also can be provoked by prolonged sitting on hard surfaces or poorly designed bicycle seats.

Sacral Plexus Nerves in the Lower Limb   The major motor nerves of the lower limb are the **gluteal nerves**, **femoral nerve**, **obturator nerve**, and the **"sciatic" nerve**. The sciatic nerve serves the hamstring muscles and all the leg and foot muscles. This large nerve bundle exits the pelvis deep to the gluteus maximus (Fig. 6.32). This is a popular place to administer an intramuscular injection, so care must be taken to avoid hitting the sciatic nerve. Stick the needle above and outside of a line connecting the posterior superior iliac spine of the hip bone, which you can usually feel, and the greater trochanter of the femur, which you can always feel (see Fig. 6.32B).

The word "sciatic" is put in quotes because the nerve bundle called sciatic is actually two separate nerves with exclusive motor and sensory functions. In terms of muscles innervated or territories of skin sensitized, the separate **common fibular nerve** and **tibial nerve** are more appropriate names. They "peel apart" from one another, usually midway down the back of the thigh (see Fig. 6.32). There is reason to use and understand the term sciatic, however, because of the common occurrence of **sciatica**, a painful condition in which the pathway of the sciatic bundle is compromised through the pelvis and buttock, causing intermittent pain and tingling along the subsequent pathway of the two nerves.

Common Fibular Nerve   Older textbooks of anatomy may still use the name **common peroneal nerve**; however, the modern name, **common fibular nerve**, better describes the location of the muscles that the nerve serves. It is comprised of the L4-S2 ventral rami, so it incorporates part of the lumbosacral trunk. In the posterior thigh, it provides motor to the short head of biceps femoris (Fig. 6.33).

As the common fibular nerve nears the knee joint, it divides into four branches, two of which are sensory only. The **lateral cutaneous nerve** of the calf does just that, and the **fibular communicating nerve** joins a twig from the tibial nerve to form a joint sensory nerve called the **sural nerve**, which runs the length of the back of the calf, providing sensory innervation along the way.

Superficial Fibular Nerve   This branch serves the lateral compartment of the leg and provides **motor** to the fibularis longus and fibularis brevis muscles. Near the ankle, it spreads over to the dorsum of the foot to provide much of the sensation to that surface and to the tops of most of the toes (see Fig. 6.33).

Deep Fibular Nerve   This branch scoots around the head of the fibula and serves the anterior compartment leg muscles: the tibialis anterior, the extensor digitorum longus, the extensor digitorum brevis, the extensor hallucis, and when present, the fibularis tertius. The deep fibular nerve also peeks out to provide sensation to the webbing between the first and second toes.

Tibial Nerve   This slightly more extensive nerve arises from L4-S3 and, thus, includes the other major commitment of the lumbosacral trunk. It is dedicated to the muscles that enable you to "curl" the whole lower limb into its version of a "fist." It controls extension at the hip ("curling" the thigh backward), flexion at the knee, and

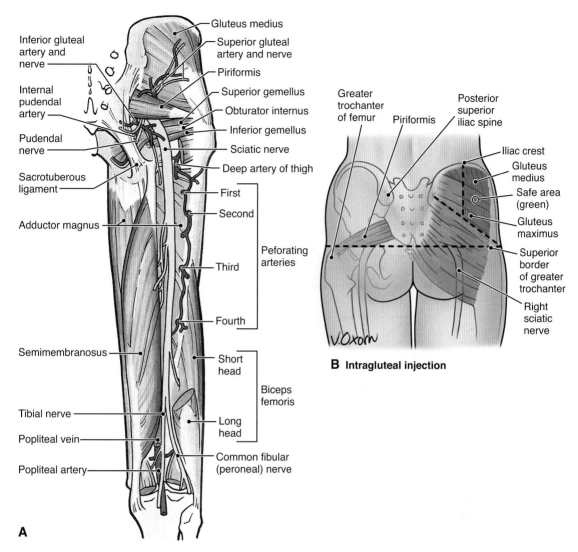

FIGURE 6.32   **Pathway of the sciatic nerve.**

The largest nerve bundle in the body, the sciatic nerve, delivers a tibial nerve fiber family to muscles and skin in the posterior thigh, leg, and foot and a fibular nerve fiber family to muscles and skin in the lateral and anterior leg (**A**). The exit of the sciatic nerve from the pelvis is clinically relevant. It can be "trapped" by the piriformis muscle or compressed against the ischium. It also must be avoided when medicine is injected in the gluteal region (**B**). A safe injection zone can be determined by feeling bony landmarks, such as the greater trochanter of the femur and the iliac crest, and aiming for the upper gluteal zone. (From Moore KL, Agur AMR. Essential Clinical Anatomy, 2nd Edition. Baltimore: Lippincott Williams & Wilkins, 2002. Figures 6.15, p. 347; Figure 6.17, p. 351.)

plantarflexion ("toeing-off"). The tibial nerve also is the only motor nerve to the sole of the foot (see Fig. 6.33).

In the thigh, the tibial nerve is a single bundle and sends motor branches to the "hamstring" muscles: the semimembranosus, the semitendinosus, and the long head of the biceps femoris. Across the knee joint, it submits a sensory branch to the sural nerve composite (see above), and it sends a small twig to serve the unusual muscle popliteus. Once into the calf, it dives into every muscle that drives you forward: the gastrocnemius, soleus, plantaris, tibialis posterior, flexor digitorum longus, and flexor hallucis longus.

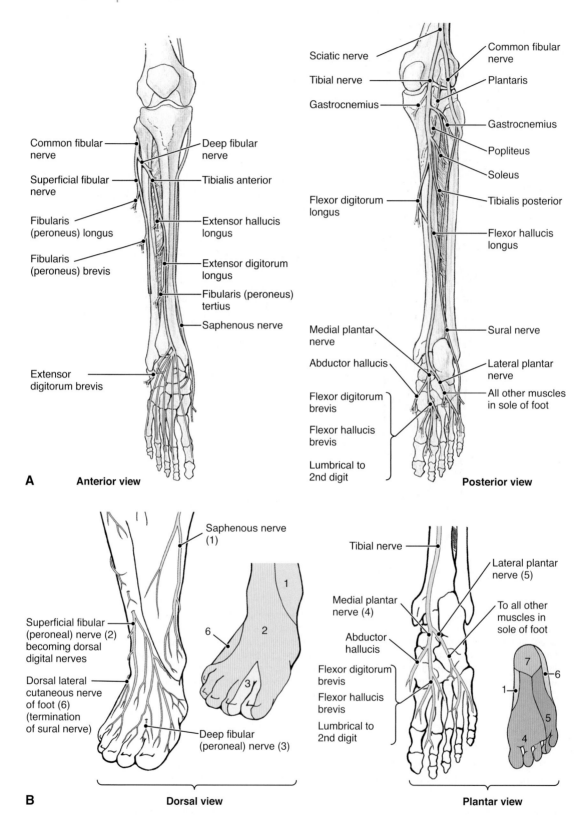

A   Anterior view

Common fibular nerve

Superficial fibular nerve

Fibularis (peroneus) longus

Fibularis (peroneus) brevis

Extensor digitorum brevis

Deep fibular nerve

Tibialis anterior

Extensor hallucis longus

Extensor digitorum longus

Fibularis (peroneus) tertius

Saphenous nerve

Posterior view

Sciatic nerve

Tibial nerve

Gastrocnemius

Flexor digitorum longus

Medial plantar nerve

Abductor hallucis

Flexor digitorum brevis

Flexor hallucis brevis

Lumbrical to 2nd digit

Common fibular nerve

Plantaris

Gastrocnemius

Popliteus

Soleus

Tibialis posterior

Flexor hallucis longus

Sural nerve

Lateral plantar nerve

All other muscles in sole of foot

B   Dorsal view

Saphenous nerve (1)

Superficial fibular (peroneal) nerve (2) becoming dorsal digital nerves

Dorsal lateral cutaneous nerve of foot (6) (termination of sural nerve)

Deep fibular (peroneal) nerve (3)

Plantar view

Tibial nerve

Medial plantar nerve (4)

Abductor hallucis

Flexor digitorum brevis

Flexor hallucis brevis

Lumbrical to 2nd digit

Lateral plantar nerve (5)

To all other muscles in sole of foot

Just above the ankle joint, the nerve must commit to one side or the other to get around the heel bone (calcaneus). In keeping with its tibial disposition, it veers to the medial side under cover of the flexor retinaculum and following the tendons of the deep calf muscles it innervates. At this point. it diverges into two named nerves.

Medial Plantar Nerve This nerve is homologous in many ways with the median nerve in the hand. It sends motor branches to the muscles that operate the big toe (abductor hallucis and flexor hallucis brevis) as well as the flexor digitorum brevis and the first lumbrical muscle of the foot. The sensory fibers of the medial plantar nerve cover the medial part of the sole of the foot and the pads and toenails of the first three-and-a-half toes (see Fig. 6.33).

Lateral Plantar Nerve This nerve is homologous in many ways to the ulnar nerve in the hand. It sends motor branches to the quadratus plantae muscle, the muscles that operate the little toe (flexor digiti minimi and abductor digiti minimi), the adductor of the big toe (adductor hallucis), and the deep muscles of the sole of the foot (dorsal and plantar interossei and the remaining three lumbricals).

Coccygeal Plexus Even the lone spinal nerve of the coccygeal region of the cord takes part in a plexus. The ventral rami of S4, S5, and Co1 work together as the **coccygeal plexus**. You probably will not see any fibers of this plexus in the cadaver, but you should remember that the coccygeal plexus provides motor innervation to the coccygeus muscle, part of the levator ani muscle group, and the skin over the coccyx. You already know this area well if you have ever slipped and landed on the "tailbone."

Patients do not present with an anatomic diagnosis in hand, of course. Instead, they present with musculoskeletal deficits, which are behaviors that display muscle weakness, regional parasthesias, or both. Mastering which spinal nerve levels primarily control which normal movements of the limbs, as illustrated in Figure 6.34, is a very useful goal of studying the spinal nerves.

The spinal nerves serve the voluntary needs of the body below the chin. Two other types of peripheral nerves must now be described: the cranial nerves, and the autonomic nervous system. In many ways, cranial nerves are identical to spinal nerves. They exit the central nervous system, and they serve the voluntary needs of the head and neck. They also, however, serve "special needs" and are particularly important targets of a physical examination or clinical evaluation. Therefore, they are an essential anatomic domain to master. The autonomic nervous system is functionally simple but structurally complex. Mastering its function is more important than mastering its pathways.

Cranial nerves

The head contains the same types of muscles and skin surfaces as the rest of the body does, so nerves that are similar to spinal nerves must emanate from the central nervous system to serve them. In some ways, the distinction between **cranial nerves** and **spinal nerves** is arbitrary, but for the most part, cranial nerves serve only tissues of the head and neck, and vice-versa. Emphasis should be placed on functions of the nerves. The anatomic pathways are best studied in the cadaver itself. In many ways, the anatomic

---

FIGURE 6.33   **Spinal nerve service to the leg and foot.**

The common fibular nerve is subject to injury as it rounds the neck of the fibula (**A**). The continuation of the tibial nerve provides motor innervation to the musculature of the calf and sole of the foot (**B**). (From Sadler TW. Langman's Medical Embryology, 9th Edition. Baltimore: Lippincott Williams & Wilkins, 2004. Figure 6.7, p. 357, Figure 6.13, p. 376.)

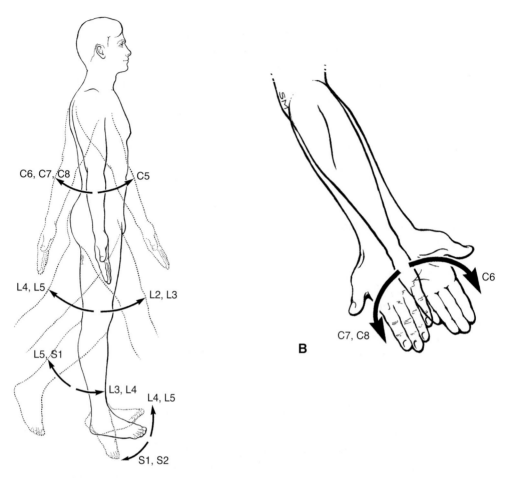

FIGURE 6.34   Certain spinal nerve levels control basic movements.

Muscles that move the limbs in the basic directions of flexion, extension (**A**), and rotation (**B**) are motored by multiple spinal levels; however, for each basic movement, such as flexing the arm, one or two spinal nerve levels dominate the motor activity (in this case, C5). (From Agur A, Dalley AF. Grant's Atlas of Anatomy, 11th Edition. Baltimore: Lippincott Williams & Wilkins, 2005.)

pathways of the nerves are less relevant clinically, because you will never be able to investigate them in a living patient as you can in a cadaver. The whole of the head, in other words, is much greater than the sum of its gross anatomy. Master first what the cranial nerves do, then where they travel.

In addition to providing general motor and sensory capacity to head and neck tissues, some cranial nerves also provide unique sensory functions. The success of animate organisms in the biology of life depends on sophisticated detection of and response to the outside world. If the headquarters of the neural tube (the brain) is to develop special detection abilities, it is logical to suppose that the structures for these abilities will be located nearby. Indeed, the "special" senses are mostly in the head. The ability to detect light waves (seeing), sound waves (hearing), chemical compounds (smelling and tasting), and equilibrium (balance) are all located in the anatomy of the head. The instruments that perform these incredible feats are nothing more than cranial nerve extensions of the brain that are exposed to the outside world in very well-protected stations.

Also, as in the rest of the body, the head benefits from subconscious, or autonomic, reactions. Delicate tissues need to be bathed in fluid. The mouth enjoys its own detergent (**saliva**) to disarm guests and to keep its own moving parts from sticking. Blood vessels need to dilate or constrict. The eyes need to focus on changing targets without much conscious processing. The sympathetic component of these reactions is head-quartered in the spinal cord and reaches the head by linking with the carotid artery circulation. The parasympathetic component of these reactions is headquartered in the brain and is routed through four of the twelve cranial nerves.

The 12 cranial nerves are as follows:

Cranial Nerve I: *Olfactory nerve*
Cranial Nerve II: *Optic nerve*
Cranial Nerve III: *Oculomotor nerve*
Cranial Nerve IV: *Trochlear nerve*
Cranial Nerve V: *Trigeminal nerve*
Cranial Nerve VI: *Abducens nerve*
Cranial Nerve VII: *Facial nerve*
Cranial Nerve VIII: *Vestibulocochlear nerve*
Cranial Nerve IX: *Glossopharyngeal nerve*
Cranial Nerve X: *Vagus nerve*
Cranial Nerve XI: *Accessory nerve*
Cranial Nerve XII: *Hypoglossal nerve*

The first two cranial nerves, the **olfactory nerve** and the **optic nerve**, smell and see (i.e., are for the special senses of smell and sight), respectively. The **oculomotor nerve** looks and manages visual resolution by constricting the pupil and bending the lens of the eye. The fourth and sixth cranial nerves (the **trochlear nerve** and the **abducens nerve**, respectively) also look by motoring two other eye muscles. The fifth cranial nerve (the **trigeminal nerve**) senses and chews; it is quite extensive and is responsible for almost all the general sensation in the head. The **facial nerve** (cranial nerve VII) expresses, both literally and figuratively. It drives salivation, lacrimation, and mucus production, as well as providing motor to all the muscles of facial expression, and it tastes from the oral part of the tongue. Cranial nerve VIII (the **vestibulocochlear nerve**) hears and balances. The **glossopharyngeal nerve** (cranial nerve IX) and the **vagus nerve** (cranial nerve X) work closely together in the head to swallow, speak, and in part, taste. The vagus nerve travels beyond the head to monitor respiration, heart rate, and digestion. Cranial nerve XI (the **accessory nerve**) moves the head via the two largest muscles attached to the head, one in the front (the sternocleidomastoid) and one in the back (the trapezius). The last cranial nerve (the **hypoglossal nerve**) wags the tongue—a behavior not to be underestimated.

This brief description does not really do justice to the cranial nerves, and much more information follows in the rest of this book. Table 6.1 shows how certain patterns in their function enable you to learn aspects of them quickly. Three of them (cranial nerves I, II, and VIII) provide only a "special" sensory function. Four of them (cranial nerves IV, VI, XI, and XII) provide only motor innervation to a total of very few mus-cles. The remaining nerves (cranial nerves III, V, VII, IX, and X) are of mixed function and substantial complexity; of them, four carry parasympathetic fibers (cranial nerves III, VII, IX, and X). Much of the clinical work with cranial nerves is testing them to see if they are working in the patient, because disabled cranial nerves can be a sign of neu-rologic trouble back at headquarters (the brain).

Cranial Nerve I: Olfactory nerve

Cranial nerve I detects smell. That is all.

This extension of the brain rests near the midline of the head, perched atop the nasal cavity. It exposes itself to the outside world in the mucosa at the upper limit of the nasal passageway (Fig. 6.35). The rest of the "external" nose is a modified pouch

TABLE 6.1 THE CRANIAL NERVES AT A GLANCE

CRANIAL NERVE	COMMON NAME	FIBER TYPE	SENSORY AREA	MUSCLES	AUTONOMIC FUNCTION
I	Olfactory	Sensory	Smell		
II	Optic	Sensory	Vision		
III	Oculomotor	Motor		Levator palpebrae superioris Superior rectus Medial rectus Inferior rectus Inferior oblique	
		Parasympathetic			Constricts pupil; Accommodates lens
IV	Trochlear	Motor		Superior oblique	
V	Trigeminal	Sensory	Head		
		Motor		Mastication muscles Mylohyoid Anterior digastric Tensor tympani Tensor veli palatini	
VI	Abducens	Motor		Lateral rectus	
VII	Facial	Sensory	Outer ear Nasal cavity Soft palate Taste (anterior 2/3 of tongue)		
		Motor		Facial expression muscles Posterior digastric Stylohyoid Stapedius	
		Parasympathetic			Tear, saliva, and mucus
VIII	Vestibulocochlear	Sensory	Hearing Equilibrium		
IX	Glossopharyngeal	Sensory	Outer ear Tongue (general sense and taste posterior 1/3) Pharynx Carotid sinus		
		Motor		Stylopharyngeus	
		Parasympathetic			Saliva secretion (parotid gland)
X	Vagus	Sensory	Outer ear Epiglottis (taste) Pharynx, larynx		
		Motor		Larynx and pharynx	
		Parasympathetic			Homeostasis, peristalsis, secretion in lungs, heart, and gut tube; visceral renal function
XI	Accessory	Motor		Sternocleidomastoid Trapezius	
XII	Hypoglossal	Motor		Intrinsic, extrinsic tongue	

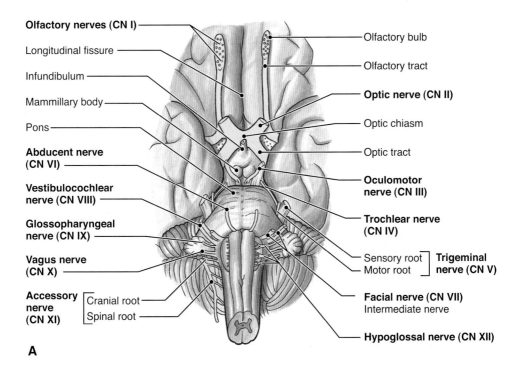

Olfactory nerves (CN I)

Longitudinal fissure

Infundibulum

Mammillary body

Pons

Abducent nerve (CN VI)

Vestibulocochlear nerve (CN VIII)

Glossopharyngeal nerve (CN IX)

Vagus nerve (CN X)

Accessory nerve (CN XI) ⎡ Cranial root ⎣ Spinal root

Olfactory bulb

Olfactory tract

Optic nerve (CN II)

Optic chiasm

Optic tract

Oculomotor nerve (CN III)

Trochlear nerve (CN IV)

Sensory root ⎤ **Trigeminal**
Motor root   ⎦ **nerve (CN V)**

Facial nerve (CN VII)
Intermediate nerve

Hypoglossal nerve (CN XII)

A

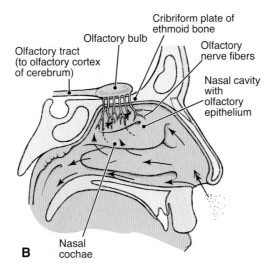

Cribriform plate of
ethmoid bone

Olfactory bulb

Olfactory tract
(to olfactory cortex
of cerebrum)

Olfactory
nerve fibers

Nasal cavity
with
olfactory
epithelium

Nasal
cochae

B

FIGURE 6.35   **Cranial nerve I (olfactory nerve).**

Cranial nerves are numbered roughly according to their appearance along the inferior brain surface (**A**). The olfactory nerve, or cranial nerve (CN) I, reaches the epithelium of the nasal passage through cribriform holes in the intervening ethmoid bone (**B**). (From Sadler TW. Langman's Medical Embryology, 9th Edition. Baltimore: Lippincott Williams & Wilkins, 2004. Figure 10.2A, p. 646; from Stedman's Medical Dictionary, 27th Edition. Baltimore: Lippincott Williams & Wilkins, 2000.)

of ectoderm that stretches off of the nasal bones and folds in on itself to form a kind of wet-lined sleeve. The lining of the sleeve moistens and eases the temperature of inspired air so that it does not stun the olfactory nerve endings. Rather, it seduces or attacks the olfactory nerve with the chemical compounds of aroma or odor.

Cranial Nerve II: Optic nerve

Cranial nerve II provides the sense of vision. That is all.

The ability to see stereoscopically and in color dominates human understanding of the world. Vision is a prized capability, and loss of vision immediately affects a person's sense of "health." Cranial nerve II is an extension of the brain, complete with the meninges that cover the central nervous system and with endings that are sensitive to certain wavelengths of light (Fig. 6.36). The optic nerve fiber endings fan out along the posterior wall of the eye globe as a **retina**. Light reaches the retina by passing through a pupillary aperture deep to the corneal surface of the eyeball. Once through this aperture, the light waves refract through a **lens**, the bending ability of which is governed by the next cranial nerve, the oculomotor nerve. Focused light waves stimulating the retina then travel back to the brain via four exclusive fiber pathways (see Fig. 6.36). Light that reflects off of objects that are directly in front of you, or in the nasal fields of vision, stimulates the lateral aspect of the retina in each eye. These retinal fibers route back through the optic nerve to the **optic tract** on the same (ipsilateral) side of the brain. By contrast, light that reflects off of objects that are in your peripheral, or temporal, fields of vision

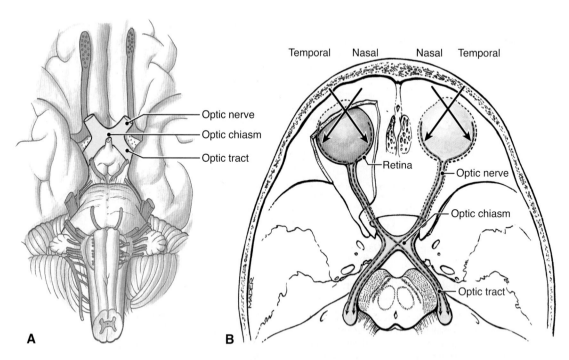

FIGURE 6.36   **Cranial nerve II (optic nerve).**

The optic nerve is dedicated to vision. Its retinal endings form a receptive dish in the back of the eyeball. Fibers that catch light from the peripheral (temporal) fields of vision actually cross to the other side of the brain through an optic chiasm. Thus, strokes or other lesions that affect vision will cause different deficits depending on where they affect the optic nerve. (From Sadler TW. Langman's Medical Embryology, 9th Edition. Baltimore: Lippincott Williams & Wilkins, 2004. Figure 10.4, p. 652.)

stimulates the medial aspect of the retina in each eye. These retinal fibers route back through the optic nerve and cross over to the opposite side in the **optic chiasm**. Thus, each side of the brain processes light signals that originate from the opposite side of the world in front of you (see Fig. 6.36). Light coming in from your right side, for example, reaches only the left side of your brain, because it stimulates the lateral aspect of the retina in the left eye (ipsilateral transmission) and the medial aspect of the retina in the right eye (contralateral transmission). Although these pathways may seem confusing, they help you to locate the position of a specific lesion or insult to the visual pathway: A patient with no ability to see out of one eye likely has a lesion in the optic nerve; a patient with limited peripheral vision likely has a lesion in the optic chiasm; and a patient with deficient perception of one side of his or her world likely has a lesion in the optic tract of the opposite side.

Cranial Nerve III: Oculomotor nerve

This cranial nerve provides motor innervation to four of the muscles that move the eyeball and one muscle that lifts the eyelid. It gives the lens of the eye the capability to accommodate its focus, and it gives the pupil of the eye the ability to constrict its aperture (limiting the amount of light that reaches the lens). This is the nerve of "looking." The muscles that move the eyeball are called **extraocular** muscles (Fig. 6.37A; see also Chapter 7). Their cell cluster origin is unclear, but they may arise from what are thought to be three clusters of myotomic cells in the mesenchyme just above the pharyngeal arches (preotic). If so, this would explain why the combination of seven extraocular muscles is driven by three different and dedicated cranial nerves (**cranial nerves III, IV**, and **VI**).

As its name implies, this nerve is primarily a motor nerve. In addition to its regular motor component to the extraocular muscles, it is one of the four cranial nerves that contain parasympathetic fibers of the autonomic system (see Fig. 6.37B). In general, parasympathetic fibers cause smooth muscles or glands to behave in a "status quo," or equilibrated, state. For the eye, this means a controlled amount of light to stimulate the optic nerve and responsive "bending" of the lens to keep the light focused on the retina as objects move closer or farther away. These are the functions of pupillary **constriction** and **accommodation**, respectively.

Parasympathetic nerves typically synapse in a ganglion near the tissue that they serve (see the discussion of autonomic nerves below). In this case, the ganglion is called the **ciliary ganglion**, and it dangles off of the oculomotor nerve near the back of the orbit. Parasympathetic fibers depart the oculomotor nerve, run through the ganglion to synapse, and then route directly into the eyeball. Some of them go to a smooth muscle called the **sphincter pupillae**, which pulls on the spindles of the iris, thus closing the aperture (**pupil**) of the opening in the middle of all the iris spindles. This action is similar to changing the aperture on a camera. It is a parasympathetic function, because the resting state of our vision is to see well with a narrow aperture.

The other parasympathetic fibers run to smooth muscle fibers of the ciliary body that surround the edges of the lens, thus bending or flattening its curvature. This keeps the incoming light focused on the retina even as the object that reflects it is moving. This is called accommodation. It is a parasympathetic action, because in a resting, "default" state, we would like to see perfectly. There is no sympathetic counteraction to accommodation (i.e., no subconscious choice to go out of focus), but for many people, the accommodation reflex needs help from the external lenses of eyeglasses or contacts.

Damage to the oculomotor nerve could result in pupils that are dilated even when stimulated by a light, because the sympathetic input to dilator pupillae is not balanced

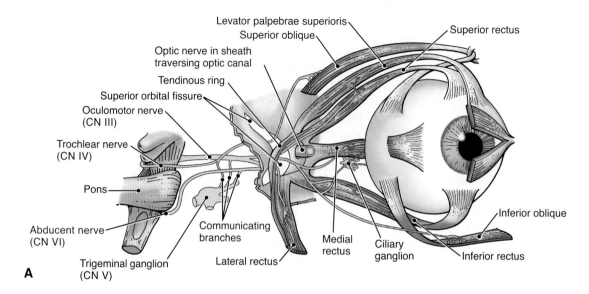

Levator palpebrae superioris
Superior oblique
Optic nerve in sheath traversing optic canal
Tendinous ring
Superior orbital fissure
Oculomotor nerve (CN III)
Trochlear nerve (CN IV)
Pons
Abducent nerve (CN VI)
Trigeminal ganglion (CN V)
Communicating branches
Lateral rectus
Medial rectus
Ciliary ganglion
Inferior rectus
Inferior oblique
Superior rectus

A

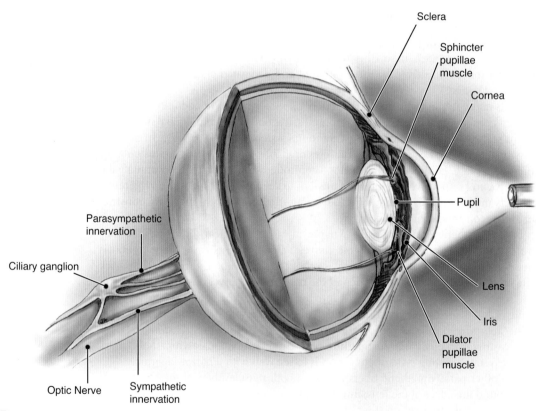

Sclera
Sphincter pupillae muscle
Cornea
Pupil
Lens
Iris
Dilator pupillae muscle
Parasympathetic innervation
Ciliary ganglion
Optic Nerve
Sympathetic innervation

B

by a working parasympathetic input to the sphincter pupillae. Likewise, the patient may be unable to accommodate focus on a moving object. Lesions that affect the motor innervation to the extraocular muscles result in a spectrum of problems characterized by the inability to move the eye medially (i.e., an uncorrected "down and out" gaze; see Chapter 7). Any of these conditions may be accompanied by "droopy lid," or **ptosis**, which is the inability to lift the eyelid fully over the pupil.

Cranial Nerve IV: Trochlear nerve

Cranial nerve IV provides motor innervation to a single eye muscle, the superior oblique muscle (see Fig. 6.37A). That is all.

The superior oblique muscle of the eye rotates the eye downward and outward. Because the nerve has such a singular role, damage to it (e.g., from a stroke) can be evaluated directly via a clinical examination. The affected patient will have difficulty gazing downward when you direct the patient's eye medially (see Chapter 7).

Cranial Nerve V: Trigeminal nerve

Cranial nerve V provides sensation from almost all head surfaces (Fig. 6.38). It also powers the muscles that you use for chewing and four muscles associated with the evolution of the jaw apparatus in mammals. It provides general sensory and general motor fibers—and a lot of them—but nothing else.

This nerve is called the trigeminal nerve because it divides into three fiber bundles after leaving the brain. These bundles are named for the general region they serve: the **ophthalmic**, the **maxillary**, and the **mandibular** (or V_1, V_2, and V_3, respectively). Only the mandibular division carries motor fibers.

The sensory distribution of the trigeminal nerve is a testament to how extensively the ectoderm wraps around the neural tube and the endoderm. Because the endoderm gives rise to separate respiratory and digestive systems, the skin of the face must adapt separately to the needs of these two intake holes (the **nose** and the **mouth**). Within the mouth, the ectoderm gives rise to cheek lining, gums, palate mucosa, hardened tooth enamel, and a loosened skin wrap for the bulging tongue.

Perhaps the most fascinating adaptation of ectoderm is the eyeball. The skin between the retina and the outside world develops into a cooperative arrangement of sclera and a translucent layer called the **cornea**. By virtue of being modified skin, these tissues need general sensation, which is provided by the trigeminal nerve.

FIGURE 6.37   **Cranial nerves III (oculomotor nerve), IV (trochlear nerve), and VI (abducens nerve).**

Cranial nerves III, IV and VI position the eyeball **(A).** This schematic figure shows the six muscles that move the eyeball and the muscle that elevates the eyelid. Cranial nerve (CN) III provides motor innervation to all but two of these muscles. Cranial nerve IV provides motor innervation to only the superior oblique muscle, and cranial nerve VI provides motor innervation to only the lateral rectus muscle. (See Chapter 7 for details of eye movement.) Cranial nerve III also constricts the pupil and bends the lens **(B).** The oculomotor nerve parasympathetically responds to light stimulation by narrowing the aperture of the pupil (sphincter pupillae). When the light level is low, sympathetic nerve fibers respond by firing the antagonistic dilator pupillae. The default tension on the lens can be relaxed when the parasympathetic impulse through the oculomotor nerve fires the ciliary muscle, which suspends the lens much like the border of a trampoline. When the circumferential muscle fires, the filaments holding the lens slacken and the lens bulges, making it easier to focus on close objects. (From Moore KL, Dalley AF. Clinically Oriented Anatomy, 5th Edition. Baltimore: Lippincott Williams & Wilkins, 2006. Figure 7.37, p. 970.)

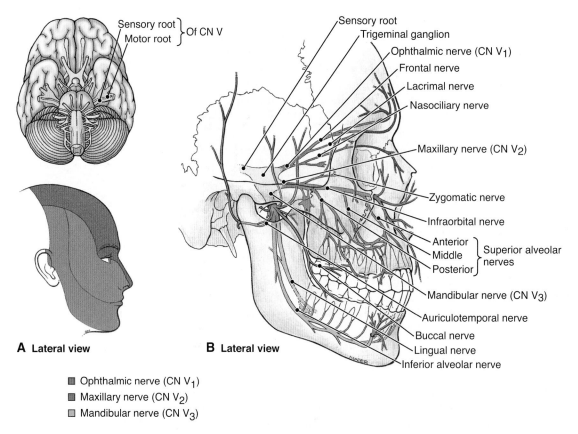

A Lateral view   **B** Lateral view

■ Ophthalmic nerve (CN V₁)
■ Maxillary nerve (CN V₂)
■ Mandibular nerve (CN V₃)

FIGURE 6.38   **Cranial nerve V (trigeminal nerve).**

Although this large cranial nerve (CN) has many peripheral branches, it has relatively few functions: general sensation from virtually all facial contact surfaces (**A**), and motor innervation to muscles of the first pharyngeal arch via the mandibular division (**B**). (From Moore KL, Dalley AF. Clinically Oriented Anatomy, 5th Edition. Baltimore: Lippincott Williams & Wilkins, 2006. Figure 9.6, p. 1140.)

The brain tissue itself does not sense pain, pressure, touch, or temperature, but its meninges do—and quite acutely. For the most part, cranial nerve V serves the meninges through fibers that travel alongside the middle meningeal artery. Occipital regions of the meninges are served by meningeal branches of cranial nerve X (the vagus nerve).

The skin of the outer ear is the only other area of the outer head that draws general sensation from nerves other than cranial nerve V. This is because the external ear derives from areas of the neck that converge on the routes of other cranial nerves (cranial nerves VII, IX, and X). The ear canal, however, and onto the tympanic membrane is ectoderm covering the exposure of the brain to the outside world and, thus, is innervated by the trigeminal nerve.

Cranial nerve V is the dedicated nerve of the first arch; thus, it provides some motor fibers to muscles that condense from the cell clusters of that arch. First arch clusters form the muscles of mastication (masseter, temporalis, medial pterygoid, and lateral pterygoid), two other muscles related to the mandible (anterior digastric and mylohyoid), and two muscles that track the uppermost reaches of the arch (tensor tympani and tensor veli palatini). Most students learn the motor innervation of the trigeminal nerve as "Muscles of Mastication plus MATT."

Cranial nerve V is large. Many of the dissectible gross nerve fibers in the head are pieces of it, and a number of them have descriptive names. The names given to the branches of the root tend to reflect where the nerve is located or headed.

Cranial Nerve V: Ophthalmic Division   This first division of trigeminal serves the eye region, the forehead above the eyes, and parts of the external and internal nose (see Fig. 6.38). As it enters the back of the orbit, cranial nerve V divides into three branches: the **frontal**, the **lacrimal**, and the **nasociliary**. The frontal nerve surfs along the top of the orbit and pushes out to the skin of the forehead through holes in the frontal bone. Here, we call the two nerve bundles the **supraorbital nerve** and the **supratrochlear nerve**, which are named for where they emerge relative to the eye. The trochlear region of the eye is toward the middle; from here, the nerves spread up to serve the forehead.

The lacrimal branch heads out alongside the orbit, eventually piercing the lacrimal gland and reaching the skin at the outside corner of the eye. It does not power the lacrimal gland (see *Cranial Nerve VII*). The nasociliary branch covers the eyeball itself and the upper part of the nose (both inside and out). Within the orbit, it plugs into the back of the eyeball and distributes to the surfaces of the eye. At the cornea, it initiates the blink reflex when something gets close to the eyeball. Other fibers skip past the globe along the inside of the orbit and enter the ethmoid bone as the **anterior ethmoidal nerve** and the **posterior ethmoidal nerve**. These will serve the air pockets (sinuses) of the ethmoid, the inner and outer skin linings of the top of the nose, and the upper eyelid.

Cranial Nerve V: Maxillary Division   This middle division also is purely sensory, and it targets the surfaces below the eyes but above the chin (roughly, the surfaces that cover the maxillary bone and its nearest neighbors). It emerges onto the skin of the face through a prominent hole in the maxilla just below the eye socket. This is called the **infraorbital foramen**, and the nerve bundle at this point is called the **infraorbital nerve**.

The zygomatic nerve branch covers the skin over the zygomatic bone and in the area under the eyeball. The lacrimal gland is in the outer part of the orbit, where the zygomatic bone sutures onto the frontal bone. The zygomatic nerve ferries a parasympathetic branch of cranial nerve VII near to this point.

As its name implies, the **sphenopalatine nerve** travels near the pterygoid plates of the sphenoid bone and the vertical portion of the palatine bone. A tiny space between these two bones is room for the **pterygopalatine ganglion**, one of the synapsing stations for parasympathetic nerves. The pterygopalatine branch of the maxillary division of the trigeminal nerve supports the ganglion, and it sends sensory fibers beyond it to targets on the soft palate and the inner lining of the nasal cavity. These nerves are named the **greater palatine nerve, lesser palatine nerve, posterior superior nasal nerves**, and **nasopalatine nerve**, based on their locations.

The bulk of the maxillary division that does not detour up as the zygomatic nerve or down through the pterygopalatine ganglion instead moves forward, toward the foramen that will allow it to reach the skin over the maxilla. This path takes it through the floor of the big maxillary sinus and perches the nerve just above the roots of the upper teeth. Branches of the maxillary division at this point shoot downward as the superior alveolar nerves to serve the sensitive tissue around the upper teeth and gums.

At last, the maxillary division reaches the skin of the face. Having spun off fibers to do the internal linings of the oral and nasal cavities, the remaining maxillary division fiber bundles exit the maxilla through the infraorbital foramen. They splay over parts of the cheek, upper lip, lower eyelid, and temporal region. What the infraorbital nerve does not cover superior to this sweep is covered by the ophthalmic division, and what it fails to cover inferiorly is handled by the mandibular division.

Cranial Nerve V: Mandibular Division   This division handles all the motor commitments of the trigeminal nerve and the sensory areas that remain on the face above the "chin-to-ear" line. This includes, importantly, the tongue surface, the lower lip, and some of the external ear. The majority of motor fibers travel to the four muscles of mastication and the muscle that bridges the floor of the mouth deep to the tongue (the mylohyoid). The routes for these motor fibers are through the infratemporal fossa, a space that is deep to the arch of the zygomatic bone. Within the fossa, muscles of mastication reach onto the mandible to pull the jaw closed and back and forth. Holes in the cranial bones transmit cranial nerves that travel forward, through the fossa, to reach the muscles and the surface structures. Here, a prominent hole is the **foramen ovale**, through which emerges the mandibular division of the trigeminal nerve. Aside from the fibers that motor the chewing muscle, the nerve ramifies into four large bundles with specific names.

The **buccal nerve** heads forward, into the skin that forms the loose cheek. This skin includes a dry outside surface (served mostly by the infraorbital nerve of the maxillary division) and a wet inside surface that runs from the upper gums to the lower gums. This skin acts as a trampoline for food particles that bounce away from the toothrow. This wet inner cheek is sensitive to pain, pressure, touch, and temperature, so it needs cranial nerve V.

The **lingual nerve** is dedicated to the surface of the front two-thirds of the tongue and brings general sensory information from it back to the brain. This surface of the tongue also is capable of detecting the chemical compounds that we call "tastes," so the lingual nerve is ideally positioned to provide these nerve endings as well—but does not. Indeed, this branch of cranial nerve V, like other branches, is simply a carrier for the special fibers that are rooted in other cranial nerves. The lingual nerve ferries a branch of cranial nerve VII called the **chorda tympani nerve** (see below) to the anterior two-thirds of the tongue so that it can serve the taste buds. Also, because it is already a taxi for this purpose, why not tack on parasympathetic fibers to the two nearby salivary glands (submandibular and sublingual)? No problem. From cranial nerve VII, via the chorda tympani bundle, the lingual nerve ferries parasympathetic fibers on their way to the submandibular and sublingual salivary glands.

Each of the divisions of cranial nerve V is destined for a hole through which it can reach the skin on the surface of the head. For the mandibular division, the **inferior alveolar nerve** is headed toward a hole in the mandible (the **mental foramen**) near the front teeth. When it emerges onto the skin of the chin, it is called the **mental nerve**. To get there, it burrows into the body of the mandible, so that it can serve, conveniently, the lower teeth along the way. It also carries some motor fibers that are destined for the mylohyoid muscle.

Because of the way in which the mandible develops, the branch of trigeminal devoted to it also serves areas behind the mandible and around the ear. The **auriculotemporal nerve** branch of the mandibular division of the trigeminal nerve runs sideways out of the foramen ovale, and it hits the skin near the ear. From there, it runs along the path of the superficial temporal artery and then spiders into the ear canal to serve the ectoderm between the external ear hole and the tympanic membrane. This pathway puts it very near the parotid salivary gland, which is innervated by cranial nerve IX. Indeed, the ganglion for the parasympathetic fibers of cranial nerve IX hangs off of the auriculotemporal nerve, and the auriculotemporal nerve ferries the fibers of cranial nerve IX from the ganglion to the gland.

Cranial Nerve VI: Abducens nerve
Cranial nerve VI provides motor innervation only one muscle of the eye, the lateral rectus. That is all.

The name of this nerve actually implies its action, which is to abduct the eye, or to move the eyes to the side (see Fig. 6.37A). If this nerve is compromised, the patient will be unable to keep the eye centered on the affected side. It will deviate medially instead.

Cranial Nerve VII: Facial nerve
Cranial nerve VII carries four modalities: general sensory, special sensory (taste), motor, and parasympathetic (Fig. 6.39). It is the dedicated cranial nerve of the second developmental arch of the head (the trigeminal nerve tracked the first arch) and, in large part, governs the way the head "expresses" and senses taste compounds. Knowledge of where the different functional components separate from one another is useful for clinical patient evaluation.

General Sensory Fibers   The only area of the head that is served by the general sensory fibers is the area around the lower part of the ear (where cranial nerve VII, IX, and X skin fibers converge). The facial nerve is in the vicinity because when the whole nerve leaves the brain, it enters the internal acoustic meatus and winds through the deep chambers of the temporal bone to reach its target tissues. This is by far the least important function of the facial nerve.

Special Sensory Fibers   The facial nerve detects taste for the anterior two-thirds of the tongue. The back of the tongue is closer to the pharynx and, thus, is in the domain of the glossopharyngeal nerve (cranial nerve IX). The taste fibers of the facial nerve bundle together as the **chorda tympani**; as the name indicates, this nerve bundle runs in a sort of tangent to the tympanic membrane at that point in the middle ear where the bundle departs from the facial nerve. Once the chorda tympani fibers slip through a crack in the temporal bone and enter the infratemporal fossa (see *Cranial Nerve V*), they can "hitch a ride" on the lingual nerve to reach the tongue.

The facial nerve also is said to provide taste capacity to the soft palate, especially in children. These nerve fibers travel a much different route, mostly in the company of parasympathetic fibers also from cranial nerve VII (see below).

General Motor Fibers   The facial nerve governs the "muscles of facial expression plus P-S-S," where P-S-S stands for posterior digastric, stapedius, and stylohyoid. All three of these muscles are related to the muscle-forming tissue cluster in the second arch of head development. The stapedius gets incorporated into the delicate function of the inner ear vibratory mechanism. The facial nerve sends a fiber its way as it routes through the inner ear toward its exit from the skull (the stylomastoid foramen).

The other two muscles anchor onto the styloid process itself, making them available to motor fibers of the facial nerve. That leaves the cluster of muscles of facial expression, which range from the scalp (to raise the eyebrows in astonishment) down to the clavicle (to stiffen the neck skin in extreme grimace). To satisfy this broad

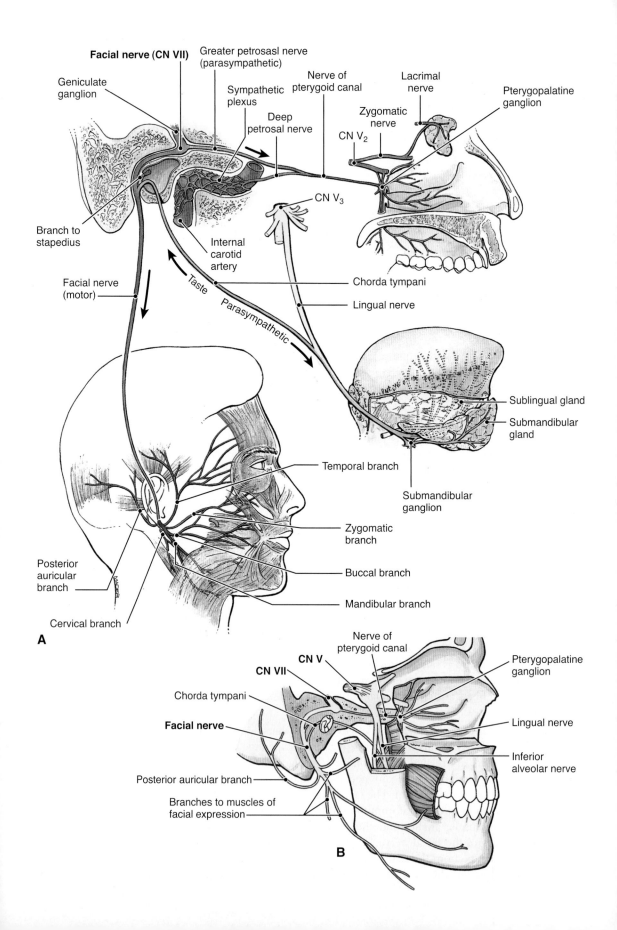

A

Facial nerve (CN VII)
Greater petrosasl nerve (parasympathetic)
Geniculate ganglion
Sympathetic plexus
Nerve of pterygoid canal
Lacrimal nerve
Deep petrosal nerve
Zygomatic nerve
Pterygopalatine ganglion
CN V₂
Branch to stapedius
CN V₃
Internal carotid artery
Chorda tympani
Facial nerve (motor)
Taste
Parasympathetic
Lingual nerve
Sublingual gland
Submandibular gland
Temporal branch
Submandibular ganglion
Zygomatic branch
Buccal branch
Posterior auricular branch
Mandibular branch
Cervical branch

B

Nerve of pterygoid canal
CN V
CN VII
Pterygopalatine ganglion
Chorda tympani
Facial nerve
Lingual nerve
Inferior alveolar nerve
Posterior auricular branch
Branches to muscles of facial expression

coverage of the superficial fascia (where the muscles are embedded), the facial nerve emerges from the stylomastoid foramen behind the lower jaw as a kind of trunk. From there, it ramifies into several branches in a fan-like design, all hidden in the substance of the parotid gland but very near the superficial fascia. Once through the substance of the parotid gland, the branches snake along the fascial plane to reach each and every expression fiber bundle.

Parasympathetic Fibers   The facial nerve is responsible for secretion in the **lacrimal gland** (tears), the wet linings of the nose and upper throat, and two salivary glands (**submandibular** and **sublingual**). These targets range from the top of the orbit to the floor of the mouth—and that is a lot of distance. To manage this, the facial nerve sends fibers toward a deep gap between the face skeleton and the brain skeleton (the **pterygopalatine fossa**), and from there, they tag along with fibers of cranial nerve V, blood vessels, or both to reach their final destination.

To reach the submandibular and sublingual salivary glands, the parasympathetic fibers leave the facial nerve deep in the ear region and join up with the chorda tympani nerve. They hang onto the chorda tympani nerve for as long as they can. Ultimately, however, that nerve is going to the tongue, and these fibers need to reach glands beneath the tongue. So, the fibers depart choroa tympani and enter a submandibular ganglion under the floor of the mouth, where they synapse. Postsynaptic fibers continue from there to the two target glands.

Parasympathetic fibers also need to reach secretory tissues in the lining of the nasal cavity and palate. To get there, fibers break off early from the facial nerve, before it has wound too deeply through the inner ear. This branch is called the **greater petrosal nerve**, and it angles forward through a gap into the small space between the pterygoid plates of the sphenoid bone and the vertical plate of the palatine bone (the pterygopalatine fossa). Here, you will find the pterygopalatine ganglion, a kind of "middle of the head cross-roads" for parasympathetic fibers of cranial nerve VII. From the pterygopalatine ganglion, parasympathetic fibers move forward in parallel to the palatine and nasal pathways of the maxillary division of the trigeminal nerve. Additionally, they may carry some taste fibers that provide taste capability to the palate.

Only the lacrimal gland is left. From the central station of the pterygopalatine ganglion, which hangs from the maxillary division of the trigeminal nerve, parasympathetic fibers reach up to ride the zygomatic branch into the floor of the orbit. From there, they ascend to the lacrimal gland in the upper outer quadrant. This represents one of the longest treks of a parasympathetic fiber after it has left its ganglion and before it reaches its target organ.

FIGURE 6.39   **Cranial nerve VII (facial nerve).**

The facial nerve provides motor innervation to all the muscles of facial expression and the three muscle derivatives of the second pharyngeal arch (posterior digastric, stapedius, and stylohyoid). It parasympathetically fires three of the four glands in the head: the submandibular and sublingual salivary glands, and the lacrimal gland (**A**). Other parasympathetic fibers stimulate mucous secretion in the nose and palate. Taste fibers from the anterior two-thirds of the tongue follow the path of the lingual branch of cranial nerve (CN) V until just before entering the cranium as a distinct chorda tympani nerve (**B**). (From Moore KL, Agur AMR. Essential Clinical Anatomy, 2nd Edition. Baltimore: Lippincott Williams & Wilkins, 2002.)

Cranial Nerve VIII: Vestibulocochlear nerve

Cranial Nerve VIII provides the special senses of hearing and balance. That is all.

The "organs" of hearing and balance are deeply embedded in the internal ear chamber of the hardest bone of the human body—the petrous portion of the temporal bone (Fig. 6.40). The nerve endings that detect fluid motion and signal balance in the brain are separate from the nerve endings that detect the vibrations of sound waves.

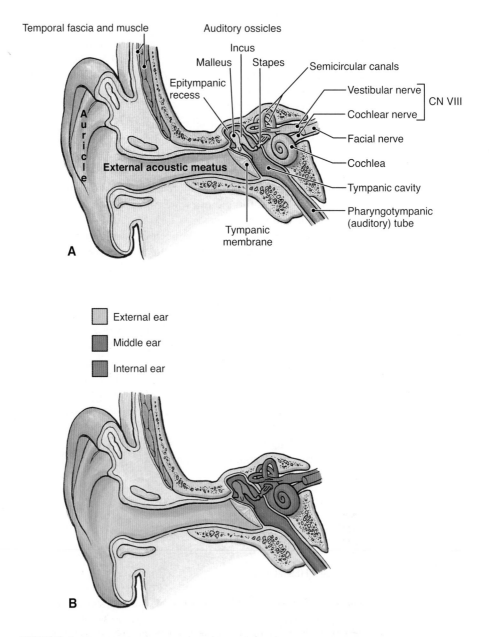

FIGURE 6.40   Cranial nerve VIII (vestibulocochlear nerve).

Hearing and balance are mostly unrelated neural phenomena, but the nerve fibers that conduct them run side by side in the bundle of cranial nerve (CN) VIII (**A**), and they end in different regions of the same bony "organ" in the internal ear chamber (**B**). (From Moore KL, Agur AMR. Essential Clinical Anatomy, 2nd Edition. Baltimore: Lippincott Williams & Wilkins, 2002. Figure 8.47, p. 578.)

Although the vestibulocochlear nerve is named as a single bundle of nerve fibers, its two functions are structurally and neurally separate. They do share the same "house" in the temporal bone, however, and the nerve endings are stimulated by the same basic phenomenon of fluid moving over exposed, hair-like filaments, causing a change in polarity that is modulated by the stimulus itself.

These delicate nerve endings must be protected. They are housed in the rock-hard petrous portion of the temporal bone, safe from direct exposure to the outside world. For sound waves to reach the nerve endings, the anatomy between the outer ear and the nerve endings must be conducive and conductive. The skin surface of the "ear" ranges from the elaborate folding of the "radar dish" of the external ear to the narrow canal and then, finally, to the tympanic membrane. As noted above, the tympanic membrane is the tightly stretched remnant of the first pharyngeal cleft and pouch. It is so tight and thin that sound waves within the "audible" part of the spectrum make it vibrate.

The vibration of the tympanic membrane is now the translated sound signal, but it is still removed from the endings of the vestibulocochlear nerve. Resident in the chamber behind the eardrum are the small remnant bones of the first and second pharyngeal arches, the ear ossicles. These tiny bones articulate with one another in an unusual chain connecting the tympanic membrane to the outer wall of the cochlea, the bony house of the auditory endings of the vestibulocochlear nerve. The vibrating tympanic membrane rattles the **malleus**, which rattles the **incus**, which taps the **stapes** bone, which drums a membrane that covers the oval window of the cochlea. This translated wave is now conducted through the fluid of the cochlea and against the exposed endings of the vestibulocochlear nerve.

The cochlea forms a spiral ducting in which the sound waves travel and a labyrinthine ducting within which balance is detected. This labyrinthine apparatus has three "opposing," semicircular ducts of fluid connected at a saccular and utricular vestibule. Because the ducts are in cardinal orientation to each other, any movement of the head can be registered. The central pools of fluid in the saccule and utricle shift with acceleration and deceleration of a level head, thus accounting for other possible displacements. Balance is the special sense of detecting the position of the head at all times. It makes perfect sense that the nerve endings sensitive to fluid displacement are encased in a deep and hardened block of bone—the inner ear, or petrous portion of the temporal bone.

Cranial Nerve IX: Glossopharyngeal nerve

Cranial Nerve IX provides a variety of services to the back of the tongue, the throat, and one of the salivary glands (Fig. 6.41). Like the facial nerve, it has several functional fiber groups, including general sensory, special sensory, motor, and parasympathetic. It is the dedicated cranial nerve of the third developmental arch of the head. In the big picture, however, its role and course are relatively simple.

The most important thing to remember about the glossopharyngeal nerve is that it works closely with the vagus nerve (cranial nerve X). Together, they form a **pharyngeal plexus** to manage swallowing, including a gag reflex in response to unwanted swallowing. It generally is assumed that the sensory arc of the gag reflex travels in the glossopharyngeal nerve. After leaving the brain, the glossopharyngeal nerve travels in close company with the vagus nerve into the jugular foramen and, from there, into the adjacent pharyngeal sleeve.

The glossopharyngeal nerve provides general sensory innervation to the outer ear, the mucous membranes of the pharynx, and the posterior one-third of the tongue. The large base of the tongue sits like an inward bulge of throat skin. Closer to the throat than to the lips, this is the domain the glossopharyngeal nerve. In one of the rare

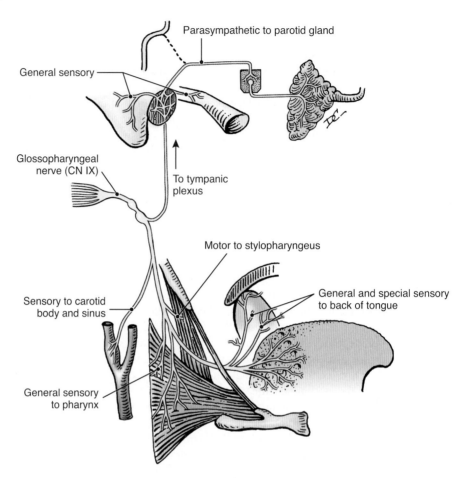

FIGURE 6.41   **Cranial nerve IX (glossopharyngeal nerve).**

Cranial nerve (CN) IX is dedicated to the derivatives of the third pharyngeal arch, which locate to the back of the oral cavity and upper pharynx. This schematic illustration displays the functional pathways of the nerve, from parasympathetic to the parotid salivary gland, to general sensation fibers from the back of the tongue and upper pharynx to taste fibers from the posterior third of the tongue and motor innervation to the one striated muscle derived from the third arch (stylopharyngeus). The one exotic function of this nerve is its reach to the base of the internal carotid artery, where it traffics messages of blood pressure and oxygen saturation back to the brain. (From Agur A, Dalley AF. Grant's Atlas of Anatomy, 11th Edition. Baltimore: Lippincott Williams & Wilkins, 2005.)

examples of efficiency in the cranial nerves, the same nerve here provides both general and special taste sensory fibers.

The glossopharyngeal nerve also trickles down the internal carotid artery (which enters the skull near to where the glossopharyngeal nerve exits) to reach the bulge in the internal carotid at the base of its emergence (the **carotid sinus**). The tissue of the artery at this point is sensitive to pressure (baroreception), and a special cluster of cells called the **carotid body** is sensitive to chemical concentrations in the blood (chemoreception). Blood pressure and oxygen saturation levels of blood heading to the brain are transmitted by the glossopharyngeal nerve. In the event of problems with either hemodynamic, the central nervous system responds by changing heart rate, force of contraction, rate of respiration, or some combination of the three.

Only one voluntary muscle appears to be linked to the third developmental arch of the head—the stylopharyngeus muscle, which is one of many accessory muscles of swallowing. The glossopharyngeal nerve provides its motor innervation. The parasympathetic fibers that leave glossopharyngeal nerve and, eventually, reach the parotid salivary gland begin as a bundle called the **lesser petrosal nerve**. They squeeze into the infratemporal fossa, form the otic ganglion dangling off of the mandibular division of the trigeminal nerve, and then follow the auriculotemporal nerve out to the side of the head, where they serve the **parotid gland**.

Cranial Nerve X: Vagus nerve

In addition to its collegial role with the glossopharyngeal nerve in the pharynx, the vagus nerve (cranial nerve X) handles all motor and sensory innervation to the larynx. It further provides general sensory innervation to the back of the meninges and the outer ear, taste from the epiglottis, and most of the vital parasympathetic function of tissues from the throat down to the descending colon (Fig. 6.42). It is essentially the nerve of swallowing, speaking, and comfortable breathing, pulsing, and digesting.

The vagus nerve arises more posteriorly from the brain than the trigeminal nerve does; this better positions the vagus nerve for general sensory innervation to the meninges of the posterior cranial fossa. The vagus nerve joins the facial, glossopharyngeal, and trigeminal nerves for some trivial sensory coverage of the outer ear. On its own and through the pharyngeal plexus, it provides some sensory innervation to the linings of the pharynx and larynx. Two named branches in this category are not part of the plexus. The **superior laryngeal nerve** departs from the ﹍gus nerve shortly after emerging through the jugular foramen, and it angles for﹍ ﹍ inward, toward the tracheal region of the neck. Just above the prominen﹍ ﹍ge, it sends an **internal laryngeal** branch through the connective ﹍ ﹍brane; this branch provides sensory innervation to the many﹍ ﹍harynx, particularly above the vocal cords.

The rest of the superior laryngeal nerve ﹍ ﹍ich angles slightly more inferiorly to penetrate ﹍ ﹍ricoid cartilage to the thyroid cartilage. This muscle ﹍ ﹍ts motor innervation is provided by this wayward branch ﹍ ﹍ is notable because all the other laryngeal muscles are innerv﹍ **﹍ent laryngeal branch** of the vagus nerve. It is called recurrent becau﹍ ﹍ splits from the vagus trunk in the thorax of the body, then recurs around a l﹍ ﹍ery to run back up into the neck alongside the trachea.

In addition to general sensation, the vagus gives the epiglottis the capacity to taste. The epiglottis is the lid that flaps down over the trachea when you swallow so that food does not inadvertently end up in the respiratory system. It derives from the base of the tongue bud within the tissue of the fourth pharyngeal arch—the domain of cranial nerve X.

As part of the pharyngeal plexus, the vagus nerve provides motor to the many subtle muscles of the pharynx and larynx. These muscles enable you to more or less "close off" the nasal cavity and respiratory tube when you swallow and narrow the back of the throat to direct food into the pharynx. The pharyngeal muscles contract in a kind of pulse that moves food toward the esophagus in a wave motion, similar to the peristalsis of the smooth muscle in the esophagus and beyond (see Chapter 7).

Parasympathetic conduct is the dominant mode of the vagus nerve. It provides parasympathetic capacity to the lungs, heart, gut tube (down to the descending colon), and kidneys. This parasympathetic activity, in general, is homeostatic, secretory, and restorative. You should not eat "on the run," for example, because the heightened

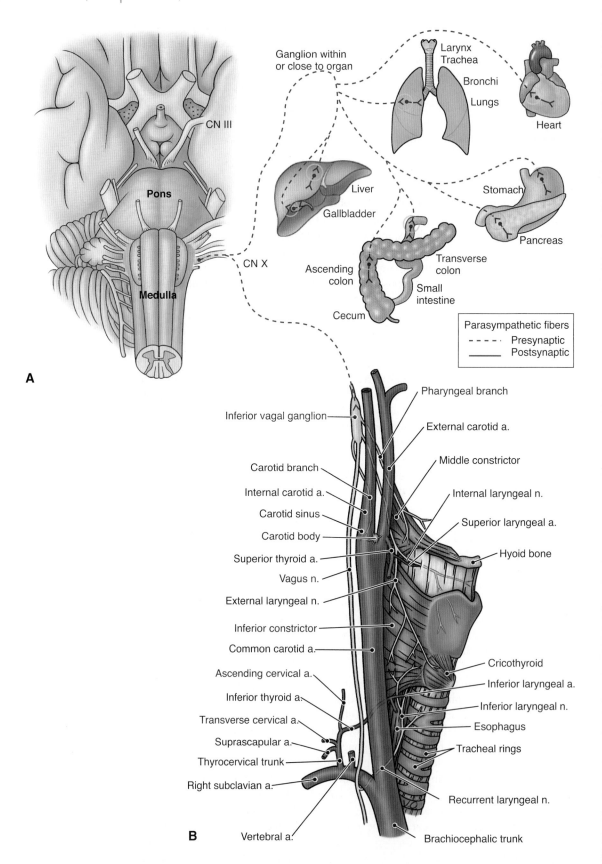

Ganglion within
or close to organ

Larynx
Trachea

Bronchi

Lungs

Heart

CN III

Pons

Liver

Gallbladder

Stomach

Pancreas

CN X

Ascending
colon

Transverse
colon

Small
intestine

Medulla

Cecum

Parasympathetic fibers	
- - - -	Presynaptic
——	Postsynaptic

A

Pharyngeal branch

Inferior vagal ganglion

External carotid a.

Carotid branch

Middle constrictor

Internal carotid a.

Internal laryngeal n.

Carotid sinus

Superior laryngeal a.

Carotid body

Superior thyroid a.

Hyoid bone

Vagus n.

External laryngeal n.

Inferior constrictor

Common carotid a.

Cricothyroid

Ascending cervical a.

Inferior laryngeal a.

Inferior thyroid a.

Inferior laryngeal n.

Transverse cervical a.

Esophagus

Suprascapular a.

Tracheal rings

Thyrocervical trunk

Right subclavian a.

Recurrent laryngeal n.

B   Vertebral a.

Brachiocephalic trunk

activity of doing something else while eating excites the sympathetic impulses of the nervous system. The body stops digesting until the other activity subsides. Resting heart rate and quiet respiration are two other major vagal domains.

As noted above, the vagus nerve bundle quickly sends fibers to do the local work as it emerges from the jugular foramen. The remaining large bundle of fibers keeps moving "south," nestled comfortably behind the large jugular vein and the carotid artery. It even gets wrapped within their protective carotid sheath of fascia. Just below the subclavian artery on the right side and below the arch of the aorta on the left, fibers peel off of the vagus nerve and head back up into the neck. These are the **recurrent laryngeal nerves** (motor and sensory to the larynx, and they have a peculiar course because of how those developmental arches of the head deal with the longitudinal folding of the embryo.

Once into the thorax, the vagus bundle sidles up to the esophagus and the aorta. From this position, it can send out plexuses, like spiderwebs, to nearby organs (e.g., the heart). To reach more distant organs, the vagus bundle typically sends out plexuses along the branches of the aorta that serve them. The plexuses include contributions from the sympathetic nerve fibers of the nervous system (see below), so the organs experience a kind of subconscious "yin and yang" control—excitability and "relax"-ability.

In the thorax, both the vagus nerve from the right side and the vagus nerve from the left side send pulmonary plexuses out along the root of the lung to serve the lung and cardiac plexuses directly to the heart. At the same time, they weave around the esophagus (and serve its smooth muscle) to form anterior and posterior vagal trunks. Then, they pass through the esophageal hiatus of the diaphragm and into the cavernous abdomen.

The vagal trunks now lose their gross identity as they cascade down the gut tube. Vagal fibers communicate back along blood vessels to the major trunks of the aorta (celiac trunk, superior mesenteric artery, etc.), where they merge with sympathetic fibers to form plexuses. These include the celiac plexus, the superior mesenteric plexus, and the hypogastric plexuses. Then, they pass back out along other branches of these trunks to the accessory organs of digestion.

The ganglia that these vagal fibers must reach before serving their organs are dispersed within the walls of the gut tube and are unnamed in gross anatomy. The vagus nerve web around the gut tube continues along the duodenum, jejunum, and ileum and then up the ascending colon and across the transverse colon. Somewhere near where the transverse colon becomes the descending colon, the vagus nerve "peters out," and parasympathetic service is taken over by nerves that emanate from the sacral region of the spinal cord (see below).

Cranial Nerve XI: Accessory nerve

Cranial nerve XI provides motor to sternocleidomastoid and trapezius muscles. That is all.

The name of this nerve refers to the fact that some nuclei that appear to be associated with it in the brainstem travel with the vagus nerve (as an "accessory"). The

---

FIGURE 6.42   **Cranial nerve X (vagus nerve).**

In addition to major parasympathetic service to the heart, lungs, and gut tube (**A**), the vagus nerve provides motor and sensory innervation to the pharynx and laryngeal derivatives of the lower pharyngeal arches. It provides motor innervation to all muscles of speaking and all constrictor and some accessory muscles of swallowing (**B**). a. = artery; CN = cranial nerve; n. = nerve. (From Moore KL, Agur AMR. Essential Clinical Anatomy, 2nd Edition. Baltimore: Lippincott Williams & Wilkins, 2002.)

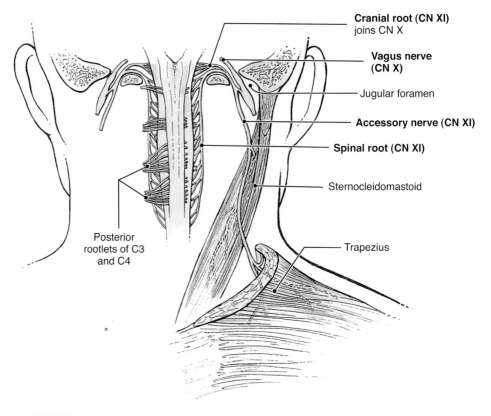

Cranial root (CN XI)
joins CN X

**Vagus nerve
(CN X)**

Jugular foramen

Accessory nerve (CN XI)

Spinal root (CN XI)

Sternocleidomastoid

Posterior
rootlets of C3
and C4

Trapezius

FIGURE 6.43   **Cranial nerve XI (accessory nerve).**

The roots of this nerve are actually in the spinal cord, but it migrates into the cranium and then out the jugular foramen, mimicking the path of a cranial nerve (CN). It provides motor innervation to the prime movers of the head (sternocleidomastoid and trapezius). (From Moore KL, Agur AMR. Essential Clinical Anatomy, 2nd Edition. Baltimore: Lippincott Williams & Wilkins, 2002. Figure 10.14, p. 666.)

fibers that provide motor to the sternocleidomastoid and trapezius actually begin as nuclei in the spinal cord; they just happen to arc up through the foramen magnum and exit the skull through the jugular foramen and, thus, look like a cranial nerve (Fig. 6.43).

Cranial Nerve XII: Hypoglossal nerve
Cranial nerve XII provides motor to all intrinsic and most extrinsic muscles of the tongue.

The name of the nerve refers to the fact that it approaches the tongue from below (Fig. 6.44). Indeed, the sweep of this nerve around the angle of the lower jaw is one of the signature views in the dissection of the carotid triangle of the neck. After leaving the brain, the nerve occupies its own foramen in the occipital bone, the **hypoglossal canal**. From there, it runs, like the wiring under a computer desk, among branches of the external carotid, the styloid process muscles, and myriad veins clustered behind the back of the lower jaw. It finally slips into the bed of the mouth between two muscles (the hyoglossus and the mylohyoid).

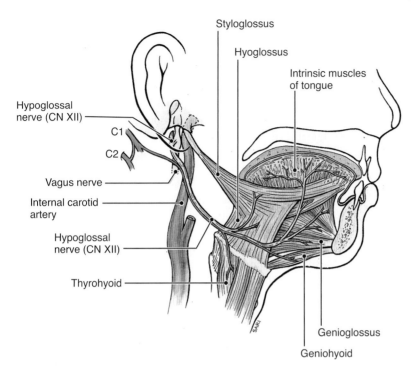

FIGURE 6.44   **Cranial nerve XII (hypoglossal nerve).**

The nerve provides motor innervation to the major muscle of the tongue, genioglossus, most of the other muscles that connect to the tongue, and all the intrinsic muscles that are embedded in the tongue surface. CN = cranial nerve. (From Moore KL, Agur AMR. Essential Clinical Anatomy, 2nd Edition. Baltimore: Lippincott Williams & Wilkins, 2002. Figure 10.15, p. 667.)

Although the tongue is anchored to the inner rim of the front of the mandible, it is an extremely mobile and "expressionable" muscular projection, because the anchoring muscle (the genioglossus) inserts on the skin of the tongue, not onto another bone. Other extrinsic muscles do the same but from other hard attachments: the hyoglossus (to the hyoid bone), the styloglossus (to the styloid process), and the palatoglossus (to the palate). In addition, some muscles are intrinsic only to the "waggable" part of the tongue and, thus, enable you to curl, flatten, or otherwise contort the tongue surface. The hypoglossal nerve innervates each of these except for the palatoglossus muscle, which is innervated by the vagus nerve.

The Autonomic Nervous System

You have learned about the general organization of the autonomic nervous system into a parasympathetic set of nerves and a sympathetic set of nerves. You have just studied the four cranial nerves that carry parasympathetic fibers (cranial nerves III, VII, IX, and X). You are aware of how the sympathetic system begins in the spinal cord (from the T1-L2 levels) and interacts with the spinal nerves to reach its own chain of ganglia (the sympathetic trunk) draped alongside the vertebral bodies. Now, we have to describe how the sympathetic and sacral parasympathetic fibers get to their destinations.

Autonomic nerves to the major organs

Autonomic responses either maintain default activity levels or heighten them. The physical nerve pathways for each type of response are separate. In general, fibers that heighten activity as needed are part of the sympathetic fiber network. Fibers that restore activity levels are part of the parasympathetic network. Restoration can be an active process (requiring parasympathetic wiring) or a passive process (simply the absence of sympathetic stimulation). Sweat glands, for example, secrete sympatheti-cally. In the resting state, the gland is inactive, so sweat glands do not receive parasym-pathetic wiring. Salivary glands, on the other hand, secrete in the "resting" state; thus, "dry mouth" is a result of anxiety and heightened activity of the sympathetic system. In this case, the gland receives both types of fibers, one of which is secretory (parasympa-thetic) and one of which is inhibitory (sympathetic). Parasympathetic wiring is more limited, and most of it is contained in the cranial nerve service to the head and the vagal service to the viscera described above. Only the sacral parasympathetic fibers remain. The sympathetic fiber network is much more extensive, and its description begins with targets in the head and then moves down the trunk.

Consider what functions the sympathetic nerves have in the head. Just as in all parts of the body, the nerves must reach smooth muscle in the arteries (for vasocon-striction), sweat glands, and the "goose bump" centers. The sympathetic system also must reach all the areas that are served by its counterpart, the parasympathetic system, such as the salivary, mucous, and lacrimal glands, as well as the muscles around the lens of the eye. To do this, the fibers will leave the sympathetic chain and track blood vessels headed to the same targets (Fig. 6.45).

To see in the dark, the retina needs to have as much light as possible pass through the lens. The pupil dilates to allow all the light around you inside. The parasympa-thetic system keeps the pupil constricted to a status-quo level; the sympathetic system dilates it for increased light flow. Because the sympathetic impulse comes from the spinal cord, a patient with severe brain damage may have pupils that are "fixed and dilated," because the sympathetic signal to dilate is unopposed by a damaged parasym-pathetic signal, which is housed in the brain.

The sympathetic system, therefore, plays a key role in the balance of subconscious function in the head, but how does it get there? Sympathetic nerve fibers emerge from the spinal cord between T1 and L2, follow a route along the ventral root into the spinal nerve, and then travel out of the nerve along a white ramus into the sympathetic chain. Once in the sympathetic chain, the fibers ascend through the chain to the inferior, middle, and superior cervical ganglia. The superior cervical ganglion is alongside the internal carotid artery very near the base of the skull. From these cervical ganglia, the sympathetic fibers jockey the carotid arteries toward every possible destination in the head and neck.

To reach the targets of the oculomotor nerve (the ciliary body and muscle), the internal carotid plexus of sympathetic fibers clings to the artery until its ophthalmic artery branch. From there, it makes a short hop off the artery and through the ciliary ganglion to mingle with the parasympathetic fibers of the oculomotor nerve, which have synapsed in the ganglion and are headed into the eyeball.

The facial nerve delivers three routes of parasympathetic service: to the lacrimal gland (an orbital vector), to the mucous glands of the nose and palate (a maxillary vec-tor), and to the submandibular and sublingual salivary glands (a mandibular vector). In each case, sympathetic fibers peel off of nearby arteries and cling to proximal bun-dles of the facial nerve as they exit the cranium and enter the pterygopalatine and infratemporal spaces behind your nasopharynx.

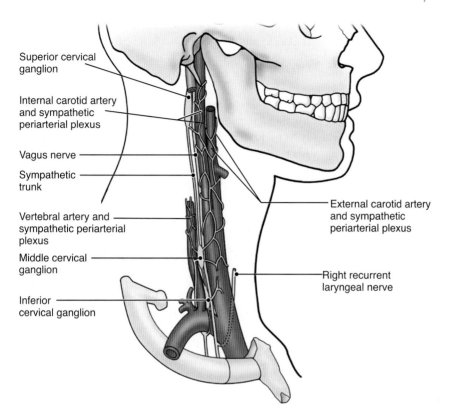

Superior cervical
ganglion

Internal carotid artery
and sympathetic
periarterial plexus

Vagus nerve

Sympathetic
trunk

Vertebral artery and
sympathetic periarterial
plexus

Middle cervical
ganglion

Inferior
cervical ganglion

External carotid artery
and sympathetic
periarterial plexus

Right recurrent
laryngeal nerve

FIGURE 6.45   Sympathetic nerves climb the carotid artery to reach the head.

The most direct route for sympathetic fibers to reach gland and smooth muscle targets in the head is
to jump onto the carotid artery system from the cervical ganglia of the sympathetic chain. (From
Moore KL, Dalley AF. Clinically Oriented Anatomy, 5th Edition. Baltimore: Lippincott Williams &
Wilkins, 2006. Figure 8.20A, p. 1080.)

Sympathetic nerves reach the parotid gland (parasympathetic service from cranial
nerve IX) by hopping off the internal carotid artery and meshing through the tympanic
plexus of cranial nerves to emerge as part of the lesser petrosal nerve. The lesser petrosal nerve then pierces the base of the skull near the foramen ovale and enters the otic
ganglion hanging off of the auriculotemporal branch of trigeminal. It routes to the
gland by tagging along with the auriculotemporal nerve, which is the part of trigeminal nerve (cranial nerve V) that provides sensation to the skin surrounding the parotid
gland.

In the neck and remaining parts of the body, the sympathetic fiber network must
reach all sweat glands, arterial smooth muscle, and the hair-erection beds. These
routes follow the same path everywhere. Sympathetic fibers track out along spinal
nerve pathways all the way to the dermis (to serve sweat glands and erector pillae muscles) or until they can jump to a neighboring artery. These routes are largely unnamed
in gross anatomy because their clinical presentations (e.g., in the event of trauma) are
less readily apparent than are the effects of damage to the spinal nerves with which they
travel (e.g., paresthesia and paralysis).

The remaining service of the sympathetic system is to the major organs and viscera
of the body (heart, lungs, digestive system, bladder, etc.). The fibers for these services

depart the chain much differently than the fibers that are busy hitting all the arterial smooth muscle, body sweat glands, and hair erectors. As a result, these fiber bundles tend to have specific descriptive names. In general, these bundles use the familiar method of reaching their target organs by tracking the blood vessels that are dedicated to the same organs.

Sympathetic fibers must help to excite the functions of the heart and lungs. These organ targets are very near the thoracic parts of the sympathetic chain, so the dedicated sympathetic fibers (typically from T1-T5) simply migrate out of the sympathetic ganglia and toward the vagus fibers collected along the esophagus. Somewhere posterior to the arch of the aorta and in front of the bifurcation of the pulmonary trunk, parasympathetic and sympathetic fibers come together as the cardiac plexus. A pulmonary plexus to serve the respiratory system comes together near the root of each lung and fully communicates with the cardiac plexus (Fig. 6.46).

The source of sympathetic fibers to serve the organs of the abdomen is in the thorax, because most of the sympathetic system is headquartered there (remember, the T1-L2 levels of the spinal cord). For dedicated organ fibers to reach the gut tube, they must depart the chain above their level of service, and they must angle down toward the midline of the body to be close to the vagus fibers they complement. This trajectory makes them grossly visible during dissection of the posterior thorax. They are called the greater thoracic splanchnic nerve, the lesser thoracic splanchnic nerve, and the least thoracic splanchnic nerve.

The **greater thoracic splanchnic nerve** typically carries fibers from the T5-T9 region of the spinal cord, and it runs a characteristic, diagonal course from the sympathetic chain "down and in" toward the aorta. The same applies to the **lesser thoracic splanchnic nerve** (T10-T11) and the **least thoracic splanchnic nerve** (T12), but as their names indicate, they are smaller in proportion and, thus, are more difficult to find. These fibers have not yet synapsed in a ganglion; rather, they are headed toward ganglia located along branches of the aorta closer to the organs they serve. These will be the celiac ganglion, the superior mesenteric ganglion, and various ganglia perched near the renal arteries and the inferior mesenteric artery (Fig. 6.47).

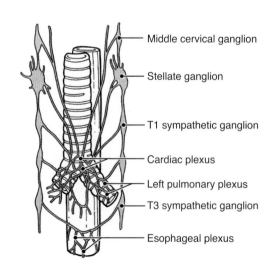

FIGURE 6.46 Autonomic nerve supply to the lungs and heart.

Smooth muscle constricts and dilates the respiratory tree and also powers the heart. Parasympathetic fibers from the vagus and sympathetics synapsing in cervical and upper thoracic ganglia coalesce into a "plexus at the nexus" at the base of the trachea. Sympathetic stimulation increases heart rate and respiratory capacity; parasympathetic stimulation restores resting heart rate and respiration. (From Moore KL, Agur AMR. Essential Clinical Anatomy, 2nd Edition. Baltimore: Lippincott Williams & Wilkins, 2002. Figure 2.37C, p. 111.)

Middle cervical ganglion

Stellate ganglion

T1 sympathetic ganglion

Cardiac plexus

Left pulmonary plexus

T3 sympathetic ganglion

Esophageal plexus

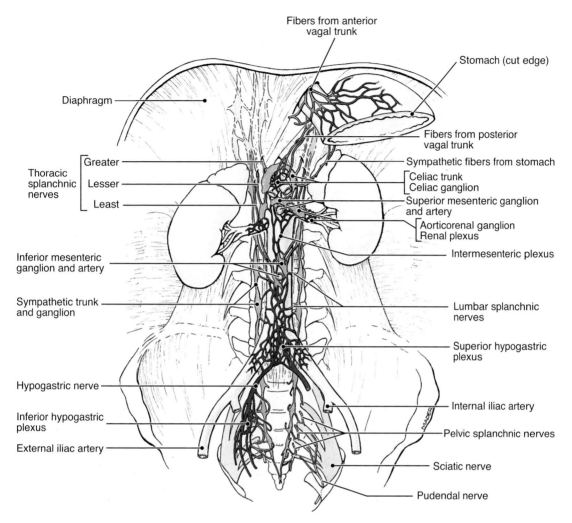

FIGURE 6.47   **Autonomic nerve supply to abdominal and pelvic viscera.**

Several plexuses of parasympathetic fibers (from the vagus nerve or the pelvic splanchnic nerves) and sympathetic fibers (all direct from the sympathetic chain via the greater, lesser, least, and lumbar splanchnic nerves) drape the abdominal aorta and its common iliac stems. Each gut tube artery has a plexus, and superior and inferior hypogastric plexuses complete the netting. In general, sympathetic stimulation arrests gut tube contraction and secretion, whereas parasympathetic stimulation restores it. Both forces interact to facilitate urination, defecation, and sexual stimulation. (From Moore KL, Agur AMR. Essential Clinical Anatomy, 2nd Edition. Baltimore: Lippincott Williams & Wilkins, 2002. Figure 3.41, p. 193.)

The first and second lumbar levels of the sympathetic system are not to be left out of the splanchnic adventure. They form lumbar splanchnic nerves that travel a much shorter distance to reach the aortic plexuses. The lumbar levels of the sympathetic system serve the lower parts of the gastrointestinal tube, the bladder, and the reproductive organs via superior and inferior hypogastric plexuses dangling off of the bifurcation of the aorta—and that concludes the extent of the sympathetic service to the organs of the abdomen and pelvis. The sympathetic chain, of course, continues down along the vertebrae toward the sacrum, providing ramus links back to each spinal nerve along the way. These are the hard-working, "soldier" fibers of the system that are destined for body wall and limb arteries, sweat glands, and piloerectors.

For the abdomen, however, we must fill in the plexuses that combine the sympathetic splanchnic nerves with the vagus fishnet coursing down the gut tube. Remember that the vagus net concludes at approximately the point where the transverse colon becomes the descending colon. This means that parasympathetic service to the rest of the gut tube and to the pelvic reproductive organs must come from the sacral source of parasympathetic nerves. In gross anatomy, these fibers rarely are seen as a discrete group, but they do get a discrete name, the **pelvic splanchnic nerves**. They emerge along with sacral spinal nerves, then depart to join the plexuses that hang off of the bifurcation of the aorta or are draped along its iliac continuation.

Superior Hypogastric Plexus

This named plexus typically is located at the most inferior part of the aorta at the point of its bifurcation into the common iliac arteries. It receives **sympathetic** fibers from the **lumbar splanchnic nerves** and routes them either to viscera (urinary or gonadal) or to the **inferior hypogastric plexus**. Like all the named plexuses along the aorta, this plexus of fibers is continuous with those above it (the mesenteric plexuses) and those below it (the inferior hypogastric plexus) (see Fig. 6.47).

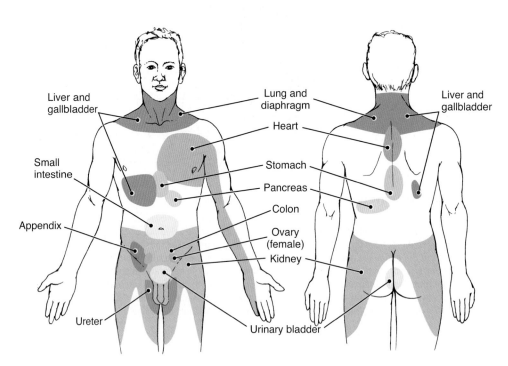

FIGURE 6.48   **Organ pain is felt in referred zones on the skin.**

Referred pain is a complex dynamic. Sensations of discomfort that originate in organ tissue often agitate somatic structures in contact with the organ, such as the pleura, pericardium, and peritoneum, which is one reason why referred liver pain tracks the C3-C5 dermatomes. Other sensations agitate adjacent bundles of spinal nerve fibers at the level where the pertinent sympathetic fibers connect to the spinal cord and, thus, are perceived along those spinal nerve dermatomes (e.g., referred pain from the kidney). (From Porth CM. Pathophysiology: Concepts in Altered Health States, 6th Edition. Philadelphia: Lippincott Williams & Wilkins, 2002.)

Inferior Hypogastric Plexus

This plexus is located along the **internal iliac artery**, which means that it is a bilateral plexus. It receives **sympathetic** fibers from the **superior hypogastric plexus** as well as **parasympathetic** fibers from the **pelvic splanchnic nerves** (S2-S4). The parasympathetic fibers will join the distribution of the sympathetic fibers for service to pelvic organs, or they will travel up the network of plexuses to gain the **inferior mesenteric artery**, which will transmit the fibers to the hindgut derivatives of the colon that they serve.

The route of autonomic nerves from these plexuses to their targets is simple. They follow the arteries that serve the same targets. These targets include the smooth muscle of the entire gut tube, bladder, vas deferens, ovary, prostate gland, uterus, vagina, urethra, and cavernous erectile tissue of the external genitals.

One of the first clinical signs of organ disturbance is **referred pain** (Fig. 6.48). Because the fibers of the autonomic system convey general rather than specific sensations of discomfort, they inform the brain of "states of being" in visceral tissues but not particular locations. Electrical activity in the visceral afferent fibers, however, can stimulate the neighboring spinal nerve fibers within the dorsal root as they pass from the sympathetic chain into the spinal cord. In these cases, the agitation may register in the brain as discomfort along the territory (the dermatome) served by the spinal nerve at that level. Because visceral pain travels in sympathetic fibers, areas of referred pain tend to be within the dermatomes of spinal nerves T1-L2. This may be why sensations of discomfort in patches of skin on the trunk correspond to disease states in particular organs, as depicted in Figure 6.48. Additionally, inflamed organs can physically irritate adjacent tissues that are innervated somatically. If an inflamed liver irritates the diaphragm, for example, the sensation will refer to the surface of the body served by the same spinal nerve levels that serve the diaphragm (C3-C5).

7

Muscle and Connective Tissues

INTRODUCTION

Mesoderm gives rise to all the tissues that enable you to move: muscles, tendons, bones, ligaments, and fascia. Some of these tissues are histologically distinct and well demarcated. Others, such as superficial fascia, are amorphous. Figuratively speaking, the mesoderm layer of the germ disc solidifies in some places, becomes elastic in others, and hardly changes in the connective spaces between them. In other words, as colonies of mesoderm cells condense into different degrees of rigidity, they never "lose touch" with one another. Histologists classify muscle cells separately from the "connective tissues" (bones, ligaments, tendons, and fascia), but muscles and connective tissues are all derived from mesoderm and are anatomically continuous with one another. Muscle cells simply have some properties, such as contractility, that are not found in the true connective tissues, so from a cellular perspective, they earn their own category.

Posture and movement require a variety of supportive tissues, from the rigid to the elastic and from dynamic muscle to static fat padding. **Bones** are often at the very core, or center, of a region. **Ligaments** strap one bone to another bone with little room for stretching. **Tendons** focus a body of muscle fibers onto a particular part of a bone. **Muscles** cross the space between two or more bones and alter that space by contracting. The tendons then transfer that force onto the bones, which move as a result but are guided by the limits imposed by the ligaments (and opposing muscles). Covering them all is undifferentiated **fascia**, always there and always ready to thicken as needed. It is a beautiful concert of cooperation, contention. and coordination.

FASCIA

Descriptions of fascias tend to be confusing, because fascias are simply more obvious layers of the general connective tissue packing of the body; all connective tissue in the body is continuous with all other connective tissue.

Hollinshead's Textbook of Anatomy, 5th ed., p. 21

Fascia is fascinating. It is like the leftover mesoderm after the specialized structures have formed, coating them like a blanket of construction dust. Fascia is a tissue membrane between the ectoderm and the muscle/connective tissues. Fascia is similar to the external surface of mesoderm, under the skin and above the muscles and bones. It consists of a loose, almost structureless **superficial fascia** and a defined **deep fascia** that is universal under the skin. Superficial fascia forms the dermis of the skin and contains fat in most places of the body. Because the connection between the superficial fascia and the deep fascia is so loose, a substantial amount of fat can accumulate in some places. In certain parts of the body, the superficial fascia is tightly bound to the deep fascia, and no fat is present (e.g., in the palm of the hand).

The deep fascia is multifunctional. It is made of much denser fibrous tissue, and it thickens in certain places to provide additional area for muscle attachment, to separate muscle groups from one another (thus, reducing friction heat during contraction), or to ensheath a neurovascular bundle (Fig. 7.1). Across the wrist and ankle joints, the deep fascia thickens even more, into **retinacula,** to strap the long flexor and extensor tendons in place. In further service to these muscles, the deep fascia reaches deeply to the finger and toe bones in the shape of a tunnel to confine the dedicated and hardworking tendons. You will need to learn the specific names for local thickenings of deep fascia, but you should also remember that deep fascia is a universal tissue layer under the skin throughout the body.

Remember the model of the animate life form. The mesoderm colony of cells that pours into place between the ectoderm and the endoderm gives the body both form

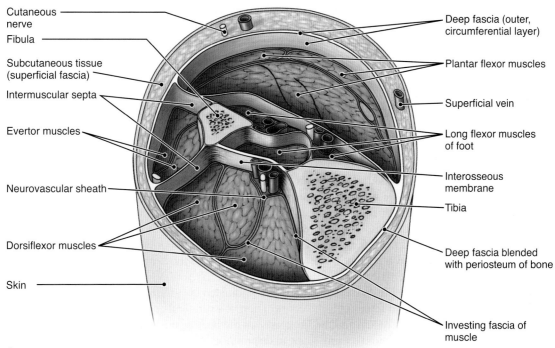

Cutaneous nerve

Fibula

Subcutaneous tissue (superficial fascia)

Intermuscular septa

Evertor muscles

Neurovascular sheath

Dorsiflexor muscles

Skin

Deep fascia (outer, circumferential layer)

Plantar flexor muscles

Superficial vein

Long flexor muscles of foot

Interosseous membrane

Tibia

Deep fascia blended with periosteum of bone

Investing fascia of muscle

A Anterosuperior view

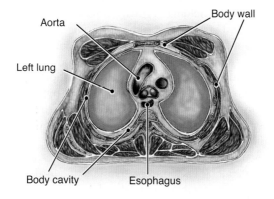

Aorta

Body wall

Left lung

Body cavity

Esophagus

B

FIGURE 7.1   **Fascia divides and supports.**

These cross-sections illustrate the structure of fascia in the body. Fascia is universal under the skin as either a superficial, fatty layer and/or a defined, deep layer. The deep layer exists everywhere and can specialize to form, among many other things, compartments for muscles (**A**). Throughout the body, the basic arrangement of an outer skin and an inner fascia, with muscles and a connective tissue (bony) framework, pertains. In the trunk, this arrangement surrounds a cavity (**B**). (Adapted from Moore KL, Dalley AF. Clinically Oriented Anatomy, 5th Edition. Baltimore: Lippincott Williams & Wilkins, 2006. Figure I.9.)

and the potential to move. The colony never separates from itself; rather, it morphs into structures along a continuum from rigid (bone) to loose (superficial fascia). In the cadaver laboratory, you will be impressed with the extent of fascia in the body and with the way it derives to serve the muscle/skin interface.

THE SKELETAL SYSTEM

Development

Recall that the mesoderm layer invades almost every available space between ectoderm and endoderm in the embryo before folding (see Figs. 1.11–1.18). We now consider how the mesoderm condenses to form tissues as rigid as bone and as elastic as muscle. In general, the paraxial mesoderm cells contribute to the vertebral skeleton, to most of the muscles that move the body, and to some of the dermal lining of the skin; the lateral plate mesoderm cells contribute to the majority of the dermis of the body "wall" (the sides and front of the "trunk") and to the bones of the limbs which are, developmentally, buds of the body wall (Fig. 7.2).

The ability to stand and move is coordinated by two major efforts of the mesoderm. The first and foremost is the construction of a vertebral column for support of the central nervous system and the "long axis" of the body against the effect of gravity. The second—folding into a trunk shape and sprouting limbs—supplements this potential.

The body can move because some soft tissues within it (muscles) pull on some hard tissues within it (bones), causing the mass to shift position in a controlled manner that converts the potential energy of gravitational pull into the kinetic energy of controlled "falling" or yielding to gravity. Bones form to give your mass a certain shape of resistance against gravity. This is the governing mechanism that underlies bone formation, and from this interplay of stability and mobility, you should be able to anticipate the anatomy of the individual bones in the body. Bones also serve other functions, such as mineral metabolism and blood cell formation, but their gross anatomy is best understood as a result of their role in position and movement.

One way to classify bone is by the process of ossification (bone growth) that it undergoes. In general, there are two types of ossification: **endochondral**, and **intramembranous**. The difference between these two types is that some bones form first as a soft (cartilaginous) model and then gradually replace the cartilage with mineral (endochondral ossification), but others form in response to the tissue that is growing "underneath" or around them (intramembranous ossification). The vast majority of bones in the body form first as cartilage models, providing a working frame that is strong enough to support you as you grow but still yielding and dynamic in the ways a growing body needs. As mentioned, these bones form through endochondral ossification, or literally "within cartilage" (Fig. 7.3). Endochondral bones tend to grow according to a basic "rod" or "cylinder" design, with modified ends to fulfill the demands of local function.

A few bones, mostly in the skull, form through intramembranous ossification (see Fig. 6.14). They harden within a bone-forming membrane or envelope, and they respond to the growth of adjacent tissue. The bones that form the upper and lateral boundaries of the braincase, for example, gradually solidify within a "cranial envelope" as the brain expands during the first 8 to 10 years of life. These bones can be said to provide a protective structure as opposed to the posture and locomotion function provided by the rest of the skeleton.

Consider the skeleton as a whole (Fig. 7.4). Some bones support the center, or trunk, or axis, of the body (the **axial skeleton**), and some bones support the limbs, or

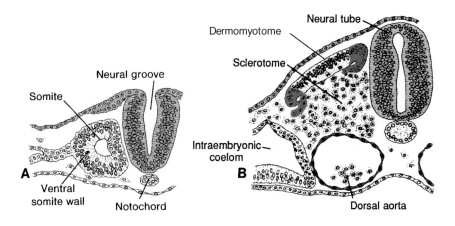

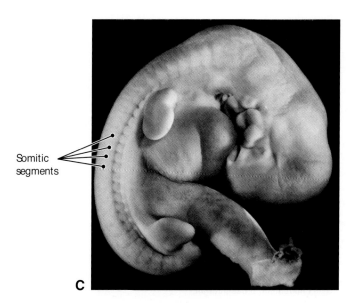

FIGURE 7.2   **Paraxial mesoderm establishes a skeleton.**

Remember that the clump of mesoderm that forms on either side of the neural tube is the paraxial mesoderm (**A**). It condenses to form segments of somites, from which the vertebrae derive (**B**). This is the beginning of the segmented axial skeleton, which is initially of equal components but eventually of specialized cervical, thoracic, lumbar, sacral, and coccygeal vertebral units (**C**). (Adapted from Sadler TW. Langman's Medical Embryology, 9th Edition. Baltimore: Lippincott Williams & Wilkins, 2004. Figure 5.19, p. 106; Figure 5.11, p. 98.)

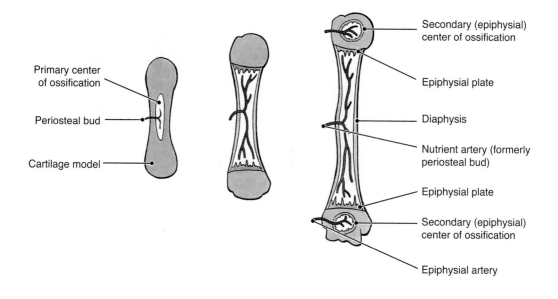

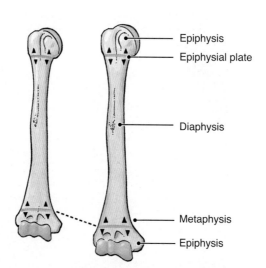

FIGURE 7.3   **Endochondral ossification.**

Mesoderm forms cartilaginous precursors of future bones. Ossification proceeds from the center to the periphery, where secondary centers facilitate growing joint articulations while allowing continued increase in size along the epiphyseal plates. (From Moore KL, Agur AMR. Essential Clinical Anatomy, 2nd Edition. Baltimore: Lippincott Williams & Wilkins, 2002. Figure 1.6, p. 15.)

FIGURE 7.4   **The skeleton in standard anatomic position.**

The axis of the body consists of the vertebral column, the skull, and the ribs that grow from the vertebrae and link to the sternum in the anterior midline. All other bones grow to support the limbs. Some, such as the clavicle and the "hip bone," anchor back to the axial skeleton. This whole-skeleton view conveys the dominant role that our appendages play in our posture and locomotion. (From Moore KL, Agur AMR. Essential Clinical Anatomy, 2nd Edition. Baltimore: Lippincott Williams & Wilkins, 2002. Figure 1.4, p. 11.)

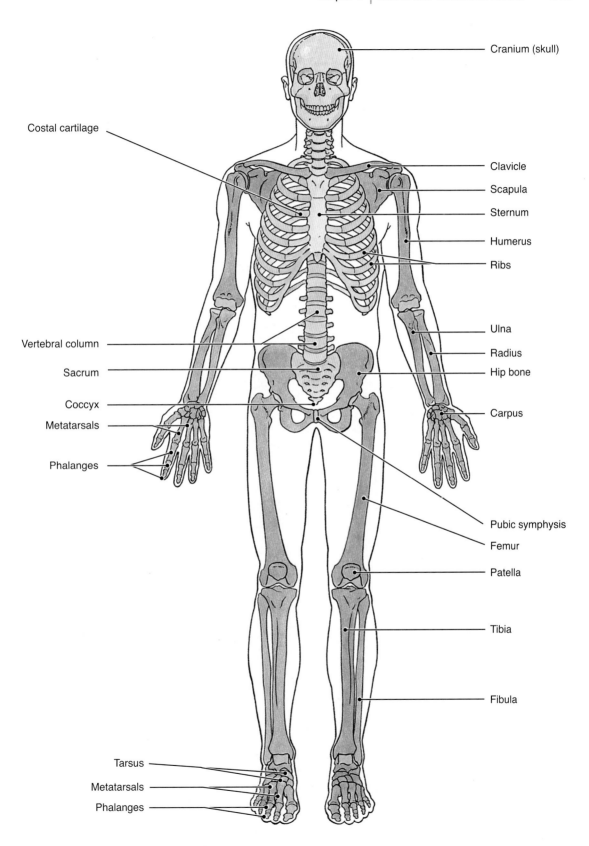

Cranium (skull)

Costal cartilage

Clavicle

Scapula

Sternum

Humerus

Ribs

Ulna

Radius

Hip bone

Vertebral column

Sacrum

Coccyx

Metatarsals

Phalanges

Carpus

Pubic symphysis

Femur

Patella

Tibia

Fibula

Tarsus

Metatarsals

Phalanges

appendices, that stick out from it (the **appendicular skeleton**). Because the appendicular skeleton makes contact with the world and is moved by some very large muscles, we are keenly familiar with its parts. By contrast, the axial skeleton is mostly abused by our sedentary lifestyles and its numerous governing muscles neglected by exercise programs. Much of the potential of physical therapy and rehabilitation, however, depends on a healthy axial skeleton, and we are all aware of the effects of age on flexibility.

The Body Axis: The Vertebrae and Vertebral Column

Animate life forms have axes, or some kind of linear arrangement that separates the intake end (generally the head end) from the outflow end (generally the tail end).

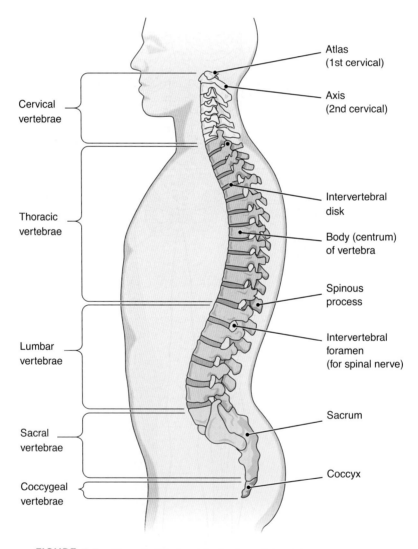

FIGURE 7.5   **The articulated vertebral column, lateral view.**

Bipedal posture "bends" the column into natural curvatures, which are called lordotic in the cervical and lumbar regions and kyphotic in the thoracic and sacral regions. (From Cohen BJ, Wood DL. Memmler's The Human Body in Health and Disease, 10th Edition. Baltimore: Lippincott Williams & Wilkins, 2004. Figure 7.10.)

Humans are no different, so the axis of the human body parallels the line connecting the mouth and the anus. In terms of bones, this axis is composed of the **vertebrae**, which collectively form the **vertebral column** (Fig. 7.5). Vertebrates have depth from front to back, so in places this axis wraps around, to reinforce the depth, in the form of the **ribs** and **sternum** (Fig. 7.6).

Developmentally, this axial skeleton is a literal axis on which the absorptive layer of tissue (the adult gut tube) hangs forward, or downward, and on which the sensory or processing layer (the central nervous system, which is shaped as the brain and spinal cord) lies. The value of protecting the central nervous system is obvious, so the axis bones grow arches devoted to surrounding it (Fig. 7.7). The upper part of the central nervous system is a more three-dimensional, voluminous expansion of the cord; as a result, an unusual type of bony growth (the intramembranous bones of the cranium) expands upward from the top of the vertebral column to house it.

Consider, then, that although you have 33 or so separate vertebrae, you really have a single type of vertebra that takes on five classes of shapes—from neck to "tail," **cervical**, **thoracic**, **lumbar**, **sacral**, and **coccygeal** (see Fig. 7.5). These vertebral regions are modified according to the role they play in maintaining upright posture and bipedal

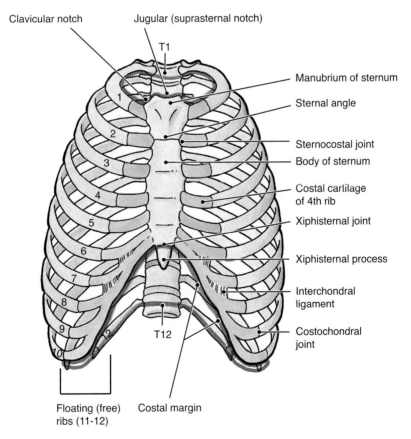

FIGURE 7.6   **Ribs and sternum, anterior view.**

The thoracic body wall adapts the costal processes of the vertebrae into a "cage" design of ribs that anchor, in some cases indirectly, to a sternum in the anterior midline. This unit as a whole is capable of some expansion during deep inspiration. (Adapted from Moore KL, Agur AMR. Essential Clinical Anatomy, 2nd Edition. Baltimore: Lippincott Williams & Wilkins, 2002. Figure 2.1A, p. 53.)

Parts:
Spinous process

Transverse process

Articular processes

Vertebral arch (lamina pedicle)

Vertebral body

Functions:
Muscle attachment and movement

Restriction of movement

Protection of spinal cord

Support of body weight

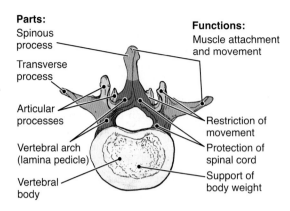

FIGURE 7.7   **Each vertebra has numerous parts, superior view.**

The elaborations away from the neural canal are lever arms and anchor points for axial muscles. (Adapted from Moore KL, Dalley AF. Clinically Oriented Anatomy, 5th Edition. Baltimore: Lippincott Williams & Wilkins, 2006. Figure 4.2A, p. 480.)

locomotion. They bear the weight of the body cumulatively from top to bottom, so it is no surprise that the sacral vertebrae, which help to transmit the weight across the hips and down into the legs, are wholly fused to one another. By comparison, the cervical vertebrae move quite loosely on one another, affording the head a wide range of motion.

A typical vertebra

The typical vertebra is one of the ingenious designs of nature. The grouping of all animals with bones is named Vertebrata, which reflects the uniform theme of this skeletal element across diverse taxa. A **vertebra** is composed of a body and a neural arch that sprouts off of the body posteriorly (or dorsally, to use the term from comparative anatomy). The neural arch begins as "tiny feet," or **pedicles**, rising off the contour of the vertebral body, and it continues as **laminae** on either side (see Fig. 7.7). The transition from pedicle to lamina is marked by a "sideways," or transverse, growth of bone called the **transverse process**. The laminae support articular surfaces that make contact with the laminae of both the vertebra above and the vertebra below. The laminae arc toward themselves, meeting in the midline as a merger called a **spinous process** (hence the terms "spine" and "spinal column"). These spines take on various lengths and angles of declination depending on where in the column they lie.

From this basic design, variations in the column accommodate differences in weight load, caliber of the spinal cord, movements to be allowed or prevented, and support of the ribs (Fig. 7.8). Thus, the cervical vertebrae tend to be small of body, long of spinous process (for all those neck muscles to support the giant head), and almost bereft of transverse projections. They also possess a hole on either side that permits the **vertebral artery** to reach the base of the brain in a well-protected route.

The thoracic vertebrae, by comparison, are somewhat thicker of body, have more steeped articular facets that are angled for reasonable side-bending but poor flexion and extension, and are possessed of remarkable transverse processes that support the ribs. This is another beautiful example of development, because the rib is nothing more than an elaborated anterior element of bony growth coming off of the pedicle. The technical

FIGURE 7.8   **Each vertebral design reflects its position.**

(**A**) The cervical, thoracic, lumbar, and sacral vertebrae develop the basic parts differently, depending on the mobility/stability trade-off in the neck, chest, abdomen, and pelvis, respectively. (**B**) The uppermost cervical vertebrae uniquely support mobility and stability of the skull as the atlas (C1) and axis (C2). (From Cohen BJ, Wood DL. Memmler's The Human Body in Health and Disease, 10th Edition. Baltimore: Lippincott Williams & Wilkins, 2004. Figures 7.11 and 7.12.)

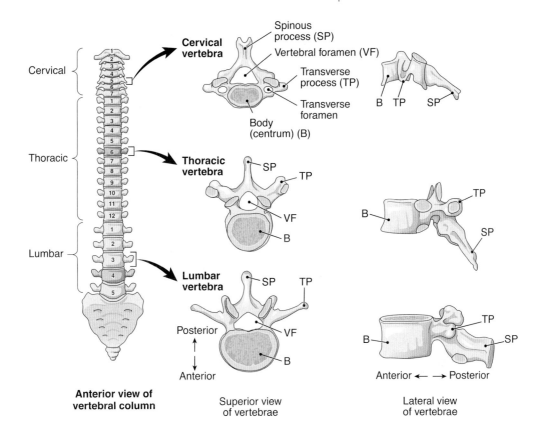

Cervical vertebra

Spinous process (SP)
Vertebral foramen (VF)
Transverse process (TP)
Transverse foramen
Body (centrum) (B)

B   TP   SP

Thoracic vertebra

SP
TP
VF
B

B
TP
SP

Lumbar vertebra

SP   TP
Posterior
VF
Anterior
B

B
TP
SP
Anterior ← → Posterior

Cervical

Thoracic

Lumbar

A

Anterior view of vertebral column

Superior view of vertebrae

Lateral view of vertebrae

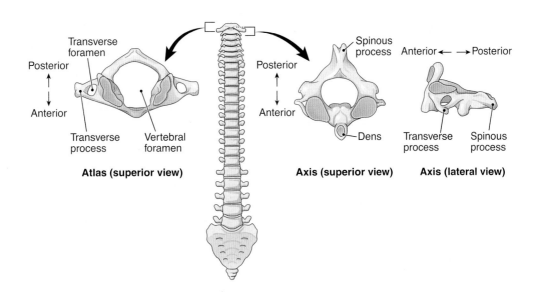

Transverse foramen
Posterior
Anterior
Transverse process
Vertebral foramen

Atlas (superior view)

Posterior
Anterior

Spinous process
Dens

Axis (superior view)

Anterior ← → Posterior
Transverse process
Spinous process

Axis (lateral view)

B

term for this is **costal process**, and in the thoracic region alone, the costal processes elongate to form ribs. In the cervical region, however, the costal processes remain stubby and help to form part of the transverse foramen through which the vertebral artery passes.

The bodies of lumbar vertebrae show the effects of increased weight-bearing, and the articular facets are rotated to be almost perpendicular to the thoracic facets. This enables this part of the column to flex and extend, but not to side-bend very easily. To your chagrin as you age, a short round of stretching exercises will confirm these potentials and limitations.

The sacral vertebrae fuse to one another during life and effectively become part of the pelvic skeleton leading to the lower limbs. The sacrum, however, remains a series of five basic vertebrae, albeit modified at the points of contact. Below the sacrum lie a variable number of coccygeal vertebrae. In many other vertebrates, these elements support the tail, or **caudal**, skeleton. In humans, they remain as a vestigial completion of the midline axis of the body.

The column is more than the sum of its parts

As a unit, the vertebral column is not a rigid axis. The joints enable some movement (see the discussion of arthrology below) and, more importantly, grow to conform to one another in a curved fashion. Two of the sections (cervical and lumbar) curve to become convex anteriorly and concave posteriorly, which is called a **lordotic curvature**. The thoracic and sacral vertebrae do the opposite, which is called a **kyphotic curvature**. Together, these curvatures give the vertebral column capacities like those of a spring for absorbing and transmitting force. These curvatures also can become abnormally exaggerated, as in the states of **lordosis** and **kyphosis** (Fig. 7.9).

The Skull

The skull image fascinates and provokes. It is one of those few universal symbols that can be recognized regardless of language. As noted above, the skull fills two main purposes: to house the central nervous system, and to give hard structure to the ports in the body that acquire energy. These two "parts" of the skull can be thought of as the **neurocranium** and the **splanchnocranium**, respectively, and they come together along midline bones that form the **basicranium**. The neurocranium has the particular feature of ossifying intramembranously, so its bones tend to be flat and shell-like and fit together along wiggly suture lines that provide an interlocking and interfingering fit. The splanchnocranium has the particular feature of housing elaborate knobs (**teeth**) for processing food and for evacuating itself with pockets of air (**sinuses**) to maintain equilibrium with atmospheric pressure (if not always effectively) as you breathe.

The brain is responsible for detecting the outside world and signaling parts of the body to respond to the information that it receives from the sensory nerves. Some of the sensory projections in the head form the core of familiar skull regions, such as the orbit and the ear canal. Together with incoming sensory nerve bundles, motor bundles also must pass from the brain to the body through holes (**foramina**, the plural of **foramen**) in the articulated skull. In addition blood vessels must either join with nerves during passage or travel through their own dedicated foramina to reach the same targets.

One other unpaired, central bone in the body is related to the skull. Suspended by numerous muscles between the sternum and the mandible is the **hyoid** bone. You can feel for it between the mandible and the thyroid ("Adam's apple") cartilage that projects against the skin of the neck. The hyoid provides a pivot point for the muscles that steer the front of the skull as you swallow (see *Muscles of Swallowing* below), and it suspends as a protective atoll of the larynx and pharynx that lie immediately deep to it.

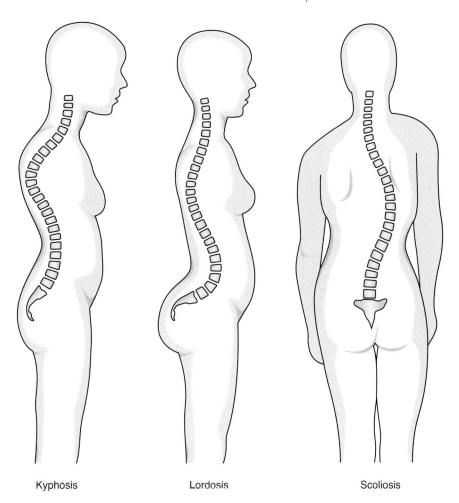

| Kyphosis | Lordosis | Scoliosis |

FIGURE 7.9 **Pathologic curvature of the spine.**

An abnormal, exaggerated curvature of the lumbar column is called a lordosis (e.g., "swayback") and of the thoracic column is called a kyphosis (e.g., "hunchback"). Lateral curvature is scoliosis, mild forms of which are very common. (From Cohen BJ, Wood DL. Memmler's The Human Body in Health and Disease, 10th Edition. Baltimore: Lippincott Williams & Wilkins, 2004. Figure 7.10.)

The skull bones fit together in joints that although technically capable of movement are virtually locked in place, thus rendering the "facial skeleton" a rigid composite rather than a jangling assortment of 10 or more interconnected bones (Fig. 7.10). Learning the names of isolated skull bones is of limited value to the clinician; the study of the cranial skeleton should be a study of the intact skull and the boundaries that it presents. In the section on the head and neck below, some of the pertinent aspects of the composite skull are demonstrated. For now, however, just think of the skull as a composite of a brain "house," capsules for its extensions (the ear, nose, and orbit cavities), and an apparatus for manipulating the opening of the gut tube, all mounted on a terminal plank of the vertebral column.

The Projections of the Body: The Limbs

For the limbs to perform as required, they are composed of a central set of long bones that are joined at the ends: the **humerus** and **ulna** in the upper limb, and the **femur**

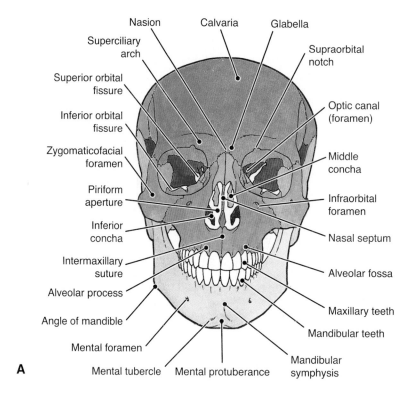

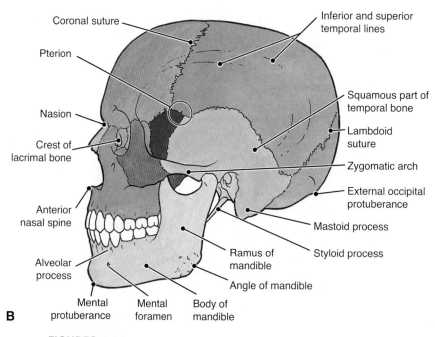

FIGURES 7.10   **The skull.**

The whole of the skull is greater than the sum of its parts, but knowing the names of the parts is essential. (**A**) Frontal view. (**B**) Lateral view. (**C**) Inferior view. (From Moore KL, Agur AMR. Essential Clinical Anatomy, 2nd Edition. Baltimore: Lippincott Williams & Wilkins, 2002. Figures 8.1 and 8.3.)

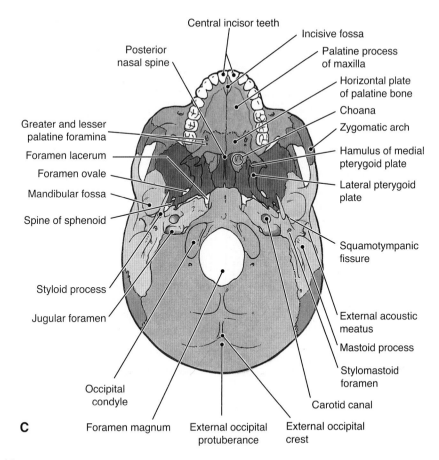

Central incisor teeth

Incisive fossa

Posterior
nasal spine

Palatine process
of maxilla

Horizontal plate
of palatine bone

Choana

Greater and lesser
palatine foramina

Zygomatic arch

Hamulus of medial
pterygoid plate

Foramen lacerum

Foramen ovale

Lateral pterygoid
plate

Mandibular fossa

Spine of sphenoid

Squamotympanic
fissure

Styloid process

Jugular foramen

External acoustic
meatus

Mastoid process

Stylomastoid
foramen

Occipital
condyle

Carotid canal

C   Foramen magnum   External occipital
protuberance

External occipital
crest

FIGURE 7.10   **The skull. *(continued)***

and **tibia** in the lower limb. The limb skeleton must anchor onto the body axis proximally, and it must elaborate distally into a contact zone with the environment. The **scapula** for the upper limb and the "hip" bone (**os coxa**) for the lower limb accomplish the anchoring part. The difference between the highly mobile scapula and the rigid pelvis reflects the very different functions of upper limbs versus lower limbs. Bones of the wrist and ankle and of the hand and foot likewise transform from a common theme according to how much contact they maintain with the environment. The demands on the lower limb, particularly its extremity (the foot), are so great that an entire field of medicine (podiatry) is devoted to it.

A highly mobile upper limb

The skeleton of the upper limb begins at the **scapula**, a rather flat bone that hovers along the back of the rib cage in a thick envelope of muscle (Fig. 7.11). It is very nearly a suspended bone, in the sense that it has no direct connection with the trunk skeleton but, rather, only a weak and oddly-angled connection to the **clavicle**, a strut-like bone that bridges the upper limb to the sternum. These bones are all about providing attachment to muscles that drive the arm and hand in activities that are displaced from the body; as such, the clavicle and scapula are not joined in a tightly wrapped or heavily ligamented joint.

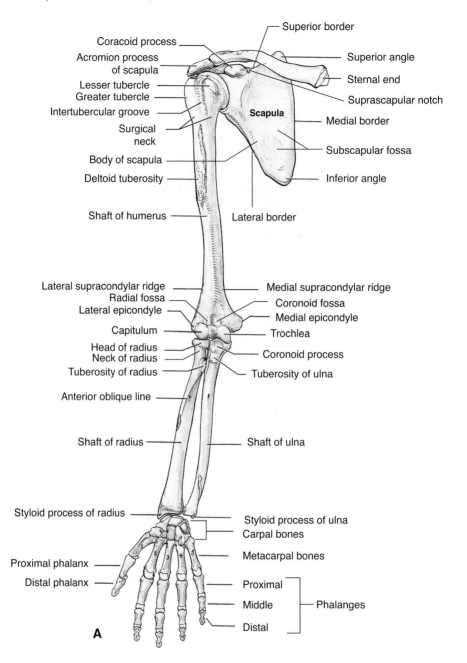

FIGURE 7.11   **The upper extremity skeleton.**

The scapula hovers against the back of the rib cage, ensheathed in a sleeve of multiple muscles that guide it back and forth against its only real joint—with the clavicle. For a bone that "anchors" the upper limb to the body wall, it is especially mobile. The humeral head is nearly spherical, providing unimpeded rotation against the scapula. The shaft tapers into epicondyles, which provide broad space for the attachment of muscles that move the forearm, wrist, and fingers. The different capitular and trochlear shapes of the condyle reflect the movements that are permitted to the radius and ulna, respectively. The forearm bones are shaped for a hinge-like motion at the humeroulnar joint and a rotating, or spinning, movement at the humeroradial joint. Note that at their distal ends, the radius dominates contact with the carpal bones, effectively governing the transmission of force across the wrist. (**A**) Anterior view. (**B**) Posterior view. (From Moore KL, Agur AMR. Essential Clinical Anatomy, 2nd Edition. Baltimore: Lippincott Williams & Wilkins, 2002. Figure 7.3, p. 408.)

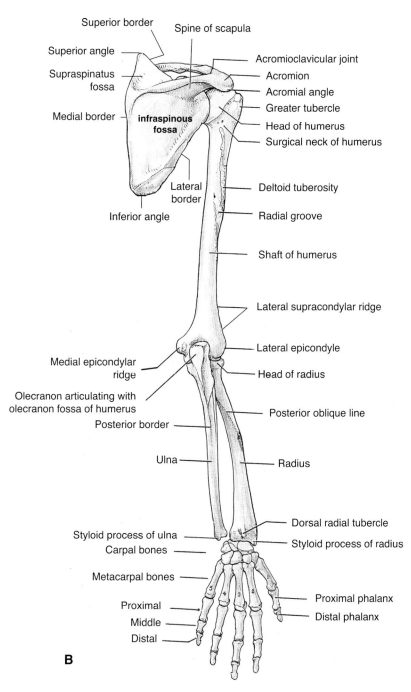

Superior border
Spine of scapula
Superior angle
Supraspinatus fossa
Medial border
infraspinous fossa
Lateral border
Inferior angle

Acromioclavicular joint
Acromion
Acromial angle
Greater tubercle
Head of humerus
Surgical neck of humerus
Deltoid tuberosity
Radial groove

Shaft of humerus

Lateral supracondylar ridge

Lateral epicondyle
Medial epicondylar ridge
Head of radius
Olecranon articulating with olecranon fossa of humerus
Posterior border
Posterior oblique line
Ulna
Radius

Dorsal radial tubercle
Styloid process of ulna
Styloid process of radius
Carpal bones
Metacarpal bones
Proximal phalanx
Proximal
Distal phalanx
Middle
Distal

B

FIGURE 7.11   *(Continued)*

Because the scapula is a source attachment for numerous muscles that control the pivoting of the joint between it and the humerus, its neatly flattened contour for gliding along the back of the ribs is elaborated with crests, angles, a notch, and a prominent spine. These deviations can be palpated in a patient or observed radiographically. The **clavicle** is shaped more uniformly. It serves the front of the body, which bears pectoral muscles to complement and counter the scapular and latissimus musculature.

The clavicle remains tubular but S-shaped along its length, and it makes end-to-end contacts with the scapula and sternum.

The bony core of the upper limb continues as the **humerus**, which is a classic long bone—cylindrical in shape but modified at either end to serve its required mobility. The upper end is part spheroid and part platform. The spheroid head of the humerus joins against a fossa of the scapula in an awkward design that is similar to putting a large ball on a small saucer. As a result, the humerus is free to move in universal motion, a hallmark of the flexibility of the human upper limb. The platforms are elevations of bone from the surface of the cylinder that receive the numerous muscles that act across the shoulder joint. Large muscles, such as the **pectoralis major** and **latissimus dorsi**, attach to the elevations (called **tubercles**), and as such, they contribute to a groove between them that is positioned conveniently for the passage of part of another muscle (the **biceps**).

The lower, or distal, end of the humerus is not spheroidal at all. It is nearly flattened into a shape that transmits force through a flap-like design. This permits powerful action in a "front-to-back," or **flexion** and **extension**, direction, but it resists dispersion of the force in other directions. This part of the humerus also is designed for a tight articulation with one bone (the **ulna**) but barely an accommodation for its neighbor (the **radius**). The result is a spool-shaped (**trochlear**) end on the ulnar side and a rounded (**capitular**) end on the radial side.

The bony core continues into the forearm as the **ulna** bone, a weak-looking stick of a cylinder with an elaborate head end for fitting against the humerus but a diminished and unmodified distal end. Parallel to the ulna is the **radius**, a more robust cylinder with the opposite emphases. The head end of the radius is simple, but the distal end is expanded and powerful. It is this very "cross-over" of command that enables the human hand to be as versatile as it is.

Force traveling through the humerus is passed along to the ulna and the radius. The ulna cannot transfer it effectively across the wrist joint, but the radius can (because it dominates the surface area of that joint; see below). The radius, however, is not "locked" into a tight joint with the humerus, so it is free to adapt to local (i.e., hand and wrist) pressures in any rotated position. It simply pivots on the stability rooted in the ulna, positioning the wrist and fingers for maximum use of the flexor muscles from the ulnar side of the forearm. Thus, the **mobile** bone of the forearm also is the **driver** of the hand, and this enables combined power and dexterity at the fingertips. Full capability in a rotated (or **pronated**) forearm is essential to fulfill the potential of a grasping hand.

The bones of the wrist and hand continue the theme of mobility. All things considered, these are simple bones that line up in a classic design of rays (the fingers) grounded against a bed of bearings (the wrist bones, or **carpals**). The individual carpals are shaped irregularly, but in the articulated state they form a close-packed system of angles that direct force into multiple hand bones (Fig. 7.12). The radius is in direct contact with two of them, the **scaphoid** and the **lunate**, which are themselves in contact with the remaining six. The thumb in particular is a marvelous design of bones that can slide, rotate, and pivot on one another before the final and simple hinge joint at the tip is activated.

Within the hand, the skeleton of each finger is similar. Beginning against the carpals will be a **metacarpal**, or ray bone, for each finger. These bones are within the palm of the hand and are easily felt by squeezing. Each metacarpal leads to a set of three true digit bones, or **phalanges**—one for each segment of the finger. Each finger has a **proximal phalanx** connected to the metacarpal, an **intermediate phalanx**, and a **distal phalanx** that bears the nail. The structure of the thumb is identical to that of the fingers except that it lacks an intermediate phalanx.

The construction of the upper limb is developed on a model of more generality and less fixation. Its attachments to the trunk are logical, familiar to our sense of self,

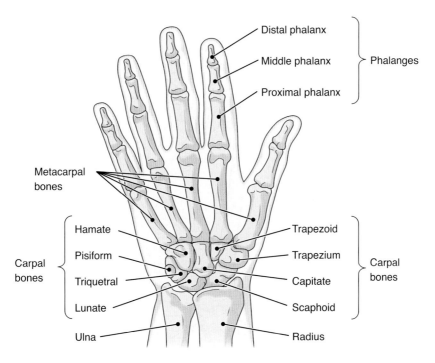

FIGURE 7.12   **The wrist and hand skeleton, anterior view.**

The wrist contains eight carpal bones, aligned in two "rows" of contact. The proximal row includes the scaphoid, lunate, triquetral, and pisiform. The scaphoid and lunate "ricochet" force delivered by the radius onward to the other carpal bones. The distal row of carpals includes the trapezium, trapezoid, capitate, and hamate bones, which are more or less dedicated to the position and movement of individual metacarpal bones. (From Cohen BJ, Wood DL. Memmler's The Human Body in Health and Disease, 10th Edition. Baltimore: Lippincott Williams & Wilkins, 2004. Figure 7.20.)

and simple in design. The bony core is minimally derived from the cylinder, or strut, model. The arm is a primary means of independent, unassisted living, and across history it has been the mechanical unit that has "built" our way of life. Gradual breakdown of the vertebral column may be tolerated as a "part of getting older," but for most patients, even minor loss of function in the upper limb is acutely distressing.

A less highly mobile lower limb

The lower limb accepts all the responsibility for posture and locomotion that the upper limb does not. As a result, it is less mobile, more robust, and significantly more specialized anatomically. The "hip bone" is the rough equivalent of the scapula and clavicle in the lower limb. This single structure is really a composite of three bones that develop separately: an **ilium**, an **ischium**, and a **pubis** (Fig. 7.13). Given the need for the lower limb to be firmly attached to the trunk these bones fuse to each other during growth to form a "single" bone that has been called the **innominate** (or "the bone with no name"). This "single" bone (formally called the **os coxa**) then forms very stable joints with the vertebral column (at the sacrum) and with its partner from the other side (at the **pubic symphysis**). Together, these three bones form the familiar pelvis and pelvic cavity, which are very much fixed entities. The ilium and ischium are not suspended in a muscular envelope like the scapula, and the pubis bones are fully melded into them and nearly into each other—quite unlike the clavicle. The pelvis, thus, forms something much more like a girdle and a true bottom to the body's trunk.

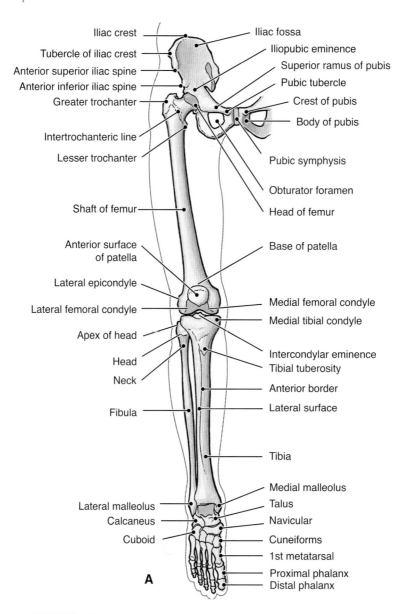

Iliac crest

Tubercle of iliac crest

Anterior superior iliac spine

Anterior inferior iliac spine

Greater trochanter

Intertrochanteric line

Lesser trochanter

Shaft of femur

Anterior surface
of patella

Lateral epicondyle

Lateral femoral condyle

Apex of head

Head

Neck

Fibula

Lateral malleolus

Calcaneus

Cuboid

Iliac fossa

Iliopubic eminence

Superior ramus of pubis

Pubic tubercle

Crest of pubis

Body of pubis

Pubic symphysis

Obturator foramen

Head of femur

Base of patella

Medial femoral condyle

Medial tibial condyle

Intercondylar eminence

Tibial tuberosity

Anterior border

Lateral surface

Tibia

Medial malleolus

Talus

Navicular

Cuneiforms

1st metatarsal

Proximal phalanx

Distal phalanx

A

FIGURE 7.13   **The lower extremity skeleton.**

The lower limb skeleton begins with the fusion of three bones (ilium, ischium, and pubis) into a single os coxa, which girdles the lower limb against the trunk. All three bones contribute to the articular socket for the femur (acetabulum). The femoral head is nearly spherical, but it lodges deeply into the acetabulum, making the degree of rotational freedom more theoretic than real. The leg skeleton is composed of a dominant tibia and a lateral fibula. The tibia alone bears the weight transmission from the femur, whereas the tibia and fibula together form the brace-like contact with the ankle. The foot skeleton is homologous to the hand skeleton in many ways: eight tarsal bones, a metatarsal for each digit, and two phalanges instead of three in the big toe. The conformation of the tarsals, however, reveals the pressure on them to dissipate weight across an arch and into a heel point and a stable toe complex. (**A**) Anterior view. (**B**) Posterior view. (From Moore KL, Agur AMR. Essential Clinical Anatomy, 2nd Edition. Baltimore: Lippincott Williams & Wilkins, 2002. Figure 6.2, p. 316.)

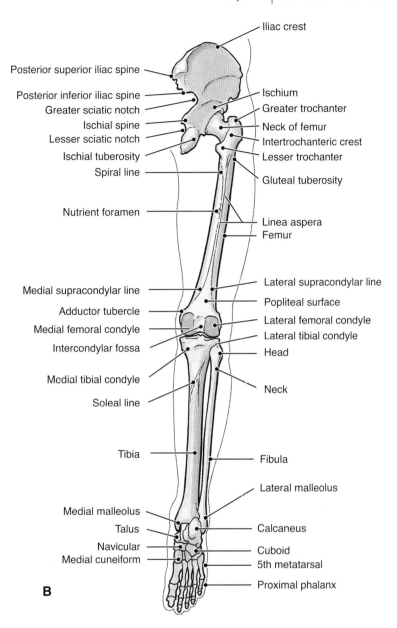

Iliac crest

Posterior superior iliac spine

Posterior inferior iliac spine
Greater sciatic notch
Ischial spine
Lesser sciatic notch
Ischial tuberosity
Spiral line

Ischium
Greater trochanter
Neck of femur
Intertrochanteric crest
Lesser trochanter
Gluteal tuberosity

Nutrient foramen

Linea aspera
Femur

Medial supracondylar line
Adductor tubercle
Medial femoral condyle
Intercondylar fossa

Medial tibial condyle
Soleal line

Lateral supracondylar line
Popliteal surface
Lateral femoral condyle
Lateral tibial condyle
Head

Neck

Tibia

Fibula

Lateral malleolus

Medial malleolus
Talus
Navicular
Medial cuneiform

Calcaneus

Cuboid
5th metatarsal
Proximal phalanx

B

FIGURE 7.13   **The lower extremity skeleton. *(continued)***

The bony core of the lower limb continues as the **femur**, which is identical in concept to the humerus but is more exaggerated at both ends. The head of the femur is nearly spherical and projects away from the shaft of the bone so much that a true "neck" is created. Because the muscle forces that pull against the top of the femur are significantly greater than those pulling against the top of the humerus, the elevations of bone at the top of the femur also are significantly larger. Here, they are called **trochanters** (as opposed to tubercles on the humerus), and by inspecting the femur, you can see and feel how substantial they are. They are the lever arms on which the muscles act to balance the heavy trunk against the strut of the lower limb during standing or movement.

The generic shape of the long bone cylinder begins to flatten out and curl back on itself near the bottom of the femoral shaft. In this anatomy—and in that of each of the three major lower limb joints—the human design for bipedal (two-legged) balance and motion displays, by far, not the most efficient and most powerful limb design in the animal world but, certainly, a logical adaptation to constraint. The "bottom," or distal, part of the femur expands into two surfaces, or **condyles**, that articulate inferiorly with the **tibia**. These condyles take the form of elaborate rocker-bottoms, convex half-wheels for the powerful flexion and extension of the leg. An important space is excavated between the condyles posteriorly so that the blood and nerve supply to the leg and foot can pass beyond the knee joint without getting pinched by it. In addition, on the sides of the condyles, as in the distal part of the humerus, small humps and ridges of bone provide attachment for muscles that drive the ankle joint. The femur, overall, is a simple bone.

In anatomy, the term **leg** generally refers to the part of the lower limb below the knee. In this sense, we should expect some parallels between the bones of the leg and the bones of the forearm, and indeed, this is the case. Both have two bones and a similar array of muscles for movement of the extremity beyond them. In the leg, however, weight and force must be transmitted with the extremity fixed against a surface. To accommodate, the leg is rotated inward (**pronated**) and the **tibia**, the equivalent of the radius bone of the forearm, is the dominant bone both proximally and distally (see Fig. 7.13). The top of the tibia is flattened out like a broad plateau on which the femur is perched. Suspended between the tibia and the femur at their joint (the knee joint) is the **patella**, a bone that grows in the tendon of the muscle group that crosses the joint. This type of bone is called a **sesamoid bone**. The tibia slightly tapers toward the ankle joint, where its contact surface forms a brace-like joint shape against the **talus** bone. All along the extent of the tibia lies the feeble **fibula**, an almost vestigial bone that provides a lateral closure of the brace-like joint at the ankle.

All the mobility that the radioulnar complex provides to the forearm and the wrist is sacrificed in the leg and ankle for the provision of a stable strut that directs the body weight into the foot in a forced posture that allows little or no rotation. This almost singular function of the leg skeleton results in one of the two bones being quite dominant (the tibia) and one being quite subordinate (the fibula). The function is further played out across the ankle joint and into the foot skeleton, which must balance the weight (often during movement) and distribute it evenly while doing so. Unlike the wrist, then, in which force is dispersed through almost all the wrist bones simultaneously, much like striking a set of billiard balls, the bones of the foot expand in size and move in position such that force tends to flow in more fixed directions.

The tibia and fibula articulate with just one bone, the **talus**, which is in a geometric plane separate from that of the other ankle bones (see Fig. 7.13). Recall that in the wrist, the radius delivers force across two bones (scaphoid and lunate) that lie side by side. The talus is perched more like the top of a dome, such that the weight of the body balanced on it can be directed from it to the rest of the dome. The talus leads to the **calcaneus** inferiorly and the **navicular** anteriorly and, so, can send force down to the "heel" of the foot and forward toward the "big toe." The big toe is aptly named because it truly dominates the structure, power, and mobility of the foot. From the calcaneus and the navicular, force can be accommodated by the adjacent **cuboid** bone and the **cuneiforms** in a conservative alignment that keeps the rays of the toes in a tight, parallel formation.

Consider the foot skeleton as a whole, because again, in this case, the whole is greater than the sum of its parts. In fact, consider the skeleton of both feet together because one of the beauties of the design of the human foot is that it forms half of a virtual geodesic dome—one of the most stable geometric constructs. Put side by side, the skeleton of the two feet conform to a near equivalent of such a dome, which makes sense given that the entire weight of the body must address the ground through them. What better design than one that maximizes its own stability and, thus, the load that it bears from above?

Look down at the outline of your two feet as you stand erect. Notice that they do not form a perfect circle, but the literal footprint would form a closed oval from the heels around the outside (lateral) edges of the foot and then back to the middle along the "ball" of the foot. This outline reflects where the bony skeleton of the foot is positioned to place the weight against the ground. The toes can rest against the ground under their own control, but much of the rest of the foot actually is elevated in a permanent **arch**. With the feet together, the parts that are arched up form the "hollow," central part of the virtual dome. These **longitudinal arches** of the feet are achieved by growth of the ankle (**tarsal**) bones into conforming shapes.

The talus sits atop the arch and directs force downward against the calcaneus, on which the talus rests. The "head" of the talus, however, which is shaped like the head of a small long bone, points forward and is locked into a receptive curve of the navicular bone, thus providing the talus with a means of sending force toward the toes independent of the calcaneus doing the same. The navicular receives the force from the head of the talus and routes it exclusively into the big toe, second toe, and third toe through three "ball-bearing" bones—the wedge-shaped **cuneiforms**. When you move, of course, body weight is balanced on the toes alone for part of the time, and this is the basic bony link by which you can manage that action.

The force delivered from the talus downward onto the calcaneus is sent mostly backward (posteriorly) to the contact that the calcaneus makes with the ground. This part of the foot skeleton is designed to hold the weight in place and to be a lever for its lift-off. The calcaneus is arched aggressively to maximize transmission of weight into the "heel" process, but it also provides a way to get force into the "lesser toes" (the fourth and fifth toes). Toward the side of the foot, the calcaneus leads to a single "ball-bearing" bone, the **cuboid**, that radiates force into the fourth and fifth toes. This is a minor amount of force compared to that being directed into the big toe, and independent movement of the fourth and fifth toes is limited (because they rest against the same single platform, the cuboid).

The foot skeleton contains one other remarkable feature related to its stressful function. Along the ray bones of the big toe (**metatarsal, proximal phalanx,** and **distal phalanx**), two loose nuggets of bone rest underneath the metatarsal-phalangeal joint. These are **sesamoid bones** and are positioned to lift the front end of the first metatarsal bone off the ground. A space exists between them for the passage of a cable, or a muscle tendon. In this case, a major muscle tendon that flexes the big toe must reach that toe by passing under the head of the metatarsal bone. If the body weight pressed the head of this bone against the ground, it would crush the tendon. Instead, the head of the bone is pressed down against the paired sesamoid bones, which then press against the ground. The tendon is spared by passing between the sesamoids; thus, you are free to "toe-off" with power as you stride. For many people, this alignment is imperfect, and its distortion over time leads to the painful development of a **bunion** (see below).

THE ARTICULAR SYSTEM

Bones form as hard tissues to make a core for support of the body, but they are only as effective as the connections they make to each other. Muscle tendons and ligaments attach to bones in such a way that they enable one bone to move against the stability of an adjacent bone, and this fundamental mechanic of animate life requires that bones somehow "fit" together. The way in which bones join together, or **articulate**, is detailed enough that many books treat the study of the **joints** (**arthrology**) as a system (the **articular system**). The common clinical problems of painful swelling of the joints (**arthritis**) warrant a closer look at their general design.

The condensed mesoderm tissue called mesenchyme, which forms the template for the bones, also exists in the small spaces between the bones and, ultimately, differentiates into the joint structures. In other words, musculoskeletal derivatives of mesoderm possess absolute continuity. The final shape and extent of rigid tissue (bone) versus elastic tissue (muscle) or connective tissue (ligaments and tendons), and so on, develops holistically, or organically, and not in separate "systems" of growth. Thus, where two bones come together, they are "joined" by a capsule and ligaments, which themselves condense from contiguous mesodermal colonies.

The particular structural/functional type of joint that occurs results from the different paths taken by this **primitive joint plate** of condensed mesenchyme. Minimal alteration of the tissue produces a joint in which the bone ends are essentially glued together (a **fibrous joint**) (Fig. 7.14). If the mesenchyme develops into cartilage between the bones (it already develops into cartilage as a precursor to the bones themselves), then this cartilage acts as a kind of buffer between the bones. Some movement is tolerated, and the cartilage mostly is a cushion between bones that are routinely forced together under great pressure (e.g., the bodies of the vertebrae). This is a **cartilaginous joint** (see Fig. 7.14). In many cases, the condensed mesenchyme evacuates until only a peripheral sheet is left and a cavity exists in the space between apposing bones. The bones retain a cartilage plate on their contacting surfaces, the peripheral sheet of mesenchyme produces a fibrous outer layer and a fluid-producing inner layer, and with a minimum of intervening tissue, the bones can move against one another very freely (a **synovial joint**) (see Fig. 7.14).

All synovial joints have a basic design that involves bringing bones close to, but not in direct contact with, one another. The friction that is created at the joint surfaces would quickly erode the bone tissue, much like putting the rim of the car tire against the road rather than wrapping an air-filled, rubber tire around it first. All synovial joints provide some amount of other connective tissue, usually **cartilage**, as a buffer between the surfaces of the bones that would otherwise make tight contact. A certain amount of very slick **fluid** also is around to facilitate further the movement of these padded surfaces against one another. This fluid must be kept in place around the joint, so typically a **capsule** of connective tissue "seals" the connection and creates an inner cavity of space. Finally, in external (and, sometimes, internal) support of the packaged fit, connective tissue bands called **ligaments** bridge the connected bones as tight tethers that resist unusual movements. Sprained ligaments disable proper joint function and are common clinical presentations.

The general design just described applies to the vast majority of joints in the body. They are designed to allow movement—sometimes, very much movement. A few joints in the body are designed to limit or resist movement and, as a result, may lack some of the packaging options. The skull, for example, is composed of many different bones that articulate with one another; however, you would rather they not move about very much. The fibrous joints between many skull bones are virtual fusions of bone and are detectable as joints only when forced apart.

Joint Types

Fibrous

Some bone-to-bone connections need to be as stable as possible. This can be achieved by eliminating the joint features that promote movement, such as fluid, cushioning cartilage, and supporting muscles. In their place are features such as an interlocking bone fit and fibrous tissue rather than cartilage between the bones.

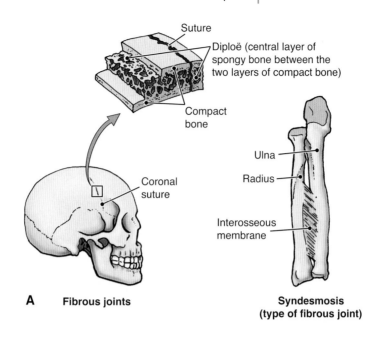

A   **Fibrous joints**

Syndesmosis (type of fibrous joint)

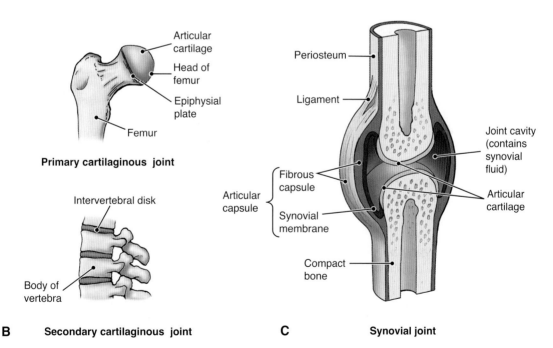

Primary cartilaginous joint

B   Secondary cartilaginous joint

C   Synovial joint

FIGURE 7.14   **The three categories of joint construction.**

(**A**) Fibrous. (**B**) Cartilaginous. (**C**) Synovial. (From Moore KL, Agur AMR. Essential Clinical Anatomy, 2nd Edition. Baltimore: Lippincott Williams & Wilkins, 2002. Figure 1.3, p. 18; and from Moore KL, Dalley AF. Clinically Oriented Anatomy, 5th Edition. Baltimore: Lippincott Williams & Wilkins, 2006. Figure I.16A, p. 27.)

The human body presents three types of fibrous joints. One type is the fit between some bones of the skull, in which the contact surface of one bone matches the contact surface of another bone in a tight-fitting, stitch-like design called a **suture**. These are called **sutural joints**, and over time, they may fuse together completely (a **synostosis**). The tooth sockets (alveoli) receive the teeth in a modified kind of fibrous joint construct called a **gomphosis**. This is the only area of the body in which bony tissue interacts with a skin derivative. The final type of fibrous joint describes what happens when bones have a side-by-side connection formed with a sheet of dense fibrous connective tissue. This type of joint is called a **syndesmosis**, which means a shared binding or fastening. The bones of the forearm and of the leg are connected by just such an **interosseous membrane**.

Cartilaginous

Many bones develop first as a hyaline cartilage precursor, which then steadily mineralizes from the center toward the periphery. This means that the "ends" of the bone are cartilaginous for longer than the "shafts" of the bone are. For a period of time during growth, the joint is functional even though the bones have not stopped growing, meaning that much of the joint in question is composed of cartilage units rather than bone units. This type of joint is called a **synchondrosis**. Because many joints go through this phase but, eventually, are composed of adult bones, this phase also is called a **primary cartilaginous phase** (to distinguish it from a **secondary cartilaginous phase**; see below).

The timing of when primary cartilaginous joints mature varies from joint to joint and from person to person, so it is possible that some joints in the body remain in this state for many years. Anatomists know of two joints that are persistent synchondroses: the joint between the sternum and first rib (the **sternocostal joint**), and the joint between the petrous portion of the temporal bone and the basilar part of the occipital bone in the head (the **petrobasilar joint**). Why these two unions persist as synchondroses is not obvious.

A few joints in the body are formed when the flat surface of one bone meets the flat surface of another bone in a position that receives tremendous compression. A substantial pad of **fibrocartilage** is wedged between the two bone surfaces, and ligaments outside of the joint ensure that any movement other than slight compression and decompression is discouraged. These joints are called **symphysis joints**, and the most obvious ones are the joints between bodies of vertebrae. The joints also are called **secondary cartilaginous joints**, because unlike synchondroses, the cartilage pad is not simply a remnant of the developing bone that eventually disappears but, rather, is a purposeful growth of cartilage designed to mediate the pressures of weight-bearing. Symphysis joints, incidentally, are found only in the midline of the body.

Synovial

In keeping with the needs of a mobile life, most joints in the body accommodate the movement of bones and minimize the friction between them. These are called **synovial joints,** which notes what they all have in common: a membrane (**synovium**) lined with fluid (**synovia**) that forms a slippery pocket between the two joint surfaces.

Synovial joints bring together ends of bones that are elaborated to reflect the type and direction of movement needed. In general, the ends of the bones involved with synovial joints are enlarged, either to allow more muscle attachment or to permit greater stability (or both). The ends that come together can be shaped alike (**homomorphic**) or in a more differential "head and socket" design (**heteromorphic**). The amount of movement that is possible is really a function of how much slipping, sliding, spinning, or rotating that the joint coverings allow. There are formal names for the shapes of synovial joints (e.g., **plane**, **saddle**, **hinge**, **pivot**, and **ball and socket**), but for now, the important thing to understand is how a typical synovial joint is constructed.

A Typical Synovial Joint

As noted above, it would be unwise to have true bone-to-bone surface connections, because movement of one bone against another would degrade the bone and cause too much heat to build up in the joint space. As a result, the surfaces of the bones that should come in contact with one another are lined with a layer of hyaline cartilage, usually called **articular cartilage**. This cartilage lacks a useful nerve and blood supply, which means that it can absorb a certain amount of punishment that never registers in the brain. As living tissue, however, it needs a nutrient supply of some kind. This is provided by **synovial fluid**. A major downside of poorly perfused tissue is that once it is damaged, it cannot heal itself effectively. Degenerative joint disease is truly degenerative.

Connective tissue surrounds the entire joint, forming a closed **capsule**. The outer bandaging of a joint is called an **articular capsule**, or a **joint capsule**, or a **fibrous capsule**. It makes the joint cavity a kind of self-enclosed system, and as connective tissue goes, it is not very elastic. It merges imperceptibly with the surface layer of bone tissue (**periosteum**), and as a barrier layer to the protected joint cavity, it is highly sensitive.

As with any sleeve-like tissue, the joint capsule has an "outer" layer and an "inner" layer. The inner layer of a synovial joint capsule is the defining feature of the joint, because it is made of a **synovial membrane** that produces and traps **synovial fluid** within the joint cavity. In this way, synovial fluid is said to "bathe" the articular cartilage, and in all measures, it provides a critical lubricant to minimize friction and heat buildup during movement. The synovial membrane is highly vascularized, and it conducts many of the physiologic exchanges that are necessary to keep the articular surfaces functioning.

Ligaments connect the bones to one another. All synovial joints are reinforced by elastic (but not very elastic) connective tissue ligaments. These may be generic capsular ligaments, or they may be large bundles of fibers that are grossly visible as a distinct unit and, so, are given specific names (typically at major joints). They typically are found outside of the joint capsule (extrinsic, or **extracapsular**, ligaments), but in a few major joints, such as the **knee joint,** ligaments are found inside of the joint capsule (intrinsic, or **intracapsular**, ligaments). In general, ligaments are placed to resist motion in undesirable directions. Ligaments have a minimal blood supply and are slow to heal when injured.

This design plan is the default arrangement in all synovial joints. These include, for example, the 14 synovial joints in the fingers and thumb of just one hand, so you can appreciate the utility and ubiquity of such a simple design. A few synovial joints, however, have special needs or unusual burdens (Fig. 7.15). In these joints, such as the **knee**, we find some of the following modifications.

Intervening Muscle Tendons and Ligaments   Muscles move bones, and in some joint cavities, the ability of one of the articulating bones to move **while in articulation** is important. Muscle fibers, therefore, may penetrate the fibrous capsule to attach to a surface of bone that lies within the joint cavity. The same is true for ligaments if the need is to stabilize the position of a bone in articulation, and in the knee joint (see below), we find both. In these cases, the synovial membrane adjusts to the presence of these "supporting cables" by winding around them. Thus, muscles and ligaments that are within the fibrous capsule (**intracapsular**) tend to lie outside of the synovial membrane (**extrasynovial**) and, therefore, are not bathed in synovial fluid.

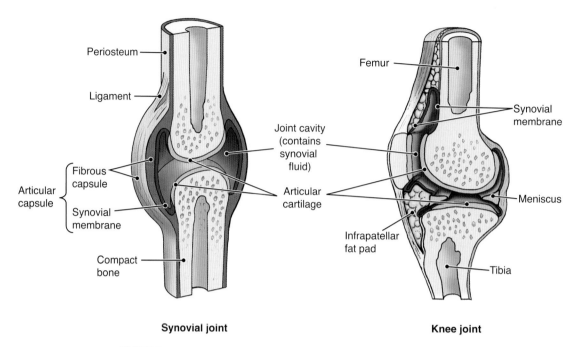

Periosteum

Ligament

Articular capsule
{ Fibrous capsule
  Synovial membrane }

Compact bone

Joint cavity (contains synovial fluid)

Articular cartilage

Synovial joint

Femur

Synovial membrane

Meniscus

Infrapatellar fat pad

Tibia

Knee joint

FIGURE 7.15   **How a real synovial joint compares to the model.**

The knee joint is an example of how the key elements of a synovial joint can derive to meet specific needs. Fat pads, extra cartilage, sesamoid bones, ligaments, and muscles can invade the joint space, and the pristine alignment of the synovial membrane can segment to accommodate them. (From Moore KL, Dalley AF. Clinically Oriented Anatomy, 5th Edition. Baltimore: Lippincott Williams & Wilkins, 2006. Figure I.16A, p. 27.)

Articular Discs and Menisci   Sometimes, the cushioning provided by the articular cartilage is not enough, and the cartilage itself needs a cushion. In these cases (and, again, in the knee joint in particular), an ingrowth of the fibrous capsule may form a plate, or pad, or **disc**, of fibrocartilage that gets crushed between the articular cartilage of the bone above and the articular cartilage of the bone below. These disks maintain a firm attachment to the outer layer of the joint capsule, so they effectively push against, but do not penetrate, the synovial membrane. Therefore, articular discs are not bathed in synovial fluid because they remain extrasynovial in position within the joint cavity. In the knee joint, the articular disc is not a complete layer but, rather is a crescent-shaped wedge that projects from the joint capsule inward. Here, because of this shape the articular disc, it is called a **meniscus** (plural, menisci).

Fluid-Lined Sacs, or Bursae, for Extra Lubrication   In some joints, friction builds up not just between articular cartilages but also in areas where tendons make sharp angles against tightly flexed joints, or in areas where a highly mobile joint, such as the shoulder joint, finds itself in an unusually extended position. Small, "pillow-like," flaccid sacs called **bursae** (singular, **bursa**) may develop in such regions. Because they are lined on the inside with synovial fluid and develop in response to friction between connective tissues, they may, in time, fuse with the synovial membrane of joint cavities, creating a sort of recess, or extension, of the joint cavity beyond its strict articulation.

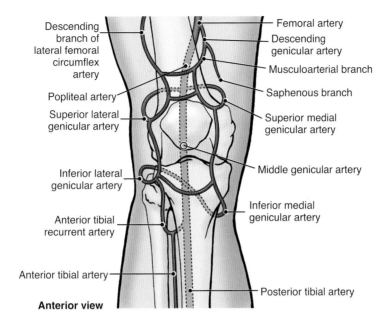

Descending branch of lateral femoral circumflex artery

Popliteal artery

Superior lateral genicular artery

Inferior lateral genicular artery

Anterior tibial recurrent artery

Anterior tibial artery

Anterior view

Femoral artery

Descending genicular artery

Musculoarterial branch

Saphenous branch

Superior medial genicular artery

Middle genicular artery

Inferior medial genicular artery

Posterior tibial artery

FIGURE 7.16   **Collateral circulation around joints.**

Synovial joints in the body occur at major musculoskeletal transitions. Central routes of circulation typically branch into collateral routes that both feed and circumvent the joint, thus providing ample alternative pathways for blood to reach tissues distal to the joint. (From Agur A, Dalley AF. Grant's Atlas of Anatomy, 11th Edition. Baltimore: Lippincott Williams & Wilkins, 2005. Figure 5.48A, p. 398.)

Joints present an obstacle to the pathway of nerves and blood vessels that must cross them to serve more distant structures. In the limbs especially, joints such as the elbow and the knee occupy almost the entire anatomic space under the skin, so neurovascular bundles somehow must find nooks and crannies to exploit to get around them. As a rule, these bundles pass along paths or zones that are collapsed rather than stretched when the joint is in flexion.

Two other general patterns apply to the regional anatomy of joints in the body. One is that the joint surfaces tend to be innervated by combinations of nerves that serve the muscles acting across the joint. With few exceptions, the specific nerve fibers are too small to be observed during a typical dissection of a cadaver. A second general pattern is that the central route of arterial flow tends to branch out and form a webbing, or **anastomosis**, around joint spaces. This means that the big "central line" of circulation stays intact as it passes across a joint, but that it is supported by smaller lines that branch off above (or before) the joint and join to (or **anastomose** with) smaller lines that branch off below (or after) the joint. The result is an elaborate mesh, or web, or plexus of arteries that form a kind of **collateral circulation** to the dominant flow (Fig. 7.16). The death of tissue, or **necrosis**, is a serious problem in joint cavities when circulation is compromised, so learning the available routes of blood flow to a joint is a very worthwhile exercise in anatomy.

Major Joints of the Body

Major joints of the body can be divided into joints of the axial skeleton, the upper limb, the lower limb, and the foot.

Joints of the axial skeleton

Vertebral Column Joints

The design of a typical vertebra suggests that together, their chain is greater than the sum of their individual parts. The joints between the vertebrae play to this theme, of course. The bindings are tight, and the movements that they permit are very conservative. The different regions of the column (cervical, thoracic, lumbar, and sacral) allow different categories and degrees of movement—for example, more in the neck than in the chest—but all regions are governed by the same basic joint configuration.

A Typical Intervertebral Joint   The bodies of adjacent vertebrae sit on top of one another like stumps (Fig. 7.17). The arches that spring from the bodies toward the back are like a chain of struts that bend, or twist, or flex, or extend, the bodies when muscles pull on them. Therefore, the typical intervertebral joint includes a close packing of the bodies onto one another and straps of ligaments that are dedicated to each type of strut along the arches. The joints between these bodies are known as **anterior intervertebral joints**.

The joints between the bodies are symphyseal joints, and their major feature is the disc between them. The intervertebral disc is composed of a fibrous perimeter (**anulus fibrosus**) and a gelatinous core (**nucleus pulposus**) that is the eventual degradation of the original notochord. With age, the nucleus pulposus tends to become fibrous; thus, you are more inclined to do cartwheels as a grandchild than as a grandparent.

The anterior and posterior surfaces of the vertebral bodies are uninterrupted—that is, they are free of projections of bone or foramina. They are ideal surfaces for a big strip of packing tape to stretch the length of the column, so the anterior intervertebral

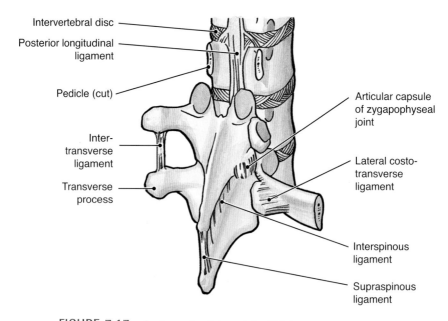

FIGURE 7.17   **Anatomy of an intervertebral joint.**

Vertebrae are joined at their bodies by a compressible symphyseal cushion and along the articular facets of the neural arches by synovial joints. The symphyseal joints are supported both in front and behind by longitudinal ligaments. The perimeter of the neural arch is bound from one vertebra to the next by the interspinous and supraspinous ligaments. (From Moore KL, Agur AMR. Essential Clinical Anatomy, 2nd Edition. Baltimore: Lippincott Williams & Wilkins, 2002. Figure 5.5c, p. 287.)

joints are supported by an **anterior longitudinal ligament** and by a **posterior longitudinal ligament**, which run essentially from the skull to the coccyx. These ligaments keep the intervertebral discs stable, and they limit the amount of flexion and extension in the column.

That leaves the vertebral arch and its articulation, the **posterior intervertebral joint**. The articular facets of adjacent vertebrae are mirror-images of one another, with subtle shifts in the angle that they make to the column from the cervical region (where swiveling is permitted) to the lumbar region (where flexing is fine but swiveling is discouraged). The arch joints, which are called **zygapophyseal joints**, are synovial.

The lamina, the pedicle, and the spine that adjoin the facet can be strapped together by ligaments wherever muscles and the spinal cord allow. Because these bony struts project from the facets in different directions, they offer a wide variety of subtle levers for the column of vertebral bodies. The ligaments associated with them therefore are more discrete in fiber bundles and more numerous. Begin along the inside lining of the arch, and note a ligament band between the laminae from one vertebra to another. This is the **ligamentum flavum** (flavum means yellow), a kind of arch that is equivalent to the anterior and posterior longitudinal ligaments. The rest of the action is all along the exterior surfaces of the arch.

Intertransverse ligaments connect the transverse processes of adjacent vertebrae, much like the more elastic intertransversarii muscles. This gives you the impression that the transverse processes are governed by an elastic muscle fiber and a much less elastic ligament fiber. The transverse process can be used like a lever to bend the column, but not too far or too fast, or else the ligament will seize control.

Interspinous ligaments are bands between the spines of adjacent vertebrae. They govern the battery of movements involving flexion and extension. **Supraspinous ligaments** surf along the tips of the spines—a minor consideration except for within the cervical region. The back of the neck is deep with muscles but shy of vertebral spines. The supraspinous ligament in this region thickens and expands like a midline curtain to provide attachment to these many levels of neck muscles. Here, the prominent flap of supraspinous ligament is called the **nuchal ligament**, or **ligamentum nuchae** (Fig. 7.18).

This basic design applies to the entire vertebral column, but with some modifications in the sacral and coccygeal region given the fusion of the sacral vertebrae and the vestigial growth of the coccygeal vertebrae. The uppermost cervical region also is quite unusual, because the cervical vertebrae must support the skull. This balancing act calls for a variation, again, on the intervertebral theme.

Atlantoaxial and Atlanto-occipital Joints   The atlas (C1) and axis (C2) vertebrae cooperatively distribute the support and positioning load that is imposed by their cranial articulation. The atlas bone (C1) effectively cups the skull; it lacks a useful body of its own. In the place of the body is the **dens**, or **odontoid process**, of the axis bone (C2). The dens of the axis is a literal axis around which the atlas can rotate, carrying the skull along with it. To accomplish this, each joint among the three bones is synovial, and the ligament arrangement is elegant and customized (Fig. 7.19).

The ligament battery that applies to the rest of the column also extends through the top two cervical vertebrae. The anterior longitudinal ligament between the atlas and the skull becomes the **anterior atlanto-occipital membrane**. The posterior longitudinal ligament becomes the **tectorial membrane** (literally, the "covering" membrane because it blankets the area of the dens and its intrinsic ligaments). The ligamentum flavum between the atlas and the skull is known as the **posterior atlanto-occipital membrane**.

FIGURE 7.18   Nuchal ligament.

In the cervical region, the midline ligament elaborates into the nuchal ligament, a curtain of connective tissue that rudders the cranium and supports several layers of neck musculature. (From Moore KL, Agur AMR. Essential Clinical Anatomy, 2nd Edition. Baltimore: Lippincott Williams & Wilkins, 2002. Figure 5.5A, p. 287.)

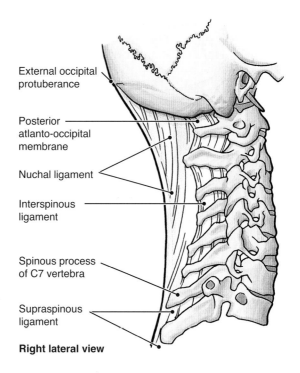

External occipital protuberance

Posterior atlanto-occipital membrane

Nuchal ligament

Interspinous ligament

Spinous process of C7 vertebra

Supraspinous ligament

Right lateral view

Because the "body" of the atlas essentially is replaced by a prong of the axis bone, the median atlantoaxial joint is a pivot type of synovial joint. Ligaments must patch the dens into position and actually enable the atlas to pivot around it. The dens is tethered to the skull as well, perhaps to reinforce its center position in this unique joint.

Witness, then, the **cruciform ligament** of the atlas, which spans longitudinally between the skull and the body of the axis and transversely between the tubercles on the lateral masses of the atlas. The longitudinal bands anchor the axis to the skull, and the transverse bands strap the dens into the alcove of the atlas. Inside this joint "cavity" are **alar ligaments**, which wing out from the dens to the skull, and an **apical ligament**, which strings down like a stalactite from the edge of the foramen magnum to the tip of the dens.

The axial skeleton also is joined to ribs, which span from the vertebrae (**costotransverse joints**) to the sternum (**sternocostal joints**). The ribs form a protective, bony cage with some capacity to support inspiration and expiration (see Fig. 7.6). Cartilage plays a large role is completing the framework of this cage, and ligaments are minor at all joints.

Joints of the upper limb

The human upper limb is a mobile unit. Here, flexibility and capability are the goals, with stability only a distant requirement. In joint anatomy, this means that bone-to-bone contact should be reduced (allowing more degrees of freedom in movement), that ligaments should be a precaution but not a restriction, and that muscle mass should dominate the tissue component across the joint.

The upper limb is so flexible that most of its bony beginning has no direct "joint" with the trunk of the body. For the most part, the scapula is free to glide and slide across the rib cage, staging the "free" part of the arm for focused movements. Only the tip of the spine of the scapula is in a negotiated joint with the trunk of the body, and

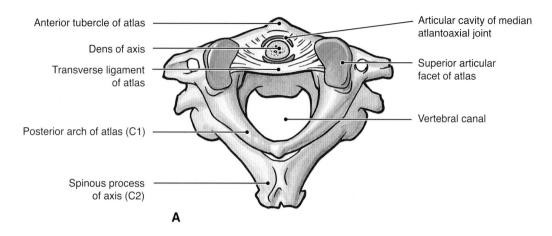

Anterior tubercle of atlas

Dens of axis

Transverse ligament of atlas

Posterior arch of atlas (C1)

Spinous process of axis (C2)

Articular cavity of median atlantoaxial joint

Superior articular facet of atlas

Vertebral canal

A

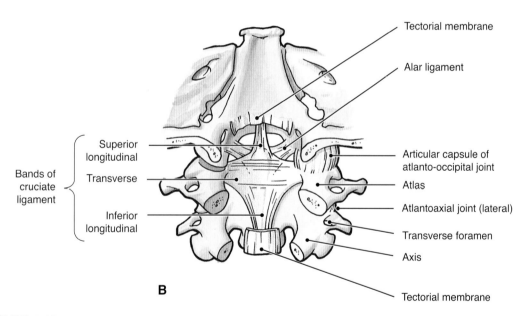

Bands of cruciate ligament

Superior longitudinal

Transverse

Inferior longitudinal

Tectorial membrane

Alar ligament

Articular capsule of atlanto-occipital joint

Atlas

Atlantoaxial joint (lateral)

Transverse foramen

Axis

B

Tectorial membrane

FIGURE 7.19   **Joining the atlas, axis, and occiput.**

(**A**) Superior view. The unusual atlantoaxial joint is supported by a transverse ligament that straps the dens of the axis against the atlas facet. (**B**) Posterior view. Delicate alar and apical ligaments tether the dens to the occipital bone. (From Moore KL, Agur AMR. Essential Clinical Anatomy, 2nd Edition. Baltimore: Lippincott Williams & Wilkins, 2002. Figure 5.7A,C, p. 289.)

even that is mediated by an independent bone, the clavicle. Given its limited strength, this **acromioclavicular joint** is a joint of position at best (Fig. 7.20).

The clavicle articulates with the trunk skeleton at the sternum (**sternoclavicular joint**) and with the scapula at the tip of the acromion process (**acromioclavicular joint**). Both are synovial joints, in which the clavicle acts in part as a "jam" between the front of the trunk and the sliding, gliding scapula. The scapula cannot slide too far

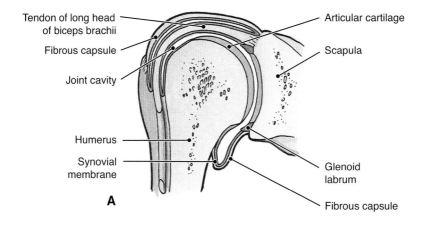

Tendon of long head of biceps brachii

Fibrous capsule

Joint cavity

Humerus

Synovial membrane

A

Articular cartilage

Scapula

Glenoid labrum

Fibrous capsule

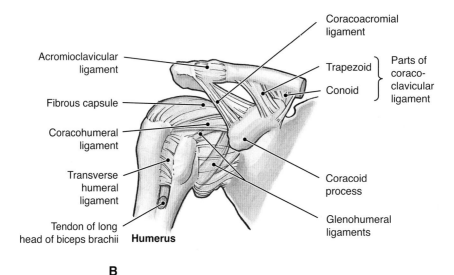

Acromioclavicular ligament

Fibrous capsule

Coracohumeral ligament

Transverse humeral ligament

Tendon of long head of biceps brachii   **Humerus**

Coracoacromial ligament

Trapezoid

Conoid

} Parts of coraco-clavicular ligament

Coracoid process

Glenohumeral ligaments

B

FIGURE 7.20   **The shoulder joints.**

(**A**) Anterior view, sectioned. Note the broad extent of the synovial cavity for the glenohumeral joint. (**B**) Anterior view, whole. The coracoacromial, coracoclavicular, and acromioclavicular ligaments span an awning over the glenohumeral joint. (From Moore KL, Agur AMR. Essential Clinical Anatomy, 2nd Edition. Baltimore: Lippincott Williams & Wilkins, 2002. Figure 7.32A,B, p. 483.)

forward, because the clavicle is jammed between it and the sternum. To absorb the impact, the sternoclavicular joint has a built-in cartilage pad between the two bones, a kind of synovial attempt to mimic a symphysis joint.

Both clavicular joints are sealed by ligament bands. The strongest ligament at the apex of the shoulder is the **coracoclavicular ligament**, which binds the clavicle to the coracoid process, a different part of the scapula altogether. This may be one way to ensure that the clavicle moves with the scapula without undue stiffening of the joint between it and the acromion process.

Glenohumeral Joint

The joint most associated with the "shoulder" is actually the **glenohumeral joint** between the scapula and the humerus. The glenoid fossa is a shallow depression that can barely receive the spherical head of the humerus (see Fig. 7.20A). This is just as well, because the glenohumeral joint is, perhaps, the most mobile synovial joint in the body. In addition, that mobility depends on the bone-to-bone contact being slight rather than "cupped." You should think of the humeral head as being "applied" to the glenoid surface because of the strong pull of the several "rotator cuff" muscles (see below).

The glenohumeral joint is our first example of a "ball and socket" type of synovial joint—even if the socket is more like an ice rink. The joint capsule must be shaped like a kind of sleeve that patches the base of the "ball" and the perimeter of the "socket." The only named ligaments of the glenohumeral joint capsule are unremarkable fiber bands that compose the anterior part of the capsule and are called, naturally, the glenohumeral ligaments (Fig. 7.21).

The accessory ligaments of the glenohumeral joint and the muscles that cross it are far more important to mechanics and movement of the joint. The accessory ligaments include the **coracoacromial ligament**, which is a good example of the power of connective tissue to assume multiple identities. This ligament connects two parts of the same bone, but rather than ossifying to be an extreme form of connective tissue, the band remains ligamentous and, thus, somewhat flexible. It hangs over the glenohumeral joint as a kind of "roof," which is a useful barrier when too much force traveling up the arm could push the head of the humerus out of the joint space.

One muscle even detours through the joint capsule on its way down the arm. The **biceps brachii**, which originates from above the glenohumeral joint, sends a bundle of tendon fibers through the joint space as it squeezes between the rotator cuff sandwich on its way to the elbow (see Fig. 7.21). To avoid intense friction against the cartilage, the tendon is blanketed by the synovial membrane, meaning that the effective joint cavity space is "uninterrupted"—that is, the synovial cavity is closed even if the joint cavity has a large tendon running through it.

Dislocations and separations of the shoulder joint are common because of the inherent weakness of the acromioclavicular joint and the lack of support inferior to the humeral head. Impact injuries may separate the acromioclavicular joint. The humeral

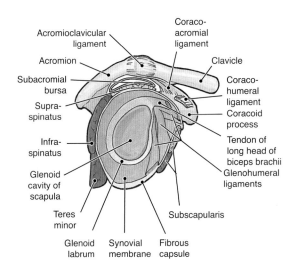

Acromioclavicular ligament
Coraco-acromial ligament
Acromion
Clavicle
Subacromial bursa
Coraco-humeral ligament
Supra-spinatus
Coracoid process
Infra-spinatus
Tendon of long head of biceps brachii
Glenoid cavity of scapula
Glenohumeral ligaments
Teres minor
Subscapularis
Glenoid labrum
Synovial membrane
Fibrous capsule

FIGURE 7.21   Inside the glenohumeral joint.

This "head-on" view of the glenoid fossa shows how muscles, rather than ligaments, secure the head of the humerus against the scapula. The ligaments of the shoulder joint, strictly speaking, are the anterior elaborations of the articular capsule (glenohumeral ligaments). (From Moore KL, Agur AMR. Essential Clinical Anatomy, 2nd Edition. Baltimore: Lippincott Williams & Wilkins, 2002. Figure 7.32C, p. 483.)

head may dislocate as a result of disproportionate extension and lateral rotation of the humerus. The strength of the rotator cuff muscles is such that a dislocated humeral head does not slide readily back into place.

The Elbow Joint

The elbow joint may be the "stiffest" joint in the upper limb, in the sense that its strongest movement is a simple but restricted flexion and extension between the ulna and humerus. The joint also allows forearm rotation (**pronation** and **supination**) of the radius. It is a joint among three bones (humerus, radius, and ulna) that functions separately between the "hinges" (humerus and ulna) and between the "pivots" (ulna and radius).

The elbow joint cavity includes the articulating parts of all three bones, even though the two allowed movements are independent of one another. The concave head of the radius fits nicely against the capitulum ("little head") of the humerus, but it mostly just spins in place here. Its main contact is between the side of the radial head and a notch on the side of the ulna. The ulna reciprocates, of course, but its main contact is an aggressive clamping of the bottom of the humerus so that it can flex and extend like a hinge (Fig. 7.22).

The elbow joint capsule wraps all three bones and both functional joints. It is uncomplicated, and it is characterized by flexibility in front and back and by strapping ligaments on the sides. These ligaments are called **collateral ligaments**; versions of collateral ligaments are common at other limb joints, such as the knee and ankle joints, where sideways bending is a bad idea.

Within the joint capsule, the **radioulnar joint** has its own dedicated ligament called the **anular ligament**. This connective tissue is C-shaped, and it connects with the side of the ulna to create a loop or a lasso of space (see Fig. 7.22A). The head of the radius fits inside, and the anular ligament acts like a sling to keep it against the side of the ulna. The cartilage that coats the top and sides of the radial head is now free to spin around against the cartilage of the ulnar notch and the inner lining of the anular ligament.

To avoid getting pinched, the major nerve (the **median nerve**) and blood vessel (the **brachial artery**) that serve the rest of the arm pass across the joint on the front side, where the elbow "gives" during forearm flexion. This **cubital fossa** is a primary location for drawing blood from a superficial vein.

The Wrist Joint

The wrist joint disperses force from the forearm into the grasping human hand. The forearm strut impacts a set of "bearings" in the wrist that transmit force in parcels to the individual fingers. The two bones of the forearm strut, however, do not articulate equally with the carpals. The radius, which is a minor component of the elbow joint, dominates the ulna at the wrist. This effectively enables the hand to be controlled by the mobile bone of the forearm without compromising the position of the forearm, which is determined by the ulna (Fig. 7.23).

The joint cavity at the wrist should include the radius, ulna, scaphoid, and lunate, but the radius so dominates the ulna that an articular disc of cartilage projects across from the bottom of the radius to block the bottom of the ulna from making contact with the wrist bones. This leaves the bottom of the ulna lodged against the radius as the distal radioulnar joint. The radius enjoys extended contact with the scaphoid and lunate as the **radiocarpal joint**.

Only two of the eight carpal bones articulate with the radius: the lunate and the scaphoid. In some sense, they traffic force and movement into the two "halves" of the hand, the dominant "thumb side" and the submissive "pinky side." The radius delivers

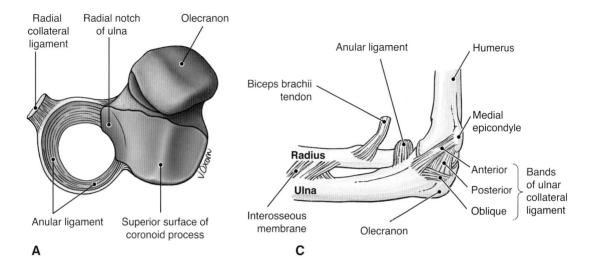

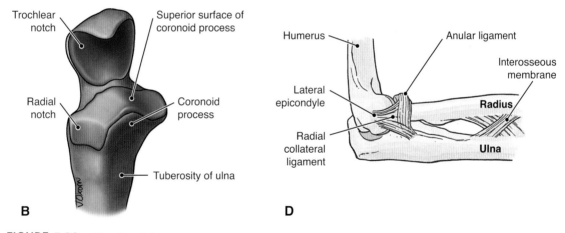

FIGURE 7.22   **The elbow joints.**

(**A**) The radius is strapped tightly to the ulna but lacks an effective articulation with the humerus (superior view). (**B**) The ulna maintains a strict hinge-joint clamp on the medial condyle of the humerus (anterior view). (**C** and **D**) The elbow joint is supported by collateral ligaments on the ulnar and radial side. The fit of the radial head against the ulna is facilitated by the anular ligament. (From Moore KL, Agur AMR. Essential Clinical Anatomy, 2nd Edition. Baltimore: Lippincott Williams & Wilkins, 2002. Figure 7.32, p. 486.)

the force through these vectors, and because it is the mobile bone of the forearm, it can position the wrist in the complete circuit of clockwise or counterclockwise positions. Thus, the wrist joint is essentially a joint of infinite positioning to stabilize the hand for power and precision movements.

The ligaments that support the articular capsule are less remarkable than the internal construction of the joint. In anticipation of the rest of the wrist and hand

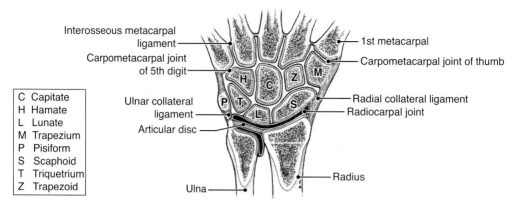

C Capitate
H Hamate
L Lunate
M Trapezium
P Pisiform
S Scaphoid
T Triquetrium
Z Trapezoid

FIGURE 7.23   **The wrist joint.**

This section of the wrist shows the synovial spaces that surround the complicated attachments of the carpal bones. Note how the ulna is separated from the carpals by an extension of the radial cartilage. The distal radius, which is free to pronate and supinate, governs transmission of force into the wrist. (From Moore KL, Agur AMR. Essential Clinical Anatomy, 2nd Edition. Baltimore: Lippincott Williams & Wilkins, 2002. Figure 7.15, p. 490.)

joints, the ligaments consist of slightly thickened bands of capsule on the sides (collateral, or medial and lateral) and/or across the front and back (ventral and dorsal) that are named accordingly.

People brace themselves against an impact or during a fall by extending their hands. This can result in a fracture of the distal radius, known clinically as a **Colles' fracture**, which is the most common fracture in adults older than 50 years. In younger adults and children, similar injuries are likely to result in a compression or fracture of the scaphoid bone, the blood supply of which is delicate enough that ischemia and necrosis may follow if the injury is not detected.

Joints of the lower limb

Our bipedal lifestyle is demanding on the joints of the lower limb. We expect to be mobile, so the joints must provide ample range of motion and some flexibility of direction. We also, however, expect to be coordinated and balanced when we move—and when at rest, for that matter. So, the designs of the lower limb joints must allow "tighter fits" than occur in their upper limb analogues.

Tighter fits are most apparent in the proximal joints. In the upper limb, the "anchor" bone, the scapula, enjoys so much mobility because it lacks a fixating joint with the trunk. In the lower limb, the equivalent of the scapula, clavicle, and sternum is the "hip bone," or **os coxa**, which is a single bone that articulates with itself anteriorly. The "hip bone" is fixed in position—so fixed, in fact, that it defines the bottom of the trunk and constrains the position and magnitude of the outflow tracks of endoderm (reproductive and digestive systems). It is such a "fixture" of the pelvic region of the body that it is easy to forget it really is three bones of the lower limb.

In keeping with a homology model, the joint between the femur and the hip should allow a global kind of rotation, similar to that of the glenohumeral joint. The knee joint should allow strong flexion and extension and, in theory, rotation of one of the leg bones on the other (it does not, however!). Like the wrist joint, the ankle joint should transfer force from a strut to bearings that govern the individual rays. By studying the upper limb joints first, you get a sense of the potential mobility of each major joint. This helps you to make sense of the unusual ways that the lower limb joints depart from the basic plan.

The pelvis presents an almost rigid girdle joining the lower extremity to the trunk. Normally, the term **pelvis** refers to the two "hip bones" (os coxae) and to the sacrum. The os coxa from one side articulates to the trunk at the sacrum and to its partner from the other side around the front (thus, forming its own equivalent of the "sternum"). Therefore, the joints are the **sacroiliac joint** in the back and the **pubic symphysis** in the front.

Sacroiliac Joint

The sacroiliac joint is a synovial joint, but it permits very little movement. This is because the bone-to-bone connection between the ilium part of the os coxa and the side surface of the sacrum is virtually a fusion of bone. The two surfaces are smashed together, and all around them is a thick articular capsule (Fig. 7.24). In addition, two big ligaments span across the joint and become major ligaments of the pelvic girdle: the **sacrotuberous ligament**, and the **sacrospinous ligament**.

The **sacrotuberous ligament** runs in a broad sweep from the back of the sacrum across to the ischial tuberosity (the part of the hip that you "sit on"). In this position, it helps to close off the **greater sciatic notch** in the ilium bone, making it a foramen instead of a notch.

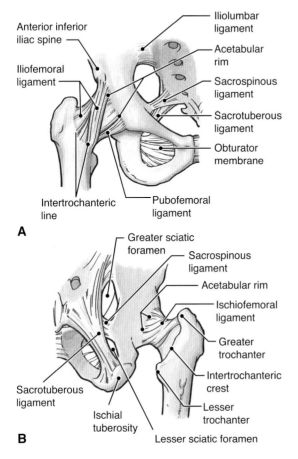

FIGURE 7.24   The sacroiliac joint.

The sacroiliac joint is plastered by comprehensive ligament patches. Supporting ligaments include the iliolumbar ligament (**A**) and the sacrotuberous and sacrospinous ligaments, which connect the sacrum to lower regions of the os coxa. In the process, they "close off" the sciatic notches into functional sciatic foramina (**B**). (From Moore KL, Agur AMR. Essential Clinical Anatomy, 2nd Edition. Baltimore: Lippincott Williams & Wilkins, 2002. Figure 6.30A,B.)

The **sacrospinous ligament** runs a shorter course from the side of the sacrum straight over to the ischial spine. With the sacrotuberous ligament, it closes off the big notch in the ilium into a **greater sciatic foramen** above and a **lesser sciatic foramen** below.

Pubic Symphysis

The pubic symphysis, the joint between the two pubis bodies, is one of the few symphyseal joints outside of the vertebral column. Although it is designed to permit less movement than a typical synovial joint, the pubic symphysis is barely reinforced by ligaments. Across the top and the bottom of the joint capsule are slight thickenings called the **superior pubic ligament** and the **arcuate pubic ligament**, respectively. These ligaments help to reinforce the pubic symphysis somewhat, but this symphysis joint definitely yields during forceful events, such as childbirth.

The projections of bone that become the pubic body (superior pubic ramus and inferior pubic ramus) are ideal "hangers" for muscles that draw the thigh inward (adductors of the thigh, much like the pectoralis major of the arm). The ^-shape underneath the pubic symphysis is well positioned to support the external muscles of the perineum; the genital anatomy essentially hangs down from the bottom of the symphysis.

Hip Joint

The hip joint is the best example of a ball-and-socket joint in the body. The nearly spherical head of the femur fits snugly in the welcoming cup of the os coxa, the **acetabulum**. Supplemented by a cartilage lip and a spanning ligament, the acetabulum extends over the "equator" of the femoral head to hold the "ball" more firmly in the "socket" (Fig. 7.25).

Unlike the mechanical requirements at the shoulder joint, those at the hip joint are stringent. The hip joint must be able to balance the body weight through this joint—and to move the body powerfully forward while keeping the body weight balanced. This is no small feat. The strength that is required comes from the deep socket holding the femoral head, the tense fibrous capsule of the joint, and muscle insertions located a good distance from the center of movement. The sacrifice, in return, is range of motion.

As with the shoulder joint, the ligaments that support the hip joint "blanket" the articular capsule and effectively sleeve the bony surfaces behind the articular surfaces of each bone. From the rim of the acetabulum come bands of ligament fibers (**iliofemoral** or **ischiofemoral**) that span across the joint in virtually full coverage, then anchor down along the buttresses of bone at the base of the femoral neck (see Fig. 7.24).

Two more interesting ligaments complete the joint. The bony acetabulum is an incomplete circumference of bone; a small notch of open space remains, giving it a nearly complete O-shape. To keep the head of the femur from popping out through this acetabular notch, a ligament spans it as a kind of trampoline. The **transverse acetabular ligament** is a tough surrogate for the bone that does not form in this region of the "socket."

Finally, the head of the femur has a kind of pit, or **fovea**, that other heads of long bones do not have. This **fovea capitis** is a well for the rope-like **ligament of the head of the femur**, also called the **ligamentum teres**, which reaches out to the margin of the acetabulum. The function of this ligament is unclear, because it seems too lax and weak to provide support.

This major joint of the body is relatively poorly perfused. Recall that the main artery serving the joint, the medial circumflex femoral artery, does not anastomose effectively with arteries serving the femoral head. Hip fractures, which occur with

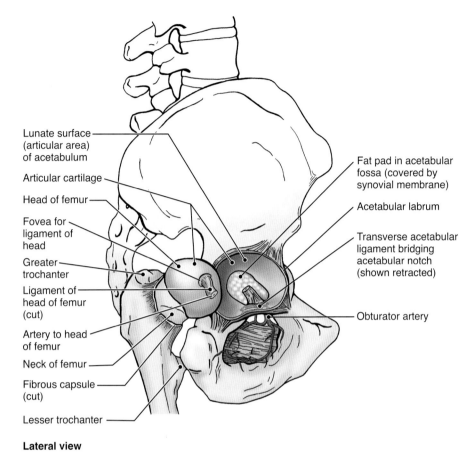

Lunate surface
(articular area)
of acetabulum

Articular cartilage

Head of femur

Fovea for
ligament of
head

Greater
trochanter

Ligament of
head of femur
(cut)

Artery to head
of femur

Neck of femur

Fibrous capsule
(cut)

Lesser trochanter

Fat pad in acetabular
fossa (covered by
synovial membrane)

Acetabular labrum

Transverse acetabular
ligament bridging
acetabular notch
(shown retracted)

Obturator artery

Lateral view

FIGURE 7.25   **The hip joint.**

The hip joint is built for stability. The deep recess of the acetabulum receives most of the spherical femoral head. The articular capsule thickens into iliofemoral and ischiofemoral "sheetwraps" (see Fig. 7.24). The head of the femur is tethered by an obscure, round ligament that ferries a tiny blood vessel from the obturator artery into the joint space. (From Moore KL, Dalley AF. Clinically Oriented Anatomy, 5th Edition. Baltimore: Lippincott Williams & Wilkins, 2006. Figure 5.51 p. 676.)

some frequency in elderly people because of osteoporosis, can entail avascular necrosis of the femoral head. In young or old patients, the ultimate result is an artificial hip replacement.

Knee Joint

The knee is the largest and most complex joint in the body. Many ligaments, both intracapsular and extracapsular, support the knee joint, which also contains two fibrous menisci to improve the fit between the tibia and the femur. The knee joint is in the midrange of both mobility and stability. It does the best it can as a hinge joint charged with the full weight of the body, enormous muscle power across it, and stress angles that no other part of the body could endure. It only has so much raw material with which to work, however, so it tends to fail.

The anatomy of the knee joint is the story of how far a synovial joint can be warped to compensate for the unusual demands of upright posture and walking. Each element of a typical synovial joint (e.g., articular capsule, ligaments, and synovial membrane) is irregular in the knee joint (see Fig. 7.15). In addition, the two big bones that abut each other do not even fit well together.

The bottom of the femur articulates with the top of the tibia, but the simplicity ends there. The condyles of the femur are "rocker-bottomed" so that the bone rolls smoothly in a flexing and extending hinge. Because the shaft approaches the knee joint at an angle, however, the contacting condyles are not symmetric. The receiving tibia is shaped like a plateau on top—an irregular plateau, of course. Unfortunately, the "wells" that receive the femoral condyles are only slightly concave. The femoral condyles cannot "dig" into a socket or fossa of any kind. Instead, they lie atop the tibia and are always at risk of sliding out of place. In between the two basins on the tibial plateau, a rise of bone, the **intercondylar eminence**, enables accessories of the knee joint to attach. These accessories, particularly the cruciate ligaments of the knee joint, are necessary to overcome the unsteady basic articulation of the femur onto the tibia (Fig. 7.26).

The knee joint includes another bony articulation, which again is unique in the body. The **patella** intervenes between the powerful quadriceps tendon and its insertion across the knee joint onto the front of the tibia. Without the patella, too much friction

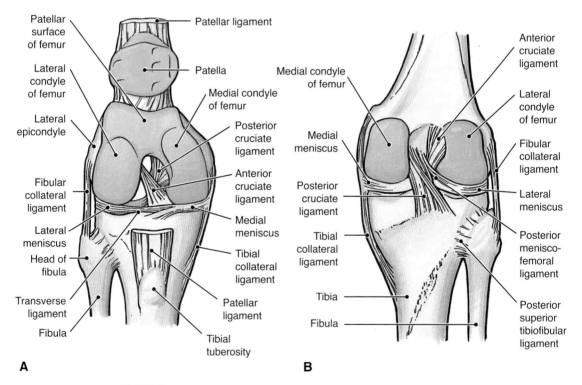

A   **B**

FIGURE 7.26   **The knee joint articular capsule and extrinsic ligaments.**

(**A**) Anterior view. The patella forms in the tendon of the quadriceps femoris muscle and is a true sesamoid bone. It helps to reduce friction across the bent knee joint, and as a kind of "extension" of the tibia, it optimizes the pull of the quadriceps muscle as it corrects a bent knee to a resting state of extension. This is the only case in the body of a tendon, a sesamoid bone, and a ligament forming a part of an articular capsule. (**B**) Posterior view. Medial and lateral collateral ligaments resist side-bending of the joint. (From Moore KL, Agur AMR. Essential Clinical Anatomy, 2nd Edition. Baltimore: Lippincott Williams & Wilkins, 2002. Figure 6.33B,C.)

heat would develop between the quadriceps tendon and the sharp angle of the knee when the knee flexes. The patella absorbs the harsh angle by abutting the femoral condyles, and it completes the mission of the quadriceps tendon through a ligament (the **patellar ligament**) that continues from it to the intended muscle insertion on the tibial tuberosity.

To deal with its vulnerabilities, the knee joint sacrifices capsule strength for extra ligaments and dedicated muscles. The joint capsule is reduced to the minimum amount of patching that is necessary to contain the synovial membrane and its fluid. As with so many other connective tissue zones, hypertrophy of one component requires hypotrophy of another. The joint capsule is extensive in range, from the femoral epicondyles down across the joint to the boundaries of the articular surfaces of the tibia, but it is relatively thin and even deficient anteriorly.

The most obvious expression of connective tissue power is the very front of the joint capsule, which is made up of the quadriceps muscle tendon, the patella, and the patellar ligament. **Rather than operating as a regular muscle tendon across a joint, this powerful knee extender actually is the joint capsule.** Thus, there is no complete, independent fibrous capsule wrapping the joint space. At least in the front, the capsule is significantly more elastic and dynamic (see Fig. 7.15). The quadriceps muscles can adjust the tension in the knee joint capsule from any position.

The knee joint is supported by extrinsic and intrinsic ligaments. The extrinsic ligaments are so small and peripheral that they seem to be feeble, but where necessary, they merge into the articular capsule in a better effort to reinforce it. On the medial side of the knee, the **tibial collateral ligament** runs from the femoral epicondyles to the tibia, just like the capsule (Fig. 7.27). It resists, but is vulnerable to, hyperextension when you endure an impact from the side, and it merges with the articular capsule at approximately its midway point. This is significant, because the medial meniscus inside the knee joint is fused to the articular capsule at the same point, effectively connecting it to the tibial collateral ligament. On the lateral side of the knee, the **fibular collateral ligament** parallels the tibial collateral ligament, but it does not attach to the articular capsule. The posterior aspect of the knee joint capsule is distinguished by the popliteus muscle, which intervenes through the articular capsule to attach to the lateral femoral epicondyle (Fig. 7.28). The capsule is reinforced centrally by the **oblique**

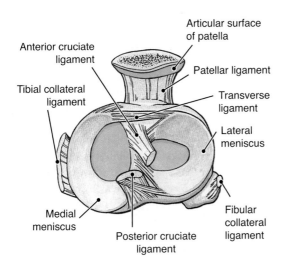

Anterior cruciate ligament

Tibial collateral ligament

Articular surface of patella

Patellar ligament

Transverse ligament

Lateral meniscus

Medial meniscus

Posterior cruciate ligament

Fibular collateral ligament

FIGURE 7.27   Inside the knee joint—menisci.

The medial and lateral menisci are another unique feature of the knee joint. They are thicker on their peripheries, which gives the tibial plateau slightly more "depth" along the edges to receive the femoral condyles. The menisci take a beating. To withstand the force, they are poorly vascularized (so as not to be chronically bruised), which means that when they tear, they generally do not heal. (From Moore KL, Agur AMR. Essential Clinical Anatomy, 2nd Edition. Baltimore: Lippincott Williams & Wilkins, 2002. Figure 6.35A.)

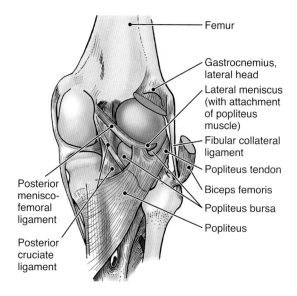

Femur

Gastrocnemius, lateral head

Lateral meniscus (with attachment of popliteus muscle)

Fibular collateral ligament

Popliteus tendon

Biceps femoris

Popliteus bursa

Popliteus

Posterior menisco-femoral ligament

Posterior cruciate ligament

FIGURE 7.28   Inside the knee joint—popliteus muscle.

The popliteus muscle is perhaps the most obvious sign that the knee joint has special needs. Because the "close-packed" position of the femur on the tibia locks when the femur spins inward, you cannot easily "unlock" the knee joint from a standing position. The popliteus muscle sneaks into the knee joint capsule and draws on the side of the lateral femoral condyle. When it contracts, it spins the femur slightly outward, unlocking the articulation and enabling the knee muscles of flexion and extension to pull effectively. (From Moore KL, Dalley AF. Clinically Oriented Anatomy, 5th Edition. Baltimore: Lippincott Williams & Wilkins, 2006. Figure 5.38B, p. 651.)

popliteal ligament, which is a connective tissue extension of the attachment of the semimembranosus muscle. Below this, on the lateral side, courses the **arcuate popliteal ligament**, which strengthens the capsule over the gap that permits the popliteus muscle to pass into and out of the capsule.

Within the capsule, two prominent ligaments bind the femur to the tibia and resist the tendency for the bones to "slide off" one another. These are the **anterior cruciate ligament** and **posterior cruciate ligament**, which are familiar to many people because of how frequently they are injured. These ligaments are named for where they attach to the tibia (see Fig. 7.27). The anterior cruciate ligament attaches to the front part of the plateau between the basins for the femoral condyles. It stretches up and back to insert on the inside surface of the lateral femoral condyle. The posterior cruciate ligament attaches on the back of the tibial plateau, again between the two condylar basins, and stretches up and forward to insert on the inside surface of the medial condyle. The ligaments "cross" one another in this maneuver and, thus, are called "cruciate" ligaments.

The cruciate ligaments team up to keep the femur and the tibia from sliding too far anteriorly or posteriorly relative to one another. The anterior cruciate ligament resists the tibia sliding too far forward relative to the femur, and the posterior cruciate ligament resists the tibia sliding too far backward relative to the femur. The cruciate ligaments are intracapsular but extrasynovial—that is, they are located inside of the boundary defined by the articular capsule, but they are not within the synovial membrane (and, thus, are not bathed in synovial fluid). For the most part, synovial membranes strictly line the articular surfaces of the bones that impact one another. This limits the synovial fluid to a space that deals with the bone-to-bone demands for lubrication. The knee is no exception. The very complicated synovial membrane (see below) snakes around the condylar basins and along the intercondylar eminence such that the two big ligaments inside the joint capsule can skirt between layers of the membrane without ever penetrating it.

Three very small ligaments complete the knee-joint battery. The **anterior meniscofemoral ligament** and **posterior meniscofemoral ligament** are small slips that run from the lateral mensicus to the posterior cruciate ligament near its origin (see Fig. 7.26). The **transverse ligament** of the knee stretches between the medial and lateral meniscus in front of the anterior cruciate ligament.

In all synovial joints, the articular surfaces of the bones are themselves covered in cartilage. This protects the bony surfaces from damage and erosion, cushions the joint, and facilitates the effect of synovial fluid in resisting friction during movement. In some joints, the impact of bone on bone is so great that even the articular cartilages are at risk. An intervening cartilage pad, independent of the articulating surfaces, can help to absorb some of the compression between the two bones. These cartilaginous pads in the knee are called menisci, with one for each condyle (a **lateral meniscus** and a **medial meniscus**). They are frequently torn and are the reason many arthroscopic surgeons are very busy (see Clinical Anatomy Box 7.1).

Given all the other irregularities of this joint, it is no surprise that the medial meniscus and the lateral meniscus are not mirror images of one another (see Fig. 7.27). They do, however, share some features in common. They are C-shaped, semi-lunar crescents of poorly vascularized cartilage. They are thick on their outer margins and paper-thin along their innermost border. They anchor into the joint complex at the "tips" of the C-shape, on the tibia plateau between the condylar basins and next to the attachments of the cruciate ligaments.

Except for the attachment to the deep surface of the articular capsule at the "apex" of the C-shape (the outermost edge), they would otherwise flap up and down between the massive femoral condyles and the tibial basins. On the medial side, this occurs at the same point that the tibial collateral ligament attaches to the capsule from the outside. The lateral meniscus has one more delicate arrangement. As the tendon of the popliteus muscle cruises by, it attaches to the edge of the meniscus, thus affecting its position as the muscle contracts.

In a typical joint, the joint capsule is lined completely by synovial membrane, and the joint cavity has a relatively uncomplicated contour. The membrane keeps the vital synovial fluid from escaping, and all contact surfaces are bathed. The knee joint is complicated, however, by various ligaments, menisci, and muscles. The only thing that is typical about its synovial membrane is that it keeps the synovial fluid trapped and bathing the contact surfaces. To achieve this, the membrane itself is quite convoluted. Realize that in such a complicated joint, the membrane that seals in the synovial fluid must warp, twist, accommodate, and slip both in and around the things that are in the way. The synovial membrane also extends into odd places to protect the cartilage as the knee tightly flexes or extends. These recesses or bursae can inflame, injuring or damaging other parts of the knee joint and resulting in painful **bursitis**.

The space behind the patella is bathed in synovial fluid (see Fig. 7.15). Because the patella migrates so far "up and down" during flexion of the joint, this central part of the synovial cavity is extensive. A **suprapatellar bursa** slips up along the shaft of the femur as high as the patella might reach in extension. An unusual muscle called the **articularis genu** binds the top of the suprapatellar bursa to the shaft of the femur so that it does not slide down into the knee joint like a loose sock. The patella is flanked by a few other bursae, including an **infrapatellar bursa** below and a **prepatellar bursa** in front. These are common locations of bursitis from chronic kneeling or crawling.

The major movement at the knee joint is flexion and extension. To complete its extension, or to commence its flexion from that point, the condyles must spin just a little bit into or out of the tibial basins. This is called "locking out" when the joint twists just a little bit so that the condyles are in the most secure position relative to the tibia in the extended knee. All joints seek a "close-packed" arrangement of their bones for

Box 7.1

COMMON KNEE JOINT INJURIES

The parts of the knee that tend to fail most often are the parts that make it an unusual synovial joint in the first place. The **menisci** are prone to tearing when the knee is twisted. Because they are vascularized only at their base, tears along their periphery rarely heal. Scraping away the torn meniscus tissue and restoring adequate function to the joint are the major goals of meniscal arthroscopic surgery.

The **cruciate ligaments** are prone to spraining or tearing when the moving body suddenly stops or when a person is tackled in a field sport. A good sense of the anatomy is key to discerning the extent of the injury when you examine the patient. Too much laxity of sliding movement in the tibia indicates a ligament that is flaccid from a sprain or tear. Testing the laxity by attempting to shift the free leg anteriorly or posteriorly while the femur is fixed can reveal which cruciate ligament is no longer working.

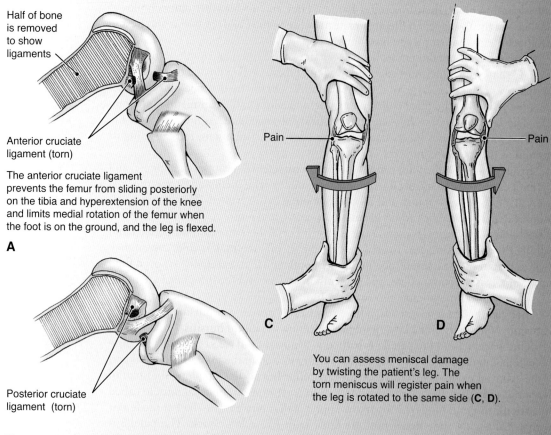

Half of bone is removed to show ligaments

Anterior cruciate ligament (torn)

The anterior cruciate ligament prevents the femur from sliding posteriorly on the tibia and hyperextension of the knee and limits medial rotation of the femur when the foot is on the ground, and the leg is flexed.

A

Pain

Pain

C

D

You can assess meniscal damage by twisting the patient's leg. The torn meniscus will register pain when the leg is rotated to the same side (**C**, **D**).

Posterior cruciate ligament (torn)

The posterior cruciate ligament prevents the femur from sliding anteriorly on the tibia, particularly when the knee is flexed.

B

Assessing knee joint injuries. (From Moore KL, Dalley AF. Clinically Oriented Anatomy, 5th Edition. Baltimore: Lippincott Williams & Wilkins, 2006. Figures B5.26 and B5.27, pp. 698–699.)

maximum stability. In the knee, the most stable position of extension requires that the medial condyle rotate "inward" (or back, as you look down at the knee) to "lock" into place.

The knee joint locks passively as a result of the momentum of walking or swinging the leg into extension. Unlocking the knee joint is more difficult—and a more active process. The joint must be unlocked so that the large muscles of flexion, such as the hamstrings, can work effectively. A special muscle called the **popliteus** is dedicated to just this purpose, and it runs right through the joint cavity (see Fig. 7.28).

The popliteus muscle attaches to the lateral condyle within the articular capsule, then pokes through an opening in the back of the capsule to insert on the tibia. A bursa follows it out of the articular capsule to pad that capsule from the friction of the contracting muscle. This is called the **subpopliteal recess**. When the popliteus contracts, it draws the lateral condyle backward, which, assuming the foot is fixed against the ground and the tibia is stable, moves the medial condyle forward. If the foot is off the ground, however, then the contracting popliteus will pull the medial part of the tibia backward. In either dynamic, the position of the medial condyle on the tibial basin reverses the "locked" position described above. Once unlocked, the bigger flexor muscles take control.

Ankle Joint

The ankle is a modified hinge joint that allows the foot skeleton to flex and extend. These movements of the foot are termed **plantarflexion** if you are moving the foot downward at the ankle joint and **dorsiflexion** if you are raising the foot upward at the ankle joint. Compared to its radiocarpal analog in the wrist, the ankle joint sacrifices range of motion to handle the demand of body weight pushing down on a "spring-loaded" and arched foot skeleton.

The ankle joint brings the bottom of the tibia and the fibula into contact with a single tarsal bone, the **talus** (Fig. 7.29). The talus rests on another single tarsal bone (the **calcaneus**), and together, they spread the force from above to the toes and to the heel. Ligaments help to strap the strut bones (tibia and fibula) to the tarsals. As with the knee and elbow, they are developed along the sides of the joint, where movement is restricted. The front and back of the joint area are dominated by powerful muscle tendons, such as the **calcaneal tendon** (Achilles tendon). The ligaments are important to learn because of the frequency of "sprained ankles." Typically, a sprained ankle means that the ligaments on either side of the joint stretch too far and too fast. This happens when the joint bends laterally or medially against its design. (See Clinical Anatomy Box 7.2). Here, the ligaments in play are called the **medial collateral ligament** and the **lateral collateral ligament**.

The medial collateral ligament protects against too much "inward" bending. It usually is called the **deltoid ligament**, because the spread of ligament fibers resembles the Greek letter delta (Δ). From the tibia, they spread down and around to reach the talus, the calcaneus, and the navicular bone in front of the head of the talus (Fig. 7.30). The lateral collateral ligaments protect against too much "outward" bending, a common sports injury when you "roll" over a foot that is planted against the ground or the court. These ligament bands are more narrow and more separated than the deltoid ligament bands. They stretch from the fibula to the talus (the **anterior talofibular ligament** and the **posterior talofibular ligament**) and to the calcaneus (the **calcaneofibular ligament**). The **anterior talofibular ligament** is not as well protected by overlying muscle tendons and retinacula, so it is the most frequently sprained or torn ligament of the ankle joint.

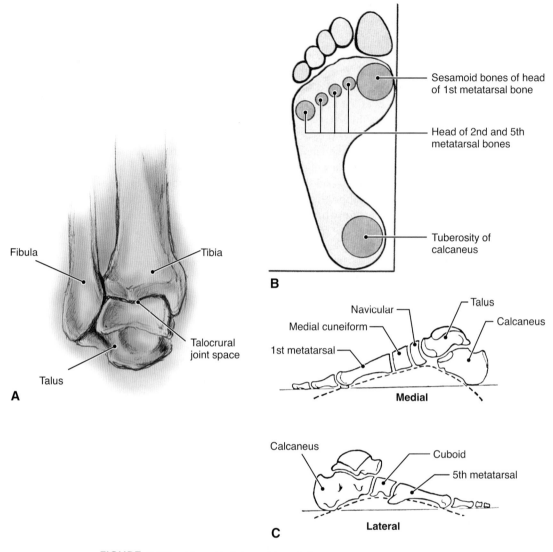

FIGURE 7.29   The ankle joint and foot skeleton.

(**A**) Anterior view. The brace-like design of the ankle joint facilitates dorsiflexion and plantarflexion movement. Strong ligaments resist side-bending here. (**B**) The talus alone receives the force of body weight through the tibia, and the arch of the foot skeleton dissipates that force to the heel point of the calcaneus and forward through the other tarsals into the toes (**C**). (Adapted from Moore KL, Agur AMR. Essential Clinical Anatomy, 2nd Edition. Baltimore: Lippincott Williams & Wilkins, 2002. Figure 6.41, p. 402.)

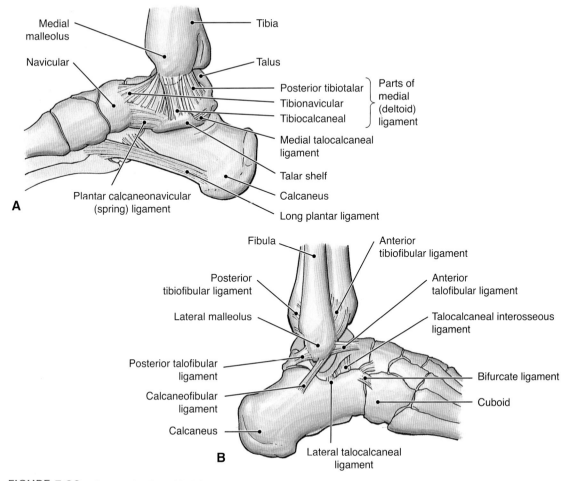

FIGURE 7.30   Support for the ankle joint.

The ankle joint is supported by a strong "composite" ligament on the medial side and three "strip" ligaments on the lateral side. The deltoid ligament on the medial side (**A**) straps the tibia to every neighboring tarsal bone, and it is so strong that tension against it tends to shear off the tibia instead of tearing the ligament. Of the lateral collateral ligaments of the ankle joint (**B**) the anterior talofibular ligament is the least supported and is prone to tearing (a "sprained ankle"). (From Moore KL, Agur AMR. Essential Clinical Anatomy, 2nd Edition. Baltimore: Lippincott Williams & Wilkins, 2002. Figure 6.37, p. 393.)

Joints of the foot

The foot skeleton enables weight that comes down through the talus to go backward, into the heel part of the calcaneus, or forward, through the navicular or the front of the calcaneus (see Fig. 7.29). Therefore, the joints of the foot begin with an alignment that puts the weight into one of three places: the heel (through the back of the calcaneus), the little toes (through the front of the calcaneus), or the big toe (through the navicular directly).

The tarsal bones involved in these joints are simple blocks, just like the carpals, except that they are warped into a platform bone (the talus) and arched intermediaries between it and the ray bones of the toes. The individual anatomic joints are clinically unremarkable. As with the carpals, the ligaments that secure the articular capsules are strap-like and named for the two bones that they connect. The talus is connected to

Box 7.2

SPRAINED ANKLE

Perhaps the most common clinical presentation involving connective tissue is the sprained ankle. Our feet contact so many uneven surfaces that we are always at risk for inverting or everting the joint too much. Sprains or tears of the lateral collateral ligaments (A) are by far more common and result from too much inversion, such as when you "roll" over the ankle joint while changing directions or when you accidentally step off of a curb.

Sprains of the medial side of the ankle joint are more rare, perhaps because of the strength of the medial collateral (deltoid) ligament. The ligament is so strong, in fact, that when the stress is too great, it is the bottom of the tibia, not the ligament, that breaks. This kind of fracture is called a **Pott's fracture. (B)**

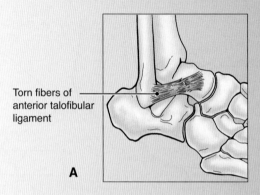

Torn fibers of anterior talofibular ligament

A

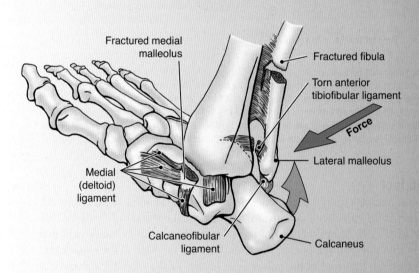

Fractured medial malleolus

Fractured fibula

Torn anterior tibiofibular ligament

Force

Lateral malleolus

Medial (deltoid) ligament

Calcaneofibular ligament

Calcaneus

B

Pott's fracture–dislocation of ankle

The sprained ankle. (From Moore KL, Dalley AF. Clinically Oriented Anatomy, 5th Edition. Baltimore: Lippincott Williams & Wilkins, 2006. Figures B5.32 and B5.33, pp. 706–707.)

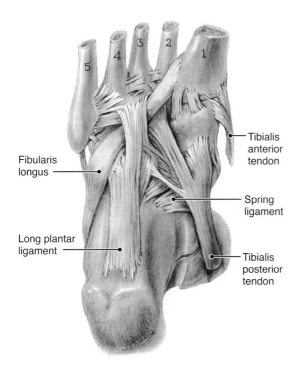

Fibularis longus

Long plantar ligament

Tibialis anterior tendon

Spring ligament

Tibialis posterior tendon

FIGURE 7.31   **Arch support, inferior view.**

Large ligaments that support the joints of the foot, particularly the composite of joints that form the foot arches, include the spring and long plantar ligaments. (Adapted from Moore KL, Dalley AF. Clinically Oriented Anatomy, 5th Edition. Baltimore: Lippincott Williams & Wilkins, 2006. Figure 5.67A, p. 709.)

the navicular, which is connected to the cuneiforms, which are connected to the three medial toes, and so on. Therefore, there must be a talonavicular joint and some naviculocuneiform joints, but the real joint action in the foot is how these anatomic joints combine their efforts to form the **functional** joints of the foot.

The major anatomic joints include the talocalcaneonavicular joint and the great tarsal joint. The **talocalcaneonavicular joint** delivers the force forward in the foot, and it is supported by the usual types of ligaments. Because it follows the arch of the foot, however, it also is supported by the powerful **plantar calcaneonavicular ligament**. Also called the **spring ligament**, the plantar calcaneonavicular ligament supports the head of the talus from below by running from the shelf of the calcaneus forward to the navicular bone (Fig. 7.31).

A single joint cavity called the **great tarsal joint** spans across the articulations of the navicular to the cuneiforms and of the cuboid to the metatarsals (see Fig. 7.13). This makes for a convoluted cavity, but having the transfer of force from the midfoot to the forefoot in one basic synovial space may help to maintain the transverse arch of the foot.

A functional joint typically includes multiple anatomic joints that act together to produce a major movement, and there are three functional joints in the foot: the functional subtalar joint, the midtarsal joint, and the tarsometatarsal joint. The **functional subtalar joint** facilitates pronation and supination of the foot. If you step down (plantarflexion) and turn your sole in toward your face (inversion), you are supinating the foot. The functional subtalar joint includes both places where the talus articulates with the calcaneus, which in fact are separate anatomic synovial joint cavities.

The **midtarsal joint** includes the **calcaneocuboid joint** and the **talonavicular joint** (see Fig. 7.29). This means that it covers the entire range of where force can go forward, from the ankle to the toes. This is the final axis for complex movement of the foot skeleton, such as pronation and supination, and it is where the greatest amount of intrinsic foot movement takes place.

The functional **tarsometatarsal joint** covers the medial and lateral tarsometatarsal joints and the tarsometatarsal part of the great tarsal joint. It mostly stabilizes the row of metatarsals against an uneven array of cuneiforms and the cuboid.

THE MUSCULAR SYSTEM

Movement in the animate world is achieved in a splendid variety of ways. Vertebrate animals achieve it using a self-contained system of bones and muscles, both of which are derived from the core tissue of mesoderm. Vertebrate movement responds to gravity, which imbues the body with the attribute of weight, or **inertia**, against which the physical elements of conscious movement act. The most rigid derivatives of mesoderm, the **bones**, form a framework for the body, and the contact areas between the bones elaborate to form **joints**. We now turn to the most elastic derivatives of mesoderm, the **muscles**, through which the property of contractility acts to move bones and, thus, the body, for which the bones are a frame.

Muscles are familiar. You know what it feels like to strain one, you see the contour of large ones as they provide a shape and curve to the skin, and you perhaps have purposely trained a set of them for years and years to perform a demanding task of precision or strength. Muscle anatomy keenly reflects the needs and potentials of the human lifestyle. Just as proper diet and exercise can enhance muscle utility, a life of inactivity can burden its elegant design.

A final concept to keep in mind is that whereas all muscles have the property of contractility, the most expressed function of some muscles is to act as a kind of superelastic ligament between bones in motion. In other words, muscles can be used to slow down or resist movement that is opposite to their contracting direction, so in this sense, muscles never act in a vacuum or in isolation.

The most basic classification of muscle is based on the histology of muscle tissue. This system considers the difference between muscles that you contract voluntarily versus those that contract because of impulses beyond your control (involuntary muscles):

- Voluntary
  - Skeletal muscle (**somatic muscle** and **striated muscle**)
- Involuntary
  - Smooth muscle (**visceral muscle**)
  - Cardiac muscle

Because of its microscopic appearance, **skeletal muscle** also is called **striated muscle**. Of the involuntary muscle types, **smooth muscle** is nonstriated, and **cardiac muscle** is striated. You are familiar with the general locations of skeletal muscles in the body, because as the name implies, skeletal muscle surrounds the skeletal framework. A few skeletal muscles actually do not attach to bone but, instead, lie in a tissue layer (the **superficial fascia**) just deep to the skin. These muscles enable you to make facial expressions and, in all aspects, are true striated, skeletal muscles. Smooth muscle is found in the "wall" of hollow organs and blood vessels as well as in secretory ducts and in association with hair follicles. The structure that is often called the **gut tube**, for example, is composed of an inner sleeve of tissue derived from endoderm and a "coating" of smooth muscle derived from mesoderm, which gives the tube structure and a pulsatile contraction. Cardiac muscle is found only in the heart, and it has the unique property of rhythmic, or myogenic, contraction.

In gross anatomy, you must learn the specific names of all the skeletal muscles. Smooth muscle and cardiac muscle are specified no further in this text but it is unwise to think of muscles as individual actors. Think instead of the activities of your body and the kind of movements those activities require. For virtually all normal activities of being, multiple muscles and joints are invoked. Paralysis of only a single muscle is unlikely; by contrast, hindrance of an activity or a capability is a major reason for going to the doctor. The "Big 4" attributes of a skeletal muscle—**origin, insertion, action,** and **innervation**—help you to infer patterns of activity. Your ultimate goal, however, is to understand the patient's weakness or inability to move. If you can describe the action of a muscle, you should be able to deduce its attachment sites with sufficient specificity. In general, the "origin" of a muscle is the attachment of lesser movement, and it usually is broader and more proximal (closer to the center of the body) than the insertion is. The "insertion" generally is more distal, and its attachment is narrower or more tendinous. (See Clinical Anatomy Box 7.3.)

Muscle Movement and Innervation

In this book, we do not explore the mechanics of muscle movement in detail. To appreciate the gross anatomy of muscles better, however, we should introduce some basic concepts of how muscles move.

It is important to distinguish between muscle **action** and when a muscle is **active.** Anatomy books and courses often emphasize muscle **action,** which generally means what happens when a muscle contracts without resistance while the body is in standard anatomic position. This is a nice attribute to know—even if it is somewhat theoretical—because in the physical examination of a patient, you can test proper muscle function by observing the empiric actions of muscles. Muscle action, however, has limited application in the real world, where the body moves in a sophisticated coordination of multiple muscle groups in multiple postures against the ground. Consider an activity such as walking, opening a door, or rising from the bed. Muscles contract in the performance of these activities, but we do not describe these activities as actions of the muscle. We say that an action of the trapezius muscle, for example, is to retract the shoulder blade, or scapula. We do not say that the action of the muscle is to open a door. Therefore, it is important that you know what actions a muscle performs, but it is more important that you understand when a muscle is active.

Movement

To extend the theme of action in isolation, consider the types of movement of which a muscle is capable. A muscle can contract in three ways: isometrically, isotonically, and eccentrically. **Isometric contraction** is when the muscle contracts just enough to match the force against it. **Isotonic contraction** is when the muscle shortens while it contracts, which is the movement we most associate with muscle action. **Eccentric contraction** is the opposite of isotonic contraction—that is, the muscle actually gets longer as it works, because the force that it is resisting is greater than its contractile force. Our muscles frequently work eccentrically in our everyday activities, but we do not think of these movements as typical actions of a muscle.

As a clinician, you will have to use very specific terms to describe the direction of movement. Some of these are obvious, but some are not. **Flexion** reduces the angle of acuity between two bones, and **extension** enlarges the same angle. Because the foot is rotated during development, these movements at the ankle joint are less obvious. **Dorsiflexion** refers to bending the "top" of the foot toward the knee, whereas **plantarflexion** refers to bending the bottom of the foot toward the ground (like stepping, or "toeing off").

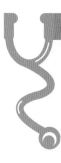

CLINICAL ANATOMY

Box 7.3

MUSCLE FIBER STRUCTURE

The basic unit of the muscle is the linear **myofibril (A)**. A myofibril is too delicate to enact much movement on its own when it contracts, so many parallel myofibrils are wrapped together by a layer of connective tissue called **endomysium**. The parallel fibril bundle is now called a **muscle fiber**. Parallel fibers form bundles themselves, wrapped this time by a **perimysium**. The bundle of parallel fibers is called a **fascicle**, or a **fasciculus**. Finally, parallel fascicles are wrapped together in a comprehensive **epimysium** to form the "muscle." It is the epimysium of a muscle bundle that condenses on itself near to bone to form a **tendon (B)**.

How much of a muscle is formed as a tendon is related to how much power that the muscle fibers are capable of exerting and to the type of movement that the power generates. Some tendons are longer than the muscle fibers that draw on them. In addition, not all tendons are shaped the same. A tendon can be broad and flat, in which case it is called an **aponeurosis**. Tendons for muscles of fine movement, such as the finger flexors, tend to be very well-defined. Tendons for muscles of stability or general movement, such as the shorter vertebral muscles, tend to be diffuse and inconstant. In gross anatomy, tendons are considered to be a part of the muscle and do not have separate names of their own.

Now think about the subsystem developmentally. Contractile tissues (muscle cells) provide the potential for movement but are not themselves equipped to grab the connective tissues. For the integration to occur, connective tissue continuous with the mesenchyme that becomes bone must "house" the muscle cells at one end and anchor to bone at the other. This is accomplished by the differentiation of mesenchyme into fibrous bands at specific areas on the periosteal layer of bone. These bands, or **tendons**, extend away from their contact with bone and grade from nearly rigid at the site of bony attachment to nearly fluid where their subdivisions finally contact muscle cells. It is as if the bony framework of the body "reaches out" with connective tissue adapters to the dynamic muscle fibers.

What makes one skeletal muscle different from another anatomically is therefore nothing more than the concentration of the subunits. The property of contractility is the same across all the shapes; it is simply played out over a relatively large, or a relatively small, tendon attachment site to bone. The body is capable of both powerful movement and precise movement not because you have sets of powerful muscle fibers and sets of precise muscle fibers but, rather, because the muscle fibers are packaged by connective tissue into cooperative bundles that produce powerful contractions or direct contractions to very specific places.

Abduction involves moving a part of the body (typically the limbs) away from the midline; **adduction** restores the same part toward the midline. Abduction of the trunk is an important movement of the hip region during walking to counter gravity. Muscles working together also are capable of rotational movement, such as the way in which the head of the humerus can spin against the scapula bone or the movement of rotating the head to indicate the universal sign for "no." A global type of rotation is **circumduction**, which is the combination of abducting, rotating, flexing, extending, and adducting joints such as the shoulder or base of the thumb (i.e., taking them through their entire range of motion).

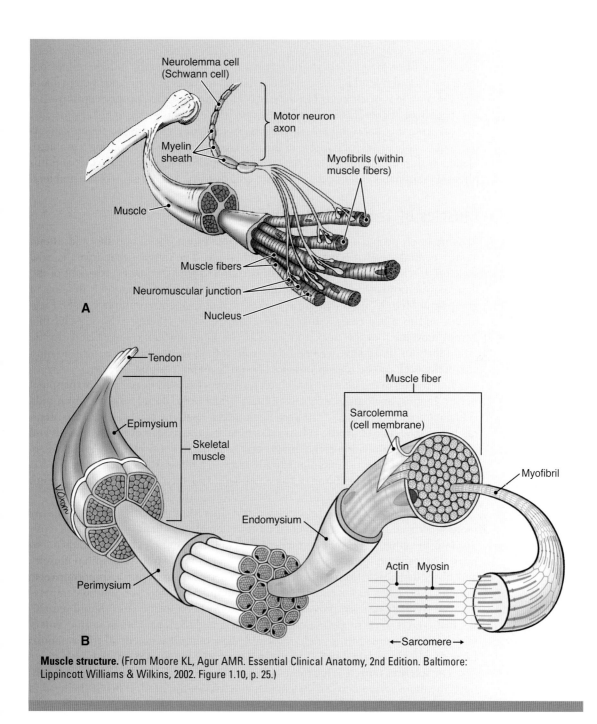

Muscle structure. (From Moore KL, Agur AMR. Essential Clinical Anatomy, 2nd Edition. Baltimore: Lippincott Williams & Wilkins, 2002. Figure 1.10, p. 25.)

Pronation involves a kind of rotation in which one bone "rolls over" another bone and "flips" a distal structure from front to back. This term applies to both the hand and the foot but principally to the hand, which can execute more powerful and precise movements when it is pronated. The position of the hands on the keyboard of a computer is a pronated position. Its opposite is **supination**, which restores a pronated joint to standard anatomic position.

Innervation

The nerve supply to a muscle usually travels next to the blood supply in a "neurovascular" bundle wrapped in fascia. The bundle typically enters the muscle from the deep side. Nerve fibers to muscle deliver a motor impulse that causes the muscle cell to contract, but they also send back sensory information to the central nervous system about how the muscle is positioned. This type of information is called **proprioception**—the key ingredient of coordination (and the reason why it is impossible to tickle yourself).

Knowing the innervation of a muscle is essential for clinical applications. Patients may not be able to describe where in the nervous system they are suffering a problem. Generally, however, patients can show you what muscles do or do not work, and this physical examination finding may lead you quickly to the true location of the problem.

Muscles of the Axial Skeleton

At some level, people are just segmented vertebrates who bend and flex and extend along a central axis that is propped up by limb buds. The muscles that drive the axial skeleton develop uniquely, for the most part, from a small, epimeric segment of the dermomyotome that is dedicated to the vertebral column. The muscles develop in groups that include fibers that cross single vertebral segments, multiple vertebral segments, and in a few cases, virtually the entire vertebral column. The muscles that govern movement of the neck and head are multiple and quite specialized. To the extent that our limbs have assumed the major role in locomotion, the intrinsic muscles of the back can be seen as muscles of posture and of position.

Innervation of the intrinsic back muscles derives from the dorsal rami of the spinal nerves. In gross anatomy, only a few of these spinal nerve dorsal rami are given individual names (see Fig. 6.22). The specific muscular anatomy of a back sprain or strain rarely is diagnosable clinically. A basic allopathic treatment plan of resting the axis and reducing the inflammation of the injury pertains to the majority of cases. A basic osteopathic treatment plan uses manipulative therapy to address where such an injury has wrenched the vertebral column out of alignment, and such manipulation may result in rapid restoration of equilibrium and muscle function.

The intrinsic back muscles display a few interesting patterns. As expected, the more superficial muscles tend to cross more vertebral units than the deep ones cross. To cover the range of possible movement directions, the muscles can be grouped into fibers that reach from a lateral origin to a medial insertion (a **transversospinal muscle**) and fibers that reach from a medial origin to a lateral insertion (a **spinotransverse muscle**) (Fig. 7.32). In the end, the vertebral column is packed with multiple muscles that can facilitate or resist movement in every directional plane. You should remember that even if some single muscles have only one directional action, no movement of the axis is governed by a single muscle. Unless otherwise noted, all innervation is from dorsal rami of spinal nerves in the region of attachment. (See Table 7.1.)

The **splenius muscle** is the most superficial muscle in the back of the neck. It connects the thoracic and cervical vertebrae to the back of the head. It bends the head to

FIGURE 7.32   **Muscles of the vertebral column.**

The intrinsic back muscles divide duty by fiber direction (**A**) and by depth (**B**). They occupy the trough between the spinous process and the transverse process (**C**) and can extend across multiple vertebral units or a single unit. (From Moore KL, Agur AMR. Essential Clinical Anatomy, 2nd Edition. Baltimore: Lippincott Williams & Wilkins, 2002. Figure 5.10, p. 295.)

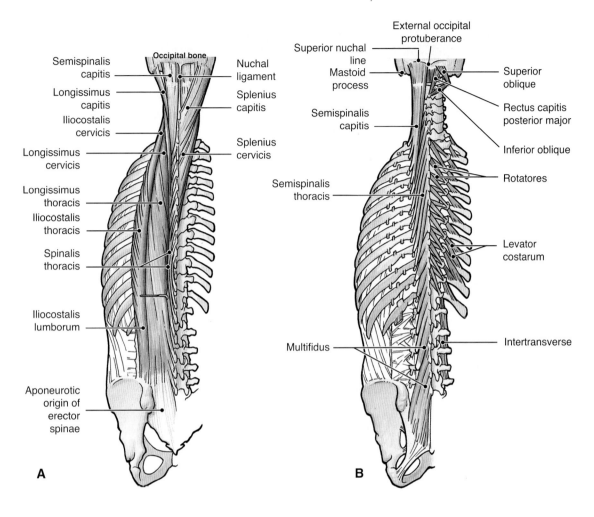

A

Semispinalis capitis
Longissimus capitis
Iliocostalis cervicis
Longissimus cervicis
Longissimus thoracis
Iliocostalis thoracis
Spinalis thoracis
Iliocostalis lumborum
Aponeurotic origin of erector spinae

Occipital bone
Nuchal ligament
Splenius capitis
Splenius cervicis

B

Superior nuchal line
External occipital protuberance
Mastoid process
Semispinalis capitis
Semispinalis thoracis
Multifidus
Superior oblique
Rectus capitis posterior major
Inferior oblique
Rotatores
Levator costarum
Intertransverse

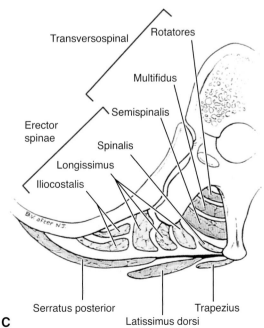

C

Transversospinal
Rotatores
Multifidus
Semispinalis
Erector spinae
Spinalis
Longissimus
Iliocostalis
Serratus posterior
Latissimus dorsi
Trapezius

B.V. after N.J.

TABLE 7.1   MUSCLES OF THE SUPERFICIAL AND DEEP VERTEBRAL COLUMN

MUSCLE	SUBUNIT	ORIGIN	INSERTION	INNERVATION	ACTION
Splenius		Nuchal ligament and spinous processes of C7-T4	Mastoid process and superior nuchal line	Dorsal rami	Unilateral: will laterally flex and rotate ipsilaterally; bilaterally: extends head
Erector spinae (spinotrans-verse) muscles					
Iliocostalis	Lumborum	Sacrum and iliac crest	Angles of lower 6 ribs	Dorsal rami	Extend and laterally bend vertebral column
	Thoracis	Angles of ribs 6–12	Upper 6 ribs	Dorsal rami	Extend and laterally bend vertebral column
	Cervicis	Angles of ribs 3–6	Transverse processes of C4-C6	Dorsal rami	Extend and laterally bend vertebral column
Longissimus	Thoracis	With erector spinae, plus lumbar vertebrae and thoracolumbar fascia	Transverse processes of thoracic vertebrae plus angles of lower 9–10 ribs	Dorsal rami	Extend and laterally bend vertebral column
	Cervicis	Transverse processes of T1-T5	Transverse/ articular processes of C2-C6	Dorsal rami	Extend and laterally bend vertebral column
	Capitis	Transverse processes of C4-T5	Mastoid process of temporal	Dorsal rami	Extend head
Spinalis	May have thoracis, cervicis, and capitis fibers	Spinous processes; cervical, thoracic, and upper lumbar vertebrae	Spinous processes of vertebrae 3–6 segments above fiber origin	Dorsal rami	Extend vertebral column and head
Transversospinal muscles					
Semispinalis		Transverse processes C4-T12	Spinous processes and occipital bone 4–6 segments above origin	Dorsal rami	Extend and contralaterally rotate vertebral column and head
Multifidus		Along articular and transverse processes in cervical, tho-racic , and sacral region	Spinous processes 2–4 segments above origin	Dorsal rami	Stabilize and rotate vertebral column

(continues)

TABLE 7.1   MUSCLES OF THE SUPERFICIAL AND DEEP VERTEBRAL COLUMN *(continued)*

MUSCLE	SUBUNIT	ORIGIN	INSERTION	INNERVATION	ACTION
Rotatores		Transverse processes, especially thoracic region	Spinous processes or lamina 1–2 segments above origin	Dorsal rami	Stabilize, extend, and rotate vertebral units
Suboccipital triangle				Dorsal ramus C1 (suboccipital nerve)	
Rectus capitis*	Posterior major	Spinous process of axis	Occipital bone just below inferior nuchal line		Ipsilateral rotation and extension of head
	Posterior minor	Posterior arch of atlas	Occipital bone just below inferior nuchal line		Extension of head
Obliquus capitis*	Superior	Transverse process of atlas	Occipital bone between nuchal lines		Ipsilateral rotation and extension of head
	Inferior	Spinous process of axis	Transverse process of atlas		Ipsilateral rotation of atlas (head)
Ventral muscles				Ventral rami, cervical spinal nerves	
Longus	Colli	Bodies of upper thoracic/lower cervical vertebrae	Bodies of upper cervical vertebrae		Bends neck forward
	Capitis	Transverse processes, middle cervical vertebrae	Occipital bone, basilar		Bends head forward
Rectus capitis	Anterior	Lateral mass of atlas	Occipital bone, basilar		Stabilizes atlanto-occipital joint
	Lateralis	Transverse process of atlas	Occipital bone, jugular process		Stabilizes atlanto-occipital joint
Scalenus	Anterior	Transverse processes C3-C6	First rib, scalene tubercle		Stabilize first rib, bend neck ipsilaterally
	Medius	Transverse processes C3-C7	First rib		Stabilize first rib, bend neck ipsilaterally
	Posterior	Transverse processes of C4-C6	Second rib		Stabilize second rib, bend neck ipsilaterally

the side (lateral flexion), and it rotates the head to the side. When acting together on both sides of the body, they bend the head backward (extension).

Just deep to the splenius is a family of spectacular muscles that range along the length of the vertebral column in a general pattern of medial origin and lateral insertion. For this reason, the three groups of three muscles each are lumped into a single muscle family called the **spinotransverse muscles**. Anatomists call the family the **erector spinae muscles**, but some clinicians combine all of the intrinsic muscles in a grouping called the **paraspinous muscles**.

The erector spinae group includes three sections of muscle fibers (**iliocostalis, longissimus,** and **spinalis**), each of which can be divided into three sets of fibers (**lumborum, thoracis, cervicis,** or **capitis**), depending on where along the vertebral column they insert. That totals nine muscle names, but really just three muscle groups and essentially one muscle family of spinotransverse fibers.

The erector spinae group is large and powerful. Because most of the fibers cross the lumbar curvature, these muscles work hard to maintain posture. As with other deep back muscles, they control posture by contracting both isotonically to restore the vertebral column and eccentrically to resist excessive flexion at the lumbar curvature. Routine activities of movement, leaning forward, and even sitting still can require the erector spinae group to pull at the vertebral column to maintain balance.

Deep to the erector spinae group are shorter muscles that run from lateral origins to medial insertions higher up the vertebral column. For this reason, the muscle family is called the **transversospinal group**. Its components are the **semispinalis muscle,** the **multifidus muscle,** and the **rotatores muscle** (see Fig. 7.32B). They do not lie side by side as the erector spinae groups do; rather, they run from superficial to deep in the well between the transverse and spinous processes of the vertebrae (see Fig. 7.32C). The deeper muscles range across fewer vertebral units. They also are not present throughout the vertebral column. The multifidus muscle is more developed in the lumbar region, and the semispinalis muscle is more developed in the neck region.

The dorsal musculature of the vertebral column is not yet complete. Some very small muscles span the distance between adjacent spinous processes of the vertebrae (**interspinales**). Some other very small muscles connect adjacent transverse processes (**intertransversarii**). In addition, a battery of 12 pairs of muscles link the transverse process of a vertebra to the rib below it (**levator costarum**).

As the occipital bone of the head begins to develop from the uppermost somite cell clusters, muscles connect it back to the vertebral column. These muscles must be homologues of the muscles you have just studied, but because of their unique position and exclusive action on the head, they have separate names. These are four the muscles of the **suboccipital triangle**, and they enable very subtle movements of the head (see Fig. 6.22). Because many other muscles apply similar actions to the head, the suboccipital muscles may be used primarily as proprioceptive organs of head position; in other words, slight shifts in the position of the head and, thus, tension on one or more of the muscles may be communicated back to the brain as position signals. These muscles may be as much guidewires and line-levelers as they are active head movers.

Each of the muscles is innervated by fibers of the same dorsal ramus—that belonging to the first cervical spinal nerve. This is one of the few dorsal rami to be given its own name (the **suboccipital nerve**). It is believed that fibers of this dorsal ramus serve only the suboccipital muscles.

The vertebral column must be supported along the front, or ventral, border as well. Most governing of posture and movement draws on the projecting levers (transverse processes and spinous processes) at the back of the column, but muscle bundles also exist along the fronts of the thoracic and cervical vertebrae (Fig. 7.33). The **longus**

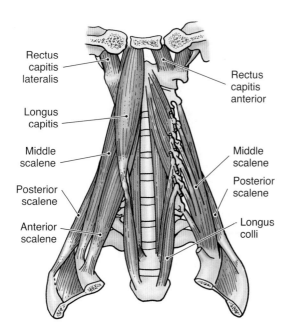

Rectus
capitis
lateralis

Longus
capitis

Middle
scalene

Posterior
scalene

Anterior
scalene

Rectus
capitis
anterior

Middle
scalene

Posterior
scalene

Longus
colli

FIGURE 7.33   **Anterior
vertebral column musculature.**

Muscles along the anterior side of
the vertebral bodies are found only
in the cervical region of the column, where they monitor position
and resist hyperextension, such as
in a whiplash injury. (From Moore
KL, Agur AMR. Essential Clinical
Anatomy, 2nd Edition. Baltimore:
Lippincott Williams & Wilkins,
2002. Figure 9.5, p. 605.)

colli muscle and **longus capitis muscle** are buried deep in the upper chest and neck, behind the respiratory and digestive systems. Although they move the vertebral column, they are innervated by ventral rami of the spinal nerves, not by dorsal rami. They may play a role in resisting excessive extension of the neck, such as occurs during a whiplash injury.

A final group of muscles, the **scalene group**, connects the neck vertebrae to the upper two ribs. These muscles are found deep in the "webbing" of the neck behind the clavicle, and they are innervated by local branches of the ventral rami of the cervical spinal nerves. They steady the upper two ribs during deep respiration, and they assist in lateral bending of the neck. The **anterior scalene muscle** and the **middle scalene muscle** are notable, because the brachial plexus of nerves passes between them on its way to the upper limb. The anterior scalene muscle also passes between the large subclavian vein in front and the subclavian artery in back.

Muscles of the Body Wall

Movement and position pertain to the entire body, not just to the limbs and the back. The body wall, which is formed by the lateral folding of the embryo, is composed mostly of a sandwich of mesoderm that takes the form of a rib cage in the thorax and three layers of muscle throughout the thorax and abdomen. Although some prominent muscles, such as the pectoralis muscle, appear to be part of the body wall, they actually are limb muscles that have migrated to anchorages on the body wall.

The muscles of the thoracic body wall are given different names than the abdominal muscles are given, but in essence, the muscles of the thoracic body wall are where they are for the same reason—to provide a closure to the body wall and to maintain the integrity of the trunk that was created by lateral folding of the embryo. In the thorax, the three-layered muscle sandwich is composed of **intercostal muscles**, so named because they are positioned, as they must be, between adjacent ribs (Fig. 7.34).

Abdominal wall muscles are somewhat simpler, in the sense that they are, in fact, the body wall. They have no ribs to incorporate and no accessory respiratory function

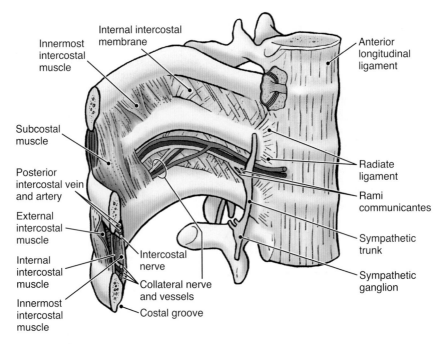

Innermost intercostal muscle

Internal intercostal membrane

Anterior longitudinal ligament

Subcostal muscle

Posterior intercostal vein and artery

External intercostal muscle

Internal intercostal muscle

Innermost intercostal muscle

Intercostal nerve

Collateral nerve and vessels

Costal groove

Radiate ligament

Rami communicantes

Sympathetic trunk

Sympathetic ganglion

FIGURE 7.34   Intercostal musculature.

The intercostal muscles are a three-layered sandwich of "elastic ligaments" between the ribs. (From Moore KL, Agur AMR. Essential Clinical Anatomy, 2nd Edition. Baltimore: Lippincott Williams & Wilkins, 2002. Figure 2.11, p. 66.)

to serve. They also insert on themselves, in the front of the body, in a thick raphe. They are of great clinical interest where they span from the side of the hip to the front of the hip, because this is the region that is most prone to a **hernia**. This vulnerability is a result of development in general and the descent of the gonads in particular. (See Table 7.2.)

Abdominal wall muscles comprise three units (Fig. 7.35). One unit serves the back of the wall and basically shuts off the gap between the lowest ribs and the top of the pelvis (the **quadratus lumborum muscle**). One unit fortifies the linear raphe from the bottom of the sternum to the top of the pelvis (the **rectus abdominis muscles**, or the "six-pack" muscles). In addition, one unit spans the side of the body wall between them as the original three-layered muscle sandwich (the **abdominal obliques**).

The quadratus lumborum effectively fills the gap between the deep muscles of the back and the musculature of the side of the abdomen. Its fascia is thick enough at the side margin that the oblique muscles can attach to it as they begin their course around and toward the front of the body. The fibers of the rectus abdominis are clumped together into more or less "squarish" blocks that are separated above and below by tendinous bands of fascia. This pattern gives lean individuals the appearance of a "washboard stomach." The lateral free border of each rectus abdominis muscle also is cinched down by a tendinous band that runs the entire length of the muscle in a semilunar line (the **linea semilunaris**) and along which the aponeuroses of the three lateral abdominal wall muscles interdigitate.

The nature of the free edges of muscles to thicken or infold is best expressed by the lower free edge of external abdominal oblique. It spans from the iliac crest to the

TABLE 7.2 MUSCLES OF THE BODY WALL

MUSCLE	UNIT	ORIGIN	INSERTION	INNERVATION	ACTION
Intercostals	External	Margins of ribs	Margins of adjacent ribs	Thoracic ventral rami	Support of thoracic body wall, assist in forced respiration
	Internal	Margins of ribs	Margins of adjacent ribs	Thoracic ventral rami	Support of thoracic body wall, assist in forced respiration
	Innermost	Margins of ribs	Margins of adjacent ribs	Thoracic ventral rami	Support of thoracic body wall, assist in forced respiration
Transversus thoracis		Back of sternum and xiphoid process	Cartilage of ribs 2–6	Thoracic ventral rami	May assist in expiration (?)
Serratus posterior	Superior	Nuchal ligament and spinous processes of C7-T2	Upper border of ribs 2–5	T1-T4 ventral rami	Elevates upper ribs during inspiration
	Inferior	Spinous processes of T11-L2	Lower border of ribs 9–12	T9-T12 ventral rami	Draws lower ribs downward during expiration
Abdominal obliques	External	External surfaces of lower 8 ribs	Iliac crest, pubic tubercle, pubic crest, and linea alba	T7-T12 ventral rami, iliohypogastric and ilioinguinal (L1 ventral ramus)	Supports abdominal cavity; flexes, bends, and rotates the trunk
	Internal	Thoracolumbar fascia, iliac crest, and inguinal ligament	Lower 3 ribs, linea alba, and pubic crest		
Transversus abdominis		Lower 6 ribs, thoracolumbar fascia iliac crest, inguinal ligament	Linea alba and pubic crest		
Rectus abdominis		Pubic crest and pubic symphysis	Xiphoid process of sternum and cartilages of ribs 5–7	T7-12 ventral rami	Flexes vertebral column and trunk
Pyramidalis		Pubic bone	Linea alba	T12 ventral ramus	Tenses linea alba
Quadratus lumborum		Lower border of rib 12, lumbar transverse processes	Iliolumbar ligament and adjacent iliac crest	Ventral rami, T12-L3	Bends trunk ipsilaterally

pubic tubercle, and its lower border is "free" of attachment. Here, the aponeurosis thickens and infolds and is called the **inguinal ligament**.

We must consider one other aspect of the trunk, its "top" and "bottom." Muscles conveniently cover the "roof" of the abdominal cavity and the "floor" of the pelvic cavity. The thoracic **diaphragm** has a tremendous origin around the circumference of the rib cage and no real insertion in the sense that it inserts on itself in a centralized tendon. When the muscle fibers contract, the dome-like shape of the diaphragm is pulled taut, or flattens out, which alters the pressure dynamics in the thoracic cavity that it effectively seals. It is a beautiful billow that makes a bellows of the lungs (Fig. 7.36).

The diaphragm gets motor innervation from the **phrenic nerve**, which is composed of the ventral rami of cervical spinal nerves 3, 4, and 5 (C3-C5), and it gets

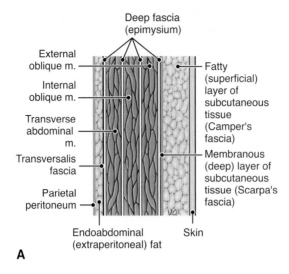

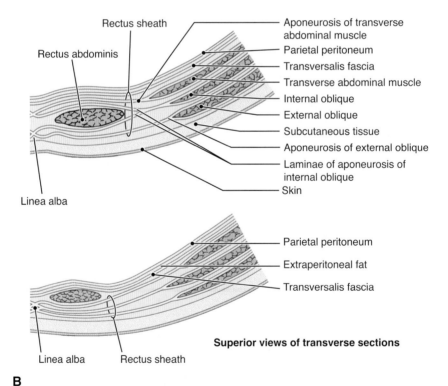

FIGURE 7.35   **Abdominal wall musculature.**

(**A**) Schematic longitudinal section. The abdominal wall muscles form a three-layered sandwich. The schematic arrangement from superficial to deep is shown here. (**B** and **C**) Schematic cross-sections. At the front and back of the abdominal wall, the muscle layering transforms into large, single muscles, such as the rectus abdominis (**D**) and the quadratus lumborum (as the wedge along the posterior limit, **C**). m = muscle.

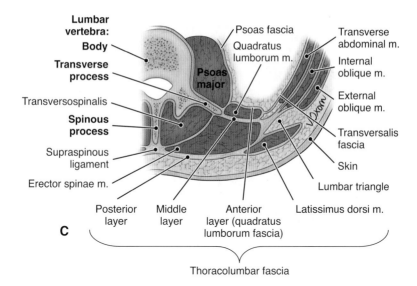

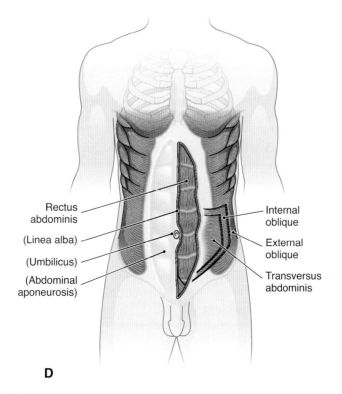

FIGURE 7.35   *(Continued)*

(From Moore KL, Agur AMR. Essential Clinical Anatomy, 2nd Edition. Baltimore: Lippincott Williams & Wilkins, 2002. Figure 3.5, p. 126; from Moore KL, Agur AMR. Essential Clinical Anatomy, 2nd Edition. Baltimore: Lippincott Williams & Wilkins, 2002. Figure 8.14; and from Cohen BJ, Wood DL. Memmler's The Human Body in Health and Disease, 10th Edition. Baltimore: Lippincott Williams & Wilkins, 2004.)

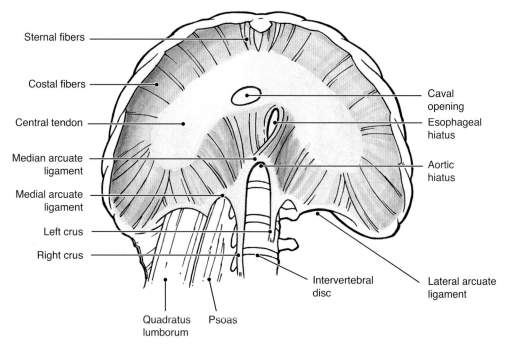

Sternal fibers

Costal fibers

Central tendon

Median arcuate
ligament

Medial arcuate
ligament

Left crus

Right crus

Caval
opening

Esophageal
hiatus

Aortic
hiatus

Intervertebral
disc

Lateral arcuate
ligament

Quadratus
lumborum

Psoas

FIGURE 7.36   **The diaphragm as seen from below.**

(From Moore KL, Agur AMR. Essential Clinical Anatomy, 2nd Edition. Baltimore: Lippincott Williams & Wilkins, 2002. Figure 3.38, p. 188.)

sensory innervation from the phrenic nerves and from local nerves of the intercostal region. This dual pattern is in keeping with how the diaphragm develops during embryonic folding, which explains why the diaphragm retains some innervation from its original home in the high cervical region of the body and some innervation from local intercostal nerves.

If the thoracic diaphragm covers the abdominal cavity from above, you might expect a similar kind of cover across the bottom. After all, what else keeps the abdominal and pelvic organs from pushing against the skin of the bottom of the trunk? Indeed, a pelvic diaphragm does span the gap between the bones of the pelvis, with some allowance for the necessary passing of reproductive and excretory structures.

The **pelvic diaphragm** (Fig. 7.37) spans the open space between the coccyx and pubic symphysis in a funnel-shaped design that suspends abdominal and pelvic viscera above while permitting the passage of their portals. The pelvic diaphragm effectively separates the **pelvic cavity** from the **perineum**, but anteriorly, just below the pubic symphysis, this separation is handled by a fascial **perineal membrane**. The muscles of the pelvic diaphragm are best appreciated as a funnel-shaped sling, with origins along the pelvic walls and insertions on the midline **central tendon of the perineum** (the **perineal body**), on a raphe connecting the perineal body to the coccyx (**anococcygeal ligament**), and/or on the **coccyx** itself.

Levator ani

This group of three muscles forms the pelvic diaphragm from the anterior border at the pubis bone to the junction of the ilium and the ischium. The name of the group implies its function. When you contract this group of muscles, you "lift" an aspect of

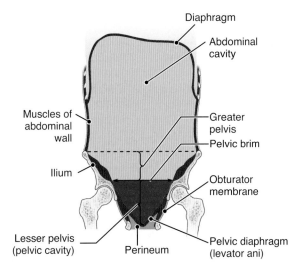

A

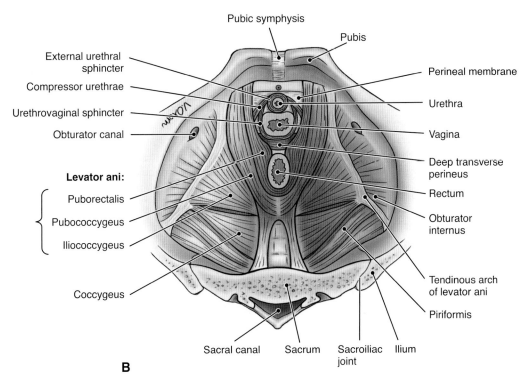

B

FIGURE 7.37   **The pelvic cavity and pelvic diaphragm.**

(**A**) Schematic coronal view of the abdominal and pelvic cavities, both of which are bounded by muscular diaphragms. (**B**) Internal, superior view. A pelvic diaphragm suspends the organs of the trunk and supports the exitway for the reproductive, urinary, and digestive system pathways. The broad, muscular band of the diaphragm is the levator ani muscle. (Adapted from Moore KL, Dalley AF. Clinically Oriented Anatomy, 5th Edition. Baltimore: Lippincott Williams & Wilkins, 2006. Figure 3.5C, p. 368; from Moore KL, Agur AMR. Essential Clinical Anatomy, 2nd Edition. Baltimore: Lippincott Williams & Wilkins, 2002. Figure 4.5C, p. 368.)

the anal canal and facilitate the passage of waste material through it. The names of the muscles in the group indicate the landmarks they span. Each is innervated by the **pudendal nerve**, which is composed of the ventral rami of sacral spinal nerves 3, 4, and 5 (S3-S5). The **puborectalis muscle** forms a U-shaped sling around the anorectal junction, anchored at the pubic symphysis. Some fibers of this muscle also surround the prostate gland in males (the **levator prostate**) or the vaginal canal (the **pubovaginalis**) and insert on the perineal body. **Pubococcygeus** is the main part of the levator ani. This sheet of fibers begins anteriorly in the midline, ends posteriorly in the midline, and therefore must encircle the channels that pierce the pelvic diaphragm: the anal canal, the urethra, the vagina, and the perineal body. The **iliococcygeus muscle** covers the side escapes of the lower pelvis by running from the obturator fascia and ischial spine to the anococcygeal ligament and the coccyx bone in the midline.

Although the **coccygeus muscle** lies in the same funnel-shaped design of the pelvic diaphragm, it is considered separately from the levator ani group, because the fibers do not surround a visceral tube or meet in the midline. Instead, they pick up where iliococcygeus muscle leaves off by connecting the lateral margin of the coccyx to the ischial spine. The coccygeus is innervated by direct branches of the S4 and S5 ventral rami, which also distinguishes it from the levator ani group.

The pelvic diaphragm is vulnerable to stretching, tearing, and other injury from excessive straining, such as during childbirth. Loss of integrity of the diaphragm results in a **prolapse** of the organ tubes that it suspends: the rectum, and the vagina. Intentional incision of the diaphragm (**episiotomy**) can reduce the risk of prolapse following traumatic childbirth, because the precut tissue can be repaired surgically with better results than can tissue that is cut traumatically.

The trunk does not just end as a canvas of skin with two (or three) holes in it. You exercise conscious control over those holes, and you achieve a kind of stiffening of the skin (**erection**) by some measure of muscle action. The following muscles interface between the end of the gut tube (the rectum and the anus) and the outside world and between the end of the reproductive system (the urinary and genital orifices) and the skin that surrounds them. These muscles do not present very often in clinical cases, but studying them is the best way to understand how you control the psychologically vital processes of urination, defecation, and sexual stimulation.

External anal sphincter

The inferior two-thirds of the anal canal is surrounded by three muscle bundles collectively called the **external anal sphincter** (Fig. 7.38). These bundles are the logical continuation of the pelvic diaphragm. The sphincter attaches to the perineal body and to the ligament between the anus and the coccyx vertebrae, which are the stable structures in front of and behind the anal orifice. Muscle tone in the external anal sphincter acts to close off the orifice in a conscious (voluntary) attempt to resist the passage of fecal matter. It is innervated by the inferior rectal branch of the **pudendal nerve**.

Sphincter urethrae

The pelvic diaphragm includes a gap for the passage of the urethra. Just inferior to where the pelvic diaphragm would be if it captured the urethra is a deep perineal space. This space includes a dedicated, voluntary muscle for squeezing the urethra that is logically called the **sphincter urethrae** (do not confuse this with the involuntary **internal urethral sphincter**). The sphincter urethrae attaches to the inferior pubic ramus and inserts on fibers of itself from the opposite side, after it has pinched the urethra. It is innervated by the **pudendal nerve**.

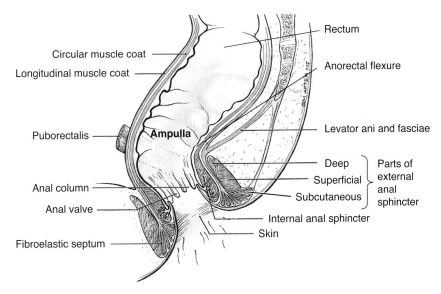

FIGURE 7.38   **Thickened sphincters constrain the anal orifice.**

The inferior limits of both the smooth muscle coat of the rectum and the striated muscle levator ani contain involuntary sphincters and voluntary sphincters, respectively. (Adapted from Moore KL, Agur AMR. Essential Clinical Anatomy, 2nd Edition. Baltimore: Lippincott Williams & Wilkins, 2002. Figure 4.22A, p. 248.)

Deep and superficial transverse perineus

Two transverse muscles behind the urethral sphincters complete the space around the urogenital ducts. One is deep, and one is superficial. The deep one attaches the ischial ramus to the perineal body and is innervated by the **pudendal nerve**. The superficial one runs along approximately the same course (but a layer closer to the skin) and also is innervated by the **pudendal nerve**.

As noted above, the reproductive system develops elaborate vasculature around where it opens to the outside world. In males, this opening is elongated forward, taking skin with it, as the **penis**. In females, this opening remains more or less flush with the skin level of the trunk, but the same rich vasculature is found all around it as well. This vasculature can make the skin over it become tight (erect) if it fills with blood that does not drain out. This process is enabled by the presence of two muscles that clamp the bottoms of the erectile bodies of blood and, thus, help to prevent blood from flowing out once it has entered. The erectile bodies are the **crus** (of the penis or clitoris) and the **bulb** (of the penis or vestibule). In males, the crus extends outward as a cavernous body (the **corpus cavernosum**), and the bulb extends along the penile urethra as the **corpus spongiosum**. Now, consider the muscles that lie just under the skin and that clamp these bodies closed (Fig. 7.39).

Ischiocavernosus

The **ischiocavernosus muscle** clamps the base of the crus. It attaches to the ischial tuberosity and ramus in a clamp-like design. When the muscle fires, it clamps the crus against the ramus, thus trapping blood that has just flowed into the crus and stiffening it like a water balloon. The muscle is innervated by the **pudendal nerve**.

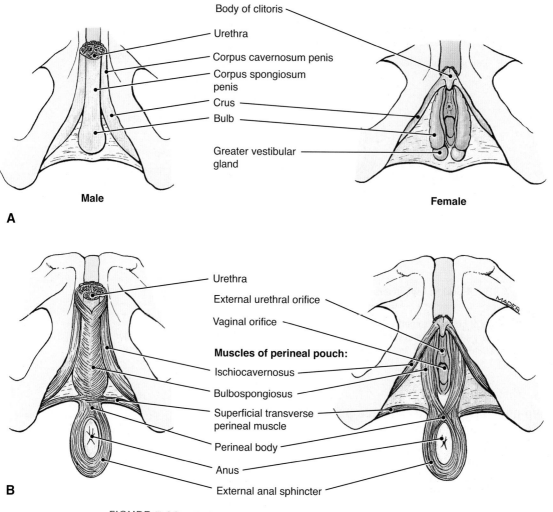

FIGURE 7.39   **Perineal muscles strap erectile tissues in place.**

Rich vascular beds develop in the phallus and urogenital folds of both males and females (**A**). Ischio-cavernosus muscles clamp the base of the corpus cavernosum erectile beds against the pubis bone (**B**). In the midline of the perineal region, a bulbospongiosus muscle surrounds the bulb of the penis in males and the bulb of the vestibule in females. Contraction of these muscles helps to restrict venous return and maintain turgidity in the erectile bodies. (From Agur A, Dalley AF. Grant's Atlas of Anatomy, 11th Edition. Baltimore: Lippincott Williams & Wilkins, 2005. Figure 3.42D,E, p. 243.)

Bulbospongiosus

The **bulbospongiosus muscle** acts on the bulb of the penis in males or on bulb of the vestibule in females. It attaches to the perineal body, and it wraps around the bulb forward in the plane of the perineum to insert on fibers of itself above the bulb. In females, this means that it effectively brackets the vestibule (the chamber that holds the urethral and vaginal orifices). In males, this means that it wraps the base of the bulb and, therefore, is contained under the skin contour at the base of the pendulous portion of the penis. When it clamps, it traps blood in the bulb, which stiffens the minor lips of the vestibule in females and the tissue that surrounds the urethra in males. It is innervated by the **pudendal nerve**.

Trunk muscles serve many functions, most of which relate to giving the volume of the body a continuous closure and controlled posture. That would be the end of the story if you were just a trunk, but the top end of the neural tube (nervous system) and the gut tube bulge out above the trunk in the form of the head and neck. The mesoderm bulges out to perform the same mesoderm roles in the head and neck as it does in the trunk: structural support of the two tubes and movement across movable joints formed by that structure.

Muscles of the Neck and Head

The whole of the head is much greater than the sum of its parts. The following muscles of the head and neck rarely, if ever, act in isolation, and knowing the litany of their origins, insertions, actions, and innervations is more of an intellectual than a surgical or a clinical exercise. The more practical goal is to consider what the head does—it looks, chews, listens, swallows, speaks, and so on—and, therefore, what neurovascular, muscular, and connective tissues likely are involved in the patient who cannot do one of those things normally. Some important "activities" that take place in the head, such as smelling, seeing, and tasting, require no overt musculature.

In general order of cranial nerve control, the functional groups of the head and neck muscles are:

- **Muscles of Looking**: The brain extends to the outside world in the form of a few special nerve endings, such as the ending of cranial nerve II, the **optic nerve**. Seeing is not looking, in the sense that the optic nerve is encased in a spherical "eyeball" that enjoys universal movements in the orbital cavity thanks to some of the most elegant muscles in the body. Dissecting them is one of the traditional exercises in a gross anatomy class, but this could never happen in a surgical or a clinical setting. Because eye movement requires three different cranial nerves, testing eye movement is a key component of any neurologic examination.
- **Muscles of Chewing**: The only movable joint in the head is the joint between the lower jaw and the temporal bone (the **temporomandibular joint**). Four large muscles act across this joint, and collectively, they enable you to masticate (chew). These muscles also are innervated by cranial nerve V, the **trigeminal nerve**.
- **Muscles of Facial Expression**: You can contort the skin of the face into an infinite number of expressions thanks to approximately two dozen separate muscle bundles that are embedded within the superficial fascia of the head and neck. These muscles are innervated by cranial nerve VII, the **facial nerve**.
- **Muscles of Hearing**: Deep in the middle part of the ear canal are very small muscles that act on the delicate malleus, incus, and stapes bone combination to control the tension in the tympanic membrane and the sensitivity of the apparatus to vibrations from sound waves. This is another "special sense zone" of the body in which the brain reaches the outside world, this time in the form of a nerve that is sensitive to sound waves (cranial nerve VIII, or the **auditory nerve**).
- **Muscles of Swallowing**: The back of the mouth is lined with a funnel-shaped series of muscles that collectively "swallow" what is in the mouth. These are the muscles of the pharynx, and they include more discrete muscle bundles that raise and lower the soft part of the roof of the mouth as well as the funnel-shaped muscles that connect the esophagus to the oral cavity.
- **The Hyoid Assembly**: The hyoid bone is the one bone in the body that does not join any other bone. Tethered to several other bones by a long list of muscles, it "floats" in the front of the neck. Together, these muscles act to facilitate movement of the "throat"

during swallowing. In some measure, they also act as a kind of binding that protects the frontal exposure of the foodway and the airway.

■ **Muscles of Speaking:** This complex act involves muscles in most of the groups just mentioned, but a few muscles function purely to move the vocal cords and cartilages of the larynx to control the expiration of air that becomes sound when you speak. These are the laryngeal muscles, and they are motored exclusively by cranial nerve X, the **vagus nerve.**

■ **Muscles of the Tongue:** The tongue is one of the most flexible structures in the body, given its many intrinsic and extrinsic muscles. The tongue plays a key role in chewing, expressing, swallowing, and speaking; as with the thumb, any loss of the tongue's ability can deeply affect a patient's sense of well-being. In gross anatomy, you will learn the extrinsic muscles (most of which are innervated by cranial nerve XII, the **hypoglossal nerve**) and how to test for their proper function.

■ **Prime Mover of the Head:** One large muscle (the **sternocleidomastoid**) that attaches to the sternum, the clavicle, and the mastoid process of the skull (hence its name) assists the many vertebral muscles to position, stabilize, and move the head. The trapezius, incidentally, can move the head in complementary directions when the upper limb is stabilized. Both the sternocleidomastoid and the trapezius are innervated by cranial nerve XI, the **accessory nerve.**

Muscles of looking

The concept of muscles working in concert is, perhaps, best expressed in the orbital cavity. Muscles that draw origin from a small purchase of bone in the back of a conical orbital cavity must reach out to grasp a globe and provide it with universal positioning power. Compounding this difficulty is the fact that while you must maintain a coordinated stereoscopic focus, the optic nerve pathway and axis of the orbit point not straight ahead but, rather, a few degrees out to the side.

The muscles of eye movement, or the muscles of looking (Fig. 7.40), which stay true to the axis of the orbit, therefore must act cooperatively to keep the eye on one side looking at the same thing as the eye on the other side. The internal arrangement and working of the orbit are not observable in the actual patient, of course. Rather, mastery of the anatomy of the orbit is a means to understand how to test the function of the cranial nerves that drive the muscles.

The **levator palpebrae superioris** is the uppermost muscle in the orbital cone. It arcs over the eyeball proper and inserts into the soft tissue of the upper eyelid. As its name implies, it keeps the eyelid elevated. By some accounts, the smooth muscle in the eyelid derives with levator palpebrae superioris making it unusual in possessing both smooth and skeletal muscle. The smooth muscle fibers are served by the sympathetic nervous system. The skeletal muscle fibers of levator palpebrae superioris are innervated by cranial nerve III (the **oculomotor nerve**).

The **superior rectus** is one of four "rectus" muscles that run in a kind of "north, south, east, and west" design, from the back of the orbital cone to the top, bottom, and sides of the eyeball. Their functions would be simple if not for the fact, as noted above, that the axis of the orbit runs obliquely rather than straight ahead. The superior rectus runs just underneath the pathway of the levator palpebrae superioris and is innervated by the same nerve, cranial nerve III (the **oculomotor nerve**).

The **inferior rectus** complements the superior rectus along the bottom of the orbit. It is innervated by a branch of cranial nerve III (the **oculomotor nerve**). The **medial rectus** runs along the inner equator of the eye globe and is innervated by a branch of cranial nerve III (the **oculomotor nerve**). The **lateral rectus** complements

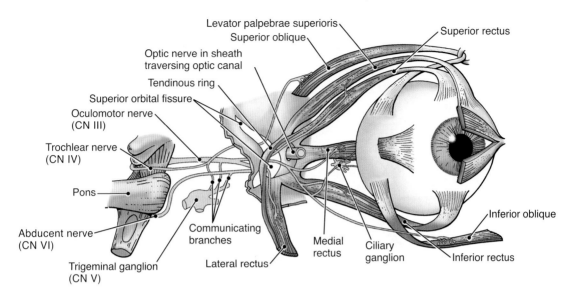

Levator palpebrae superioris
Superior oblique
Superior rectus
Optic nerve in sheath traversing optic canal
Tendinous ring
Superior orbital fissure
Oculomotor nerve (CN III)
Trochlear nerve (CN IV)
Pons
Abducent nerve (CN VI)
Communicating branches
Medial rectus
Ciliary ganglion
Inferior oblique
Trigeminal ganglion (CN V)
Lateral rectus
Inferior rectus

FIGURE 7.40   **The muscles of looking.**

The "eyeball" is an extension of the brain at the end of the optic nerve, which is able to detect changes in light waves. The position of the eyeball is controlled locally by the extraocular muscles. Most of these muscles originate from rigid connective tissue at the back of the bony orbit, which is shaped like a cone. From there, they project forward, beyond the "equator" of the eyeball globe, and insert into its sclera. (From Moore KL, Dalley AF. Clinically Oriented Anatomy, 5th Edition. Baltimore: Lippincott Williams & Wilkins, 2006. Figure 7.37, p. 970.)

the medial rectus on the outer equator but is innervated by its own dedicated cranial nerve, cranial nerve VI (the **abducens nerve**).

Two other extraocular muscles run in less cardinal directions and, in concert with the rectus muscles, enable the eyeball to look forward instead of perpetually toward the outsides of the field of vision. The **superior oblique** runs along the upper and inner part of the orbital cone, and it must overshoot the eyeball and then return toward it to gain access away from the coverage of the rectus muscles. In the upper inner corner of the orbital cavity is a pulley-loop of connective tissue through which the superior oblique passes before it turns back toward the eyeball. This **trochlea** becomes a fulcrum for contraction of the superior oblique, so its pull on the eyeball is actually leveraged from in front of the center of the ball. The superior oblique inserts behind the center point of the eyeball on its upper surface (and, thus, well behind the insertion of the superior rectus, under which it tucks). It has its own dedicated innervation from cranial nerve IV (the **trochlear nerve**).

The **inferior oblique** is the partner of the superior oblique, but it runs a less complicated course that begins in the anterior part of the orbital cone. From a medial attachment in the front part of the floor of the orbit, it runs "sideways" underneath the eyeball to insert behind the center point on the outer margin, tucked just underneath the passing of lateral rectus. The inferior oblique is innervated by a branch of cranial nerve III (the **oculomotor nerve**). Because of their "sideways" insertions on the eyeball, the obliques can, if necessary, "spin" the eyeball around its own axis.

Eye movements can be learned by studying a diagram of vectors. If the concept of a vector troubles you, just follow the arrows in Figure 7.41 and memorize Table 7.3.

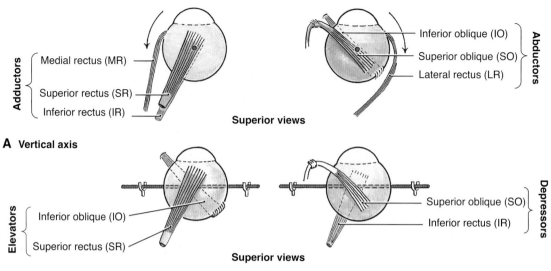

A Vertical axis

B Horizontal axis

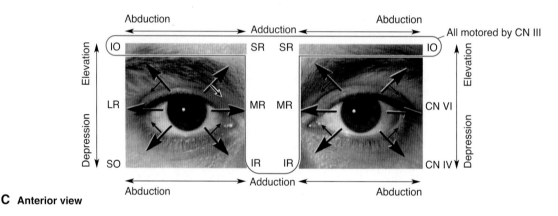

C Anterior view

FIGURE 7.41   **Basic eye movements.**

(**A and B**) These illustrations add an equator (red bar) and a center point (red dot) to a right eyeball to show how the muscles act in reference to the axis of the optic nerve. The eye focus is straight ahead, but no muscle actually runs straight back from the pupillary aperture. The important thing to remember is which cranial nerve governs which eye movement. (**C**) Muscles involved in specific changes of eyeball position. From this diagram, you can deduce that the oculomotor nerve governs all inward and upward gaze, while individual cranial nerves specialize in "downward" and "outward" gazing. CN = cranial nerve. (Adapted from Agur A, Dalley AF. Grant's Atlas of Anatomy, 11th Edition. Baltimore: Lippincott Williams & Wilkins, 2005. Figure 7.8, p. 649.)

Muscles of chewing

The jaw joint is a terrific combination of hinge, gliding, and swivel joints all packaged into one. You can, of course, open and close the mouth with power. You also can glide the lower jaw forward, however, and with some effort and pain tolerance, you can swivel the lower jaw from side to side. You rarely execute these moves discretely; rather, when you chew, you employ all three types of movement. The muscles that move the lower jaw against the skull are positioned to enable these movements (Fig. 7.42). All of these muscles are innervated by cranial nerve V (the **trigeminal nerve**).

TABLE 7.3   MUSCLES OF EYE MOVEMENT

MUSCLE	ORIGIN	INSERTION	INNERVATION	ACTION
Levator palpebrae superioris	Sphenoid bone inside orbital cone	Skin of upper eyelid	Oculomotor nerve (cranial nerve III)	Lifts the upper eyelid
Superior rectus	Common tendinous ring around optic canal	Eyeball sclera "north"	Oculomotor nerve (cranial nerve III)	Elevates, adducts and slightly intorts the eyeball
Inferior rectus	Common tendinous ring around optic canal	Eyeball sclera "south"	Oculomotor nerve (cranial nerve III)	Depresses, adducts, and slightly intorts the eyeball
Medial rectus	Common tendinous ring around optic canal	Eyeball sclera "inner side"	Oculomotor nerve (cranial nerve III)	Adducts eyeball
Lateral rectus	Common tendinous ring around optic canal	Eyeball sclera "outer side"	Abducens nerve (cranial nerve VI)	Abducts eyeball
Superior oblique	Sphenoid bone inside orbital cone	Eyeball sclera deep to superior rectus	Trochlear nerve (cranial nerve IV)	Abducts, depresses, and slightly intorts eyeball
Inferior oblique	Anterior floor of orbit	Eyeball sclera deep to inferior rectus	Oculomotor nerve (cranial nerve III)	Abducts, elevates, and slightly extorts eyeball

The **masseter** is the thickest of the muscles of mastication. It runs a short course from the bridge of bone just below the "temple" (the **zygomatic arch**) to the angle of the lower jaw on the outside surface. When you fire this muscle, you forcefully bring the back teeth into occlusion. The masseter is the essential muscle for mashing and pounding food between the molars.

The **temporalis** has a very broad expanse of origin along the side of the cranium, like an exaggerated, giant sideburn. The fibers converge as they pass forward and down

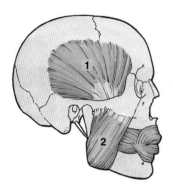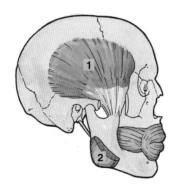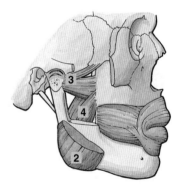

FIGURE 7.42   **Muscles of chewing.**

The muscles of mastication include two powerful muscles for closing the jaw—the temporalis(1) and the masseter (2)—and two deeper positional muscles—the lateral pterygoid (3) and the medial pterygoid (4)—for gliding the mandible back and forth and from side to side. The temporomandibular joint includes an articular disc to pad the chronic impact of the mandible against the temporal bone. The mobility of the lower jaw requires that the joint space allow forward and backward gliding, some of which is passive and some of which is actively monitored and directed by the lateral pterygoid muscle. (From Moore KL, Agur AMR. Essential Clinical Anatomy, 2nd Edition. Baltimore: Lippincott Williams & Wilkins, 2002. Figure 8.7.)

behind the zygomatic process. They insert on a very small area of the mandible, the **coronoid process**, with some fibers feeling their way down along the internal surface of this "lever" of the mandible. When the temporalis fires, it governs the true hinge movement of the jaw joint—that is, it "slams the door shut." The temporalis drives the front of the lower jaw into the front of the upper jaw; in other words, it brings the incisors into occlusion. Because some of its fibers travel virtually straight forward, the temporalis also can retract the mandible from its forward position when the jaw is gaping open.

The **lateral pterygoid** and **medial pterygoid** are internally positioned muscles. They arise from the lateral pterygoid plates of the complex sphenoid bone in the center of the skull. As their names imply, one of them arises from the lateral surface of this plate, and one of them arises from the medial surface. They enable the head of the mandible to slide forward when the mouth opens, and they swing the jaw from side to side to maximize the effect of grinding the tooth surfaces together. The pterygoids act in concert with the powerful masseter and temporalis to enable very subtle changes in jaw position during speaking and chewing. The lateral pterygoid attaches to the capsule of the jaw joint and is a chief protruder of the mandible. The medial pterygoid attaches to the angle of the mandible, but on the opposite side from the masseter. The medial pterygoid assists in protrusion of the jaw and is the principal swiveler of the jaw to the opposite side. (See Table 7.4.)

Muscles of facial expression

The skeleton of the face supports seeing, smelling, and eating the world around you. These abilities require entryways to the body. The same muscles that act to open, close, widen, or narrow those passageways also express feelings, attitudes, intentions, and emotions. Numerous muscles that are embedded in the skin of the face, with no bony attachment, contract to move the skin into the infinite myriad of facial expressions. Together, they are called **muscles of facial expression** (Fig. 7.43). These muscle purse the lips, raise the eyebrows, flare the nostrils, blow out the cheeks, smile, frown, squint, grimace, and many other things.

All muscles of facial expression are innervated by cranial nerve VII (the **facial nerve**). The facial nerve bundle that serves these muscles exits the stylomastoid foramen

TABLE 7.4   MUSCLES OF MASTICATION

MUSCLE	ORIGIN	INSERTION	INNERVATION	ACTION
Masseter	Zygomatic arch	Gonial angle of mandible	Mandibular division of trigeminal nerve (cranial nerve V)	Forcefully clamps the lower jaw against the upper jaw at a force point near the crushing molar teeth
Temporalis	Side of cranium	Coronoid process of mandible		Forcefully "snaps" the jaw shut in a swinging motion, bringing the front of the jaw into occlusion
Lateral pterygoid	Lateral surface of lateral pterygoid plate	Head of mandible and temporo-mandibular joint capsule		Slides the head of the mandible forward within its hinge joint, enabling you to protrude your jaw
Medial pterygoid	Medial surface of lateral pterygoid plate	Inner surface of gonial angle of mandible		Protrudes mandible and swivels it toward the opposite side as a positioner for the crushing effect of the masseter

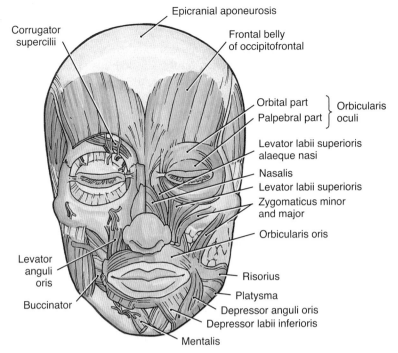

Anterior view

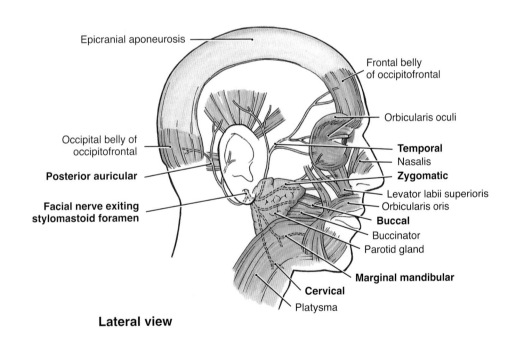

Lateral view

Bold = Branches of facial nerve

FIGURE 7.43   **Muscles of facial expression.**

Muscles of facial expression are embedded in the superficial fascia of the facial skin. They run in virtually every direction and enable you to express very subtle differences in temperament. Some muscle bundles are discrete enough to be named, such as the orbicularis oculi. All facial expression muscles are innervated by cranial nerve VII, the facial nerve. (**A**) Anterior view. (**B**) Lateral view. (From Agur A, Dalley AF. Grant's Atlas of Anatomy, 11th Edition. Baltimore: Lippincott Williams & Wilkins, 2005. Figure 7.1, p. 603.)

deep to the parotid gland and is vulnerable to compression or damage. Such localized trauma paralyzes all muscles of facial expression on the affected side. This condition, known as Bell's palsy, leaves the patient with a characteristic "masked," or expressionless, side of the face.

The muscles of facial expression canvas virtually the entire dermal zone of the face and neck. Those with discrete responsibility for major functions should be incorporated into routine neurologic examination. The **orbicularis oris** rims the lips and enables you to squeeze the lips together to speak and eat. The **orbicularis oculi** likewise rims the orbit and enables you to squint and wrinkle the brow; it is the major reaction muscle in the blink reflex. The **occipitofrontalis** actually runs the length of the skull, from the eyebrow line to the back of the head, and it enables you to "shorten up" the scalp, the major effect of which is to raise the eyebrows.

The **zygomaticus major** and **zygomaticus minor** angle down from the zygomatic area of the cheek to lift the upper lip. The **levator anguli oris** and **levator labii superioris** also do this, but from slightly different angles, and with the result that you can express many emotions by raising the corners and border of the upper lip using the fine motor control afforded by these muscles.

The **nasalis** reaches onto the nares, or the nostrils, from a sideways vantage. It helps you to flare or dilate the nasal opening. The **depressor labii**, **depressor anguli oris**, **mentalis**, and **risorius** act on the corner of the mouth and the lower lip, and they complement the muscles of the upper lip. For every smile, there is a potential frown or pout.

The **buccinator** is a powerful muscle of facial expression. It is effectively the substance of the cheek, running from where the pharynx commences in back (the **pterygomandibular raphe**) to where the orbicularis oris begins in front. It controls the position of the cheek skin, which is important for expelling air while speaking or singing (or, especially, playing the trumpet), for sucking air or liquid through tightened lips, and for bouncing pieces of food back toward the center of the mouth from the pouch between the cheek and gum.

The **platysma** is a strange muscle of expression because it is in the neck. It runs from the jawline down across the clavicle line, and when it tightens, the skin of the neck stiffens.

Muscles of hearing

Just as muscles play a role in vision, muscles play a role in hearing. The ability to hear relies on bones that have become very small over evolutionary time (the **malleus, incus,** and **stapes**) and on the elastic fibers (muscles) that move and stabilize them. Sound waves impact the ear drum (the **tympanic membrane**), which jiggles these three bones against a chamber of pressurized fluid (Fig. 7.44). The vibration is detected by cranial nerve VIII (the **vestibulocochlear nerve,** or **auditory nerve**), and the impulse is "translated" by the brain as sound. Two muscles are active in this process—but only to the extent that they work to dampen very loud sound to protect both the "surface" of sound (the tympanic membrane) and the "receiver" of sound (the oval window of the cochlea).

The **tensor tympani** inserts into the handle of the malleus bone from a broad origin along deep surfaces of the sphenoid bone and auditory tube. When it contracts, it draws the handle of the malleus toward the tympanic cavity, which tenses the tympanic membrane. This makes it more difficult for sound to vibrate the tympanic membrane, which is protective in environments of very loud sound. It is innervated by cranial nerve V (the **trigeminal nerve**).

The **stapedius** is a smaller muscle located deep within the middle ear cavity and inserting on the neck of the stapes bone. When it contracts, it tilts the anterior part of the base of the bone toward the tympanic cavity, which reduces movement of

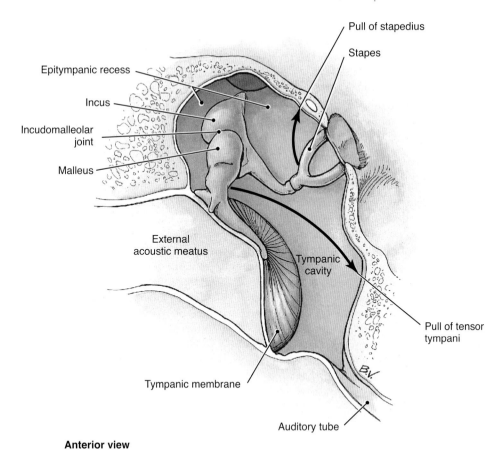

Anterior view

FIGURE 7.44   **Muscles of hearing.**

Hearing actually does not require muscles, but two small muscles help to blunt the impact of very loud sounds by dampening ossicle vibration. Their effect, rather than their actual position, is illustrated here. The tensor tympani steadies the malleus against dramatic vibrations of the tympanic membrane. As a derivative of the first pharyngeal arch, it is innervated by the trigeminal nerve. The stapedius lessens the vibration of the stapes bone against the oval window, which also blunts the effect of intense sound waves. As a derivative of the second pharyngeal arch, it is innervated by the facial nerve. (Adapted from Agur A, Dalley AF. Grant's Atlas of Anatomy, 11th Edition. Baltimore: Lippincott Williams & Wilkins, 2005. Figure 7.81A, p. 700.)

the footplate. This dampens the effect of loud sound rapping on the fluid-filled chambers of the cochlea. It is innervated by cranial nerve VII (the **facial nerve**).

Hearing loss is a common clinical problem in elderly patients that often is caused by a "freezing up," or fixation, of these "chain-link" ear ossicles. When establishing the diagnosis of problems in the middle ear, you must be able to determine if nerve damage has resulted in muscle paralysis (thus affecting sensitivity in the tympanic membrane), if the bones have fused together (**otosclerosis**), or if the deficit is in the inner ear or cranial nerve itself.

Muscles of swallowing

Terrestrial vertebrates breathe in air as a means of absorbing energy from the environment. In the neck and below, the airway lies anterior to the gut tube, which matches its initial position. As the head develops, however, the common chamber for air and food (the **throat**) is partitioned into an entryway/exitway for air and one for, mostly, food (the **nasal cavity** and the **oral cavity**, respectively). The nasal cavity is positioned closer to the brain (all the better for the cranial nerve I, the **olfactory nerve**, to reach the outside world), which means that inspired air must pass through the back of the oral cavity on its way to the front of the neck and thorax. The two passageways intersect, and this requires a separating flap of some kind. This flap is called the **epiglottis**. A few muscles embedded between the soft part of the roof of the mouth and the sides of the oral cavity encourage food to go where it should and not into the respiratory route. These muscles facilitate swallowing after you move what you are chewing to the back of your mouth and before you are beyond the swallowing "point of no return."

As with other parts of the head, the emphasis here is on the activity (swallowing) and how it is achieved. The individual muscles and their actions are much less significant than their cooperative function. The ultimate clinical application is to know what nerves govern the detection and swallowing of food and, thus, how to evaluate problems with swallowing (**dysphagia**).

The **superior constrictor**, **middle constrictor**, and **inferior constrictor** make up the bulk of the funneling throat muscles (Fig. 7.45). Think of them as hanging down off of the bottom of the skull like a soccer net. The constrictors are attached to the bone surfaces that surround the back of the oral cavity (the pterygoid plates of the sphenoid bone, the mylohyoid line of the mandible, and even a tubercle on the occipital bone near the foramen magnum). The constrictors on the right side insert on the constrictors on the left side in the same kind of midline raphe that you have seen for the mylohyoid muscle and the muscles of the abdominal wall. The superior constrictor weaves into the middle constrictor, which weaves into the inferior constrictor, which weaves into the esophagus, and in so doing, skeletal muscle eventually weaves into smooth muscle.

The middle constrictor attaches to the stylohyoid ligament and the greater and lesser horns of the hyoid bone. Therefore, when you move the hyoid bone, you drive some of the swallowing apparatus, and vice versa. Having three overlapping constrictors instead of one long sleeve enables blood vessels and nerves to slip into the back of the pharynx. Moreover, three overlapping constrictors sequence the swallowing reflex among a starter sleeve (superior constrictor), a trigger for the hyoid bone (middle constrictor), and a true funnel for the esophagus (inferior constrictor).

All three constrictors are innervated by the pharyngeal plexus, that combination of motor and sensory service of cranial nerve IX (the **glossopharyngeal nerve**) and cranial nerve X (the **vagus nerve**). They contract somewhat involuntarily during swallowing (which may be why the process is called a reflex). Their ability to receive a bolus of food and direct it into the esophagus instead of the trachea depends on some tiny accessory muscles embedded in the mucuous membranes of the roof of the mouth (soft palate), the internal access to the ear canal (auditory tube), and the base of the tongue.

The **palatoglossus** was mentioned above as a muscle that defines the arch at the back of the mouth between the soft palate and the tongue. The **stylopharyngeus** runs from the busy styloid process downward and between the superior and middle constrictors on its way to fanning out along the surface of other pharyngeal muscles and the thyroid cartilage. It is a notable muscle in cadaver dissection exercises because a bundle of cranial nerve IX (the **glossopharyngeal nerve**) fibers runs along with it.

The **salpingopharyngeus** runs under the membrane that covers the opening of the auditory tube (also known as a **salpinx**) and heads downward to blend in with the palatopharyngeus muscle. The **palatopharyngeus** tents backward from the soft palate into the receptive blanket of the pharyngeal constrictors (Fig. 7.46).

The palatoglossus, stylopharyngeus, salpingopharyngeus, and palatopharyngeus are innervated by the **pharyngeal plexus**. The stylopharyngeus is believed to be innervated

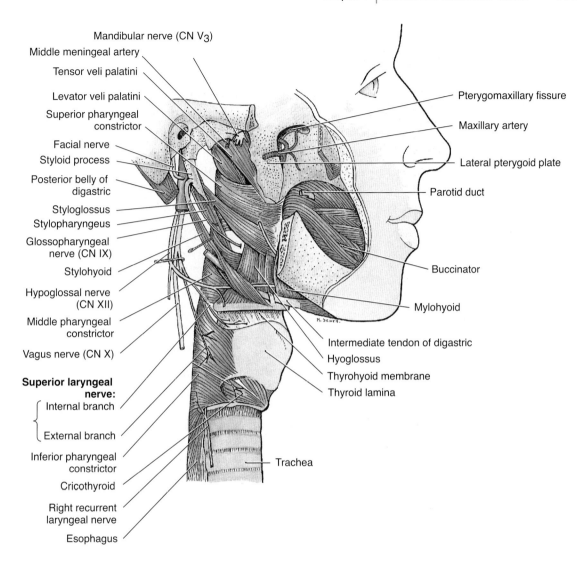

Mandibular nerve (CN V$_3$)

Middle meningeal artery

Tensor veli palatini

Levator veli palatini

Superior pharyngeal constrictor

Facial nerve

Styloid process

Posterior belly of digastric

Styloglossus

Stylopharyngeus

Glossopharyngeal nerve (CN IX)

Stylohyoid

Hypoglossal nerve (CN XII)

Middle pharyngeal constrictor

Vagus nerve (CN X)

Superior laryngeal nerve:

Internal branch

External branch

Inferior pharyngeal constrictor

Cricothyroid

Right recurrent laryngeal nerve

Esophagus

Pterygomaxillary fissure

Maxillary artery

Lateral pterygoid plate

Parotid duct

Buccinator

Mylohyoid

Intermediate tendon of digastric

Hyoglossus

Thyrohyoid membrane

Thyroid lamina

Trachea

Lateral view

FIGURE 7.45   **Muscles of swallowing—I.**

The transition between mouth and esophagus is sleeved by three constrictor muscles: the superior, the middle, and the inferior. They are anchored to all the nearby bones at the base of the skull as well as to the floating hyoid bone. They contract from the top down, and at some point, the continuation is involuntary. CN = cranial nerve. (From Agur A, Dalley AF. Grant's Atlas of Anatomy, 11th Edition. Baltimore: Lippincott Williams & Wilkins, 2005. Figure 8.7, p. 767.)

just by the glossopharyngeal nerve that runs along with it. When these muscles contract, they bring the two things they link closer together. This generally results in a tightened border to the back of the mouth so that food is directed toward the central canal of the pharynx, not into a blind pouch or alley along the sides of the back of the mouth.

The **tensor veli palatini** accomplishes just what it claims—it tenses the soft palate. It does this by reaching onto the palatine aponeurosis of the soft palate (where several

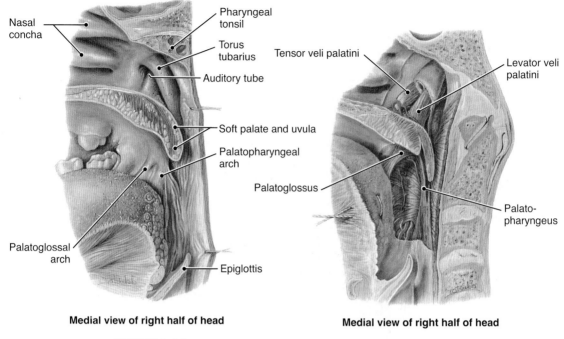

Nasal concha

Pharyngeal tonsil

Torus tubarius

Tensor veli palatini

Auditory tube

Levator veli palatini

Soft palate and uvula

Palatopharyngeal arch

Palatoglossus

Palato-pharyngeus

Palatoglossal arch

Epiglottis

Medial view of right half of head   **Medial view of right half of head**

FIGURE 7.46   **Muscles of swallowing—II.**

More specialized muscles conspire to hike up the soft palate and raise the back of the tongue to move food into the pharynx. These muscles lie just under folds in the mucous membranes. Among them are the palatoglossus, salpingopharyngeus, palatopharyngeus, tensor veli palatini, levator veli palatini, and stylopharyngeus (see Fig. 7.45). (Adapted from Agur A, Dalley AF. Grant's Atlas of Anatomy, 11th Edition. Baltimore: Lippincott Williams & Wilkins, 2005. Figure 8.32A,C, pp. 774–775.)

of the muscles described above also claim attachment to the palate) from a secure position on the wing of the sphenoid bone above and including the cartilaginous arch of the auditory tube. It is innervated by cranial nerve V (the **trigeminal nerve**), through fibers that also serve the nearby medial pterygoid muscle of mastication.

The **levator veli palatini** is a neighbor living behind the tensor veli palatini. It approaches the soft palate at a slightly different angle, which allows this muscle to lift up the palate flap as much as draw it tight. It is innervated by cranial nerve X (the **vagus nerve**). Together, the palatini muscles and the accessory pharyngeal muscles assure that the soft palate blocks the nasal cavity during swallowing so that food particles do not end up in the back of the nose. When the mucous membranes that blanket most of these muscles are irritated or inflamed, such as when you have a head cold, swallowing can be uncomfortable.

As with most regions of the head, your major priority is to master the functions of the different cranial nerves that are active in the area. Cranial nerves V (the **trigeminal nerve**), IX (the **glossopharyngeal nerve**), X (the **vagus nerve**) and XII (the **hypoglossal nerve**) all supply motor fibers to the many muscles involved in swallowing. Most of the preparatory, or initial, aspects of swallowing are governed by the trigeminal and hypoglossal nerves. By contrast, most of the "inevitable," or cascading, or "downward" aspects of swallowing are governed by the pharyngeal plexus (motor innervation supplied by the vagus nerve). A characteristic effect of a deficit in the vagus nerve is deviation of the uvula from unilateral paralysis of a levator veli palatine muscle (Fig. 7.47), which is easily seen during a clinical examination. (See Table 7.5.)

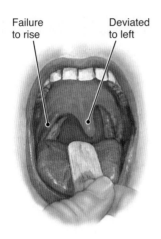

Failure to rise

Deviated to left

FIGURE 7.47   **A vagus nerve lesion can manifest as a deviated palate.**

Paralysis of the soft palate musculature from a vagus nerve lesion will leave the palate margin flaccid and the uvula deviated when you ask the patient to say "Ahhh." Inspecting a patient for signs of healthy cranial nerve activity is a central theme of the neurologic examination. (From Bickley LS and Szilagyi P. Bates' Guide to Physical Examination and History Taking, 8th Edition. Philadelphia: Lippincott Williams & Wilkins, 2003.)

TABLE 7.5   MUSCLES OF SWALLOWING

MUSCLE	ORIGIN	INSERTION	INNERVATION	ACTION
Superior constrictor	Pterygomandibular raphe, mylohyoid line of mandible	Median raphe of the pharynx and bottom of the skull (occipital bone)	Vagus nerve (cranial nerve X) and pharyngeal plexus	Constricts walls of the pharynxx during swallowing
Middle constrictor	Stylohyoid ligament and hyoid bone	Median raphe of the pharynx	Vagus nerve (cranial nerve X) and pharyngeal plexus	Constricts walls of the pharynx during swallowing
Inferior constrictor	Thyroid cartilage and side of cricoid cartilage	Median raphe of pharynx	Vagus nerve (cranial nerve X) and pharyngeal plexus	Constricts walls of the pharynx during swallowing
Palatoglossus	Palatine aspect of soft palate	Side of tongue	Vagus nerve (cranial nerve X)	Elevates back of tongue
Stylopharyngeus	Styloid process	Back of thyroid cartilage, between superior and middle constrictors	Glossopharyngeal nerve (cranial nerve IX)	Elevates pharynx and larynx during swallowing and speaking
Salpingopharyngeus	Cartilaginous part of pharyngotym- panic tube	Side of pharynx along with palatopharyngeus	Vagus nerve (cranial nerve X) and pharyngeal plexus	Elevates pharynx and larynx during swallowing and speaking
Palatopharyngeus	Hard palate and palatine aponeurosis	Side of pharynx and back of thyroid cartilage	Vagus nerve (cranial nerve X) and pharyngeal plexus	Elevates pharynx and larynx during swallowing and speaking
Tensor veli palatini	Pterygoid plate, sphenoid, and pharyngotympanic tube	Soft palate	Mandibular division of trigeminal nerve (cranial nerve V)	Tenses soft palate and opens pharyngotympanic tube during swallowing and yawning
Levator veli palatini	Pharyngotympanic tube and petrous part of temporal bone	Soft palate	Vagus nerve (cranial nerve X) and pharyngeal plexus	Elevates soft palate during swallowing and yawning

TABLE 7.6   THE HYOID ASSEMBLY

MUSCLE	ORIGIN	INSERTION	INNERVATION	ACTION
Infrahyoid unit			Ansa cervicalis (C1–C3 ventral rami)	
Sternohyoid	Sternum	Hyoid		Tethers and depresses hyoid
Omohyoid	Scapula	Hyoid		Tethers and depresses hyoid
Sternothyroid	Sternum	Thyroid cartilage		Depresses larynx during swallowing
Thyrohyoid	Thyroid cartilage	Hyoid		Links larynx to hyoid for mutual movement during speaking and swallowing
Suprahyoid unit Mylohyoid	Mandible	Midline raphe and hyoid bone	Mylohyoid nerve (a branch of cranial nerve V, trigeminal nerve)	Elevates the hyoid bone, floor of mouth, and tongue during swallowing and speaking
Geniohyoid	Genial tubercles of mandible	Hyoid	C1 ventral ramus	Pulls hyoid bone upward and forward during swallowing
Stylohyoid	Styloid process of temporal	Hyoid	Facial nerve (cranial nerve VII)	Elevates and retracts the mandible in a cooperative rocking with geniohyoid during swallowing
Anterior belly of digastric	Mandible	Tendon to body and greater horn of hyoid	Mylohyoid nerve (a branch of cranial nerve V, trigeminal nerve)	With posterior belly of digastric, it elevates hyoid apparatus or depresses mandible against a steadied hyoid bone
Posterior belly of digastric	Digastric groove of temporal	Tendon to body and greater horn of hyoid	Facial nerve (cranial nerve VII)	With anterior belly of digastric, it elevates hyoid apparatus or steadies it during swallowing

The hyoid assembly

The hyoid assembly is summarized in Table 7.6.

Infrahyoid Group

Several muscles anchor the hyoid bone to surrounding structures (the thyroid cartilage, the sternum, and of all things, the scapula). These muscles are all strap-shaped and are called the **infrahyoid strap muscles**. They share a motor innervation from fibers of the upper cervical spinal nerves (C1-C3), which reach the muscles in a looping web called the **ansa cervicalis** (Fig. 7.48).

The **sternohyoid** lies close to the midline and just under the skin. The name says it all—it connects the sternum to the hyoid bone, and when it shortens, it draws the hyoid bone down (a necessary ripple motion in the act of swallowing or opening the mouth against resistance).

The **omohyoid** is probably the most peculiar muscle in the body. Its superior belly runs from the undersurface of the hyoid bone (next to the attachment of sternohyoid) down through a sling of connective tissue on the clavicle and first rib, then back as an inferior belly to the upper border of the scapula. The bellies act in concert and, presumably, act to depress the hyoid bone.

The **sternothyroid** lies deep to sternohyoid and reaches up only to the thyroid cartilage below the hyoid bone. From the same patch of attachment arises the origin of the **thyrohyoid muscle**, which completes the course upward to the underside of the hyoid bone. Acting in unison, these muscles mimic the action of the sternohyoid, with the extra effect of moving the thyroid cartilage as well. When thyrohyoid acts alone, it

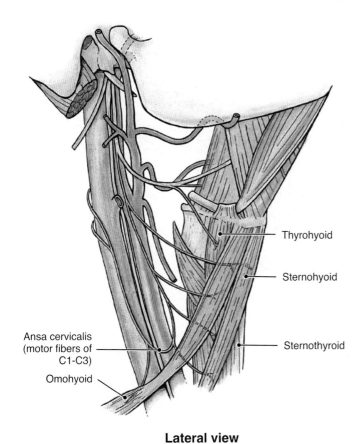

Lateral view

FIGURE 7.48   **Muscles of the hyoid assembly.**

A number of small muscles overlie the respiratory and alimentary tubes. The superficial muscles are the long ones. The omohyoid runs from the shoulder blade to the hyoid. The sternohyoid runs from the sternum to the hyoid. Deep to them lay two muscles of half the length. The sternothyroid runs from the sternum to the thyroid cartilage. The thyrohyoid runs from the thyroid cartilage to the hyoid bone. The strap-like design continues from the hyoid bone to the mandible in the form of the geniohyoid (not shown). These muscles are innervated by a loop of cervical plexus nerves called the ansa cervicalis, indicating that they are not directly or primarily involved in swallowing. (Adapted from Agur A, Dalley AF. Grant's Atlas of Anatomy, 11th Edition. Baltimore: Lippincott Williams & Wilkins, 2005. Figure 8.10A, p. 741.)

can perform the very important function of drawing the thyroid cartilage toward the hyoid bone during swallowing. This approximation lowers the chance that food particles will fall into the airway deep to the thyroid cartilage. Both the sternothyroid and the thyrohyoid are innervated by fibers of the upper cervical spinal nerves, but the fiber that reaches the thyrohyoid travels along the route of cranial nerve XII (the **hypoglossal nerve**) across the neck until it shoots off to reach the muscle. The **nerve to thyrohyoid** is thus a dissectable nerve fiber that is separate from the ansa cervicalis and is vulnerable to damage during neck surgeries. It is a challenging nerve to find during the neck dissection in anatomy class, which makes its discovery all the more satisfying.

Suprahyoid Group

Several muscles complete the arc of the hyoid assembly by spanning the possible ranges between the upper surface of the hyoid bone and the framework of the skull above. These are collectively called the **suprahyoid muscles**. They function to "stiffen" the barrier between the food tube and the skin of the neck or, more simply, to facilitate the swallowing reflex by "roller-coastering" the floor of the mouth (Fig. 7.49).

The **mylohyoid** is a kind of diaphragm or trampoline muscle that fans out from the body of the hyoid bone upward to the rim on the inside surface of the body of the mandible. The mylohyoid from one side attaches to the mylohyoid from the other side in a midline raphe, thus making the muscle an effective bed or diaphragm for the bottom of the oral cavity. Remember that the hyoid bone sits almost at the same level as the lower jawline, so the mylohyoid fibers run almost straight forward. When the

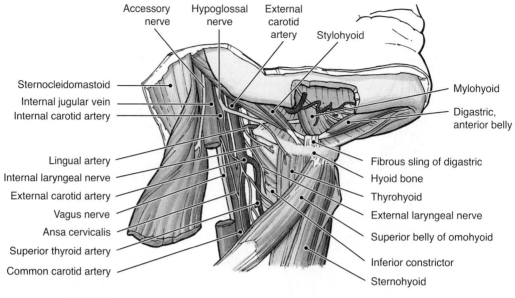

FIGURE 7.49   **Muscles of swallowing—III.**

The muscles above the hyoid bone include the mylohyoid muscle, which closes off the floor of the oral cavity just like a diaphragm, and the anterior belly of the digastric muscle. Together with posterior partners, such as posterior digastric and stylohyoid (see Fig. 7.45), they hike the hyoid assembly in a rolling fashion to commence the voluntary phase of swallowing. (Adapted from Moore KL, Agur AMR. Essential Clinical Anatomy, 2nd Edition. Baltimore: Lippincott Williams & Wilkins, 2002.)

muscle contracts, it stiffens the floor of the oral cavity and effectively raises it during the swallowing reflex. The mylohyoid is innervated by the **mylohyoid nerve**, which is a branch of cranial nerve V (the **trigeminal nerve**, or the nerve of mastication).

The **geniohyoid** also connects hyoid to mandible, but with fibers that form a bundle instead of a sheet. These bundles run from the spines on the inside surface of the center of the mandible back to the body of the hyoid bone, all on top of the mylohyoid sheet. The muscle is innervated by a fiber of the first cervical spinal nerve, conveyed to the muscle along the route of cranial nerve XII (the **hypoglossal nerve**).

The **stylohyoid** is a virtual string of muscle from the styloid process of the skull to the body of the hyoid bone at the base of its greater horn. Before it can get onto the hyoid bone, however, it must split to allow the **digastric muscle** to pass through (see below), which makes its attachment look more like two slips of muscle fiber. The stylohyoid lifts and pulls back on the hyoid bone in something of a "tug of war" with the geniohyoid muscle. The muscles actually work in sequence during the swallowing reflex. The stylohyoid is innervated by cranial nerve VII (the **facial nerve**) because it derives from the embryonic tissue block in which this nerve is located.

The **digastric** has two bellies, as its name implies. The **anterior belly** runs from the lowest edge of the mandibular symphysis back toward the hyoid body, where it then runs through the split in the stylohyoid. After surfing the top of the hyoid body, the **posterior belly** arcs backward, toward a groove between the mastoid process and the styloid process on the skull. The digastric muscle hikes up on the hyoid bone; if the hyoid position is fixed by a stronger combination of other muscles, it depresses the mandible. The digastric muscle is interesting because its anterior belly is innervated by cranial nerve V (the **trigeminal nerve**), but its posterior belly is innervated by cranial nerve VII (the **facial nerve**).

Paralysis of an individual hyoid apparatus muscle is uncommon. Difficulty swallowing (dysphagia) can result from a wide variety of extrinsic and intrinsic causes and is not uncommon. If muscles of the hyoid assembly are implicated in the problem, it may be the result of a deficit in one or more of the cranial nerves involved (trigeminal, facial, and hypoglossal).

Muscles of speaking

A psychological sense of well-being depends on being able to communicate, and speaking is a predominant mode of communication. We speak by forcing out air through narrowings and twistings of our anatomy, so knowing the anatomy of speech is important for helping patients with dysarthria, or difficulty speaking. Just as the pharynx is the chamber that leads from the oral cavity to the digestive system, the larynx is the portal that leads from the oral cavity to the respiratory system and through which expelled air is channeled to make purposeful sounds. (See Table 7.7.)

The larynx itself is formed by cartilages that connect the trachea to the bottom of the oral cavity. These cartilages expand to form a large hollow, thanks to the cricoid and thyroid cartilages. The ligaments that bind the cricoid cartilage to the thyroid cartilage are the vocal ligaments; together with the fold of mucous membrane that coats them, these ligaments form a vocal cord (Fig. 7.50). The suspension of the vocal folds against the lining of the larynx enables them to vibrate when air is forced through the larynx, resulting in sound waves. The gross anatomy is slightly more complicated, but the basic modification of the trachea into a "voicebox" is fairly simple.

The muscles of the larynx can be defined as those that manipulate the whole apparatus by moving the neck (**extrinsic muscles**) and those that manipulate specific cartilages and folds to operate the larynx itself (**intrinsic muscles**). The extrinsic muscles have been described above (the hyoid apparatus muscles). Now, consider the intrinsic muscles, all of which are innervated by cranial nerve X (the **vagus nerve**).

TABLE 7.7   MUSCLES OF SPEAKING

MUSCLE	ORIGIN	INSERTION	INNERVATION	ACTION
Cricothyroid	Cricoid cartilage	Thyroid cartilage	External laryngeal branch of vagus (cranial nerve X)	Tensions vocal cords for a dynamic range of sounds
Posterior cricoarytenoid	Posterior surface of cricoid cartilage	Muscular process of arytenoid cartilage	Recurrent laryngeal branch of vagus (cranial nerve X)	Abducts vocal cords to maximize vocal inlet (rima glottidis)
Lateral cricoarytenoid	Arch of cricoid cartilage	Muscular process of arytenoid cartilage	Recurrent laryngeal branch of vagus (cranial nerve X)	Adducts vocal cords to close off the rima glottidis and enable phonation
Transverse arytenoid	Arytenoid cartilage	Opposite arytenoid cartilage	Recurrent laryngeal branch of vagus (cranial nerve X)	Helps to close rima glottidis
Oblique arytenoid	Arytenoid cartilage	Opposite arytenoid cartilage	Recurrent laryngeal branch of vagus (cranial nerve X)	Helps to close rima glottidis
Thyroarytenoid	Thyroid cartilage	Muscular process of arytenoid cartilage	Recurrent laryngeal branch of vagus (cranial nerve X)	Slackens or relaxes vocal cords to enable modulation of sound

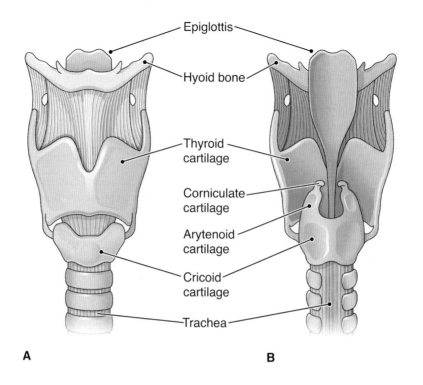

Epiglottis

Hyoid bone

Thyroid
cartilage

Corniculate
cartilage

Arytenoid
cartilage

Cricoid
cartilage

Trachea

A

B

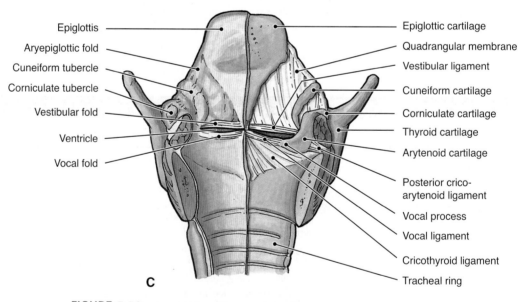

Epiglottis

Aryepiglottic fold

Cuneiform tubercle

Corniculate tubercle

Vestibular fold

Ventricle

Vocal fold

Epiglottic cartilage

Quadrangular membrane

Vestibular ligament

Cuneiform cartilage

Corniculate cartilage

Thyroid cartilage

Arytenoid cartilage

Posterior crico-
arytenoid ligament

Vocal process

Vocal ligament

Cricothyroid ligament

Tracheal ring

C

FIGURE 7.50   **Laryngeal cartilages and membranes.**

(**A**) Anterior view. (**B**) Posterior view. (**C**) The opened larynx as viewed anteriorly. The vocal cords run
from the arytenoid cartilages anteriorly to the back facing of the large thyroid cartilage. By virtue of
a free upper edge, they vibrate as air is expelled. Because allergies and gastroesophageal reflux
are so common and can affect vocal cord behavior, each fold of mucuous membrane is clinically
relevant. (From Cohen BJ, Wood DL. Memmler's The Human Body in Health and Disease, 10th Edition.
Baltimore: Lippincott Williams & Wilkins, 2004. Figure 18.03; from Moore KL, Agur AMR. Essential
Clinical Anatomy, 2nd Edition. Baltimore: Lippincott Williams & Wilkins, 2002. Figure 9.16B, p. 625.)

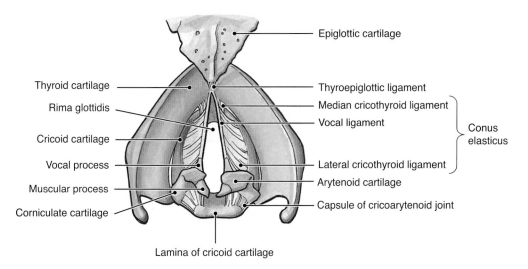

FIGURE 7.51   **Laryngeal connective tissue, superior view.**

Speaking is a function of passing air forcefully through the space between the vocal cords and then closing them tightly. Failure of muscles to push the vocal cords tightly together, or structural polyps or growths on the cord, can lead to a hoarse or whispery sound. (From Moore KL, Agur AMR. Essential Clinical Anatomy, 2nd Edition. Baltimore: Lippincott Williams & Wilkins, 2002. Figure 9.16, p. 625.)

The intrinsic muscles alter the length, tension, and distance separating the vocal cords (Fig. 7.51). The vocal cords are attached to the cricoid cartilage below (via an elastic cone of tissue), to nothing but a mucous membrane above (which is why you can see them in a laryngoscope), and to movable cartilages in back. The action therefore is mostly along the back and sides of the cricoid and thyroid cartilages. The intrinsic muscles are mostly paired muscles, and all of them except the cricothyroid muscle lie in the space between the cartilage framework of the larynx and the mucous membrane that coats it.

The **cricothyroid** is a relatively large intrinsic muscle that connects the cricoid cartilage to the prominent thyroid cartilage just above it (Fig. 7.52). By running from the lower cartilage in front to the higher cartilage in back, the cricothyroid pulls the cricoid cartilage up and back, which **tenses** the vocal cords. Because of its size and power, the cricothyroid is the chief tensor of the vocal cords. Cranial nerve X (the **vagus nerve**) reaches the cricothyroid as an **external laryngeal branch** of the **superior laryngeal nerve**, which means that it is slightly exposed in the neck and vulnerable to compression by a tumor or to being cut during surgery.

The Arytenoid Levers
You change the aperture of the larynx by bringing the vocal cords closer together or by keeping them apart. The cartilages that link to the vocal cords are delicate and a little strange in appearance. Chief among them is the **arytenoid cartilage**, which sits atop the back of the cricoid cartilage and can crank the vocal cords together into a complete closure. Several muscles govern this process, just as several muscles govern the hyoid bone. They all have "arytenoid" in their name.

The **posterior cricoarytenoid** is a broad muscle that is attached to the fat back of the cricoid cartilage. Its fibers converge around the side of the cricoid cartilage to insert on a muscular process of the arytenoid cartilage. This muscle is the only one that fully

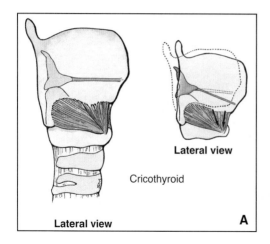

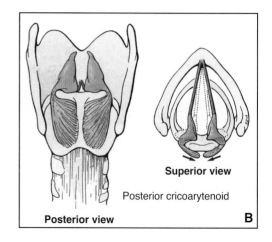

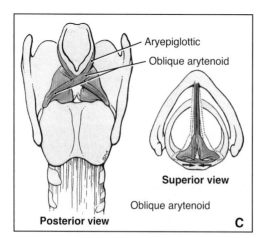

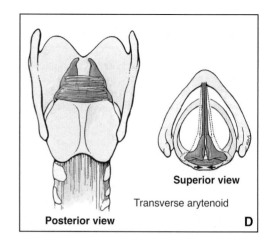

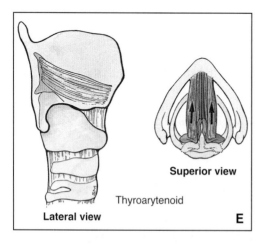

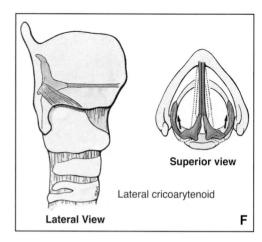

FIGURE 7.52 **Muscles of speaking.**

(**A**) The cricothyroid is the primary tensor of the vocal cords. (**B**) The posterior cricoarytenoid is the primary abductor of the vocal cords, which is necessary for maximum inspiration. (**C–F**) Numerous muscles conspire to appose the vocal cords. (From Agur A, Dalley AF. Grant's Atlas of Anatomy, 11th Edition. Baltimore: Lippincott Williams & Wilkins, 2005. Figure 8.8, pp. 784–785.)

abducts the vocal cords, which keeps the larynx open. This is necessary to take a deep breath. Like all the arytenoid levers, it is innervated by the **recurrent laryngeal branch** of cranial nerve X (the **vagus nerve**).

The **lateral cricoarytenoid** comes to the same attachment from the opposite direction. It begins along the side of the cricoid cartilage and tangents back and up to reach the muscular process of the arytenoid. Therefore, when it contracts, it rotates the arytenoids toward themselves, which slams the vocal cord attached to one arytenoid into the vocal cord attached to the other arytenoid. This is called **adduction** of the vocal cords, and it gives resonance to the voice (otherwise, the voice is hoarse).

The **transverse arytenoid** is the only unpaired intrinsic muscle. It stretches from one muscular process to the other muscular process in a space that is parallel to and just above the fat back of the cricoid cartilage. Rather than rotate the arytenoids, however, it simply pinches them closer together. When the arytenoids are already rotated toward each other, thus closing the larynx, the transverse arytenoid assures that the wide gap in the very back of the larynx is pinched closed.

The **oblique arytenoid** makes an X-shape across the back of the transverse arytenoid. Rather than attaching directly to the arytenoid cartilage at the top of each limb of the X-shape, the oblique arytenoids continue "up-slope," along the margin of the mucous membrane fold of the epiglottis. In this position, the fibers are called the **aryepiglottic muscle**. And in this way, they help to tense the perimeter of the vocal inlet, help the transverse arytenoids to pinch those cartilages together, and help to bend the epiglottis downward over the vocal inlet.

The **thyroarytenoid** is a flat band of muscle that straps the inside of the looming thyroid cartilage to the arytenoid cartilages that hover in the back of the space protected by the same thyroid cartilage. The fibers are virtually parallel to the vocal cords themselves, but they attach to that busy muscular process that sticks out from the arytenoid cartilage. When the fibers contract, they have the dual capacity to pull the arytenoid apparatus forward (which would put **slack** in the vocal cords) and to powerfully swivel the arytenoid cartilages toward themselves (which contributes to the closing of the aperture, or **adduction** of the vocal cords).

The vocal cord itself is a kind of muscle as well. Running from the side of the thyroepiglottic muscle into the vocal fold of mucous membrane and along that line back to the vocal process of the arytenoid cartilage is the **vocalis muscle**. This delicate muscle gently pulls on the vocal cord from the side as a kind of tension gauge.

Obviously, these muscles are more important as a composite than as singular actors on the lever of the vocal cords. As a clinician, you must evaluate their capacity and the tissue vigor of the larynx membranes. Learning these tiny laryngeal muscles individually is a great exercise in the mechanics of position and contraction, but do not lose sight of the forest for the trees as you master the anatomy of speech.

Muscles of the tongue

The tongue is a big weave of "muscle fun" (Fig. 7.53). Some of the muscles are intrinsic to what you feel as the tongue, and others anchor on bones around the oral cavity and insert into a median septum or edge of the intrinsic muscles (and, thus, are called extrinsic muscles). (See Table 7.8.) With one exception, all the muscles of the tongue are innervated by a dedicated cranial nerve (cranial nerve XII, the **hypoglossal nerve**).

The intrinsic muscles consist of a superior and inferior longitudinal, a transverse, and a vertical longitudinal family of fibers that range out from a midline septum of fibrous tissue. They embed the tongue with the ability to "express itself," to contort and roll or flatten regardless of where the tongue is positioned. They are not dissectable from one another in the gross anatomy laboratory and are all innervated by cranial nerve XII.

FIGURE 7.53   **Muscles of the tongue–I.**

The tongue is almost all muscle—and almost all of that is genioglossus. The fan-like muscle has a micro-origin from small tubercles on the mandible and a macroinsertion along the intrinsic longitudinal musculature, just under the skin of the tongue. Contraction of the "lower" fibers of the muscle protrudes the tongue. Paralysis of the muscle on one side causes the protruded tongue to deviate to the same side. (Adapted from Moore KL, Agur AMR. Essential Clinical Anatomy, 2nd Edition. Baltimore: Lippincott Williams & Wilkins, 2002.)

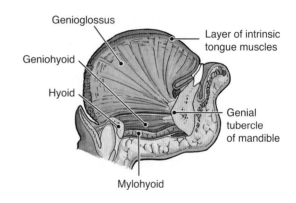

The **genioglossus** forms the bed of the tongue and is the largest of the tongue muscles. It cuts a distinctive profile in a sagittal view of the tongue. Its fibers fan out from a dense attachment on the inside of the mandibular symphysis (the same genial tubercles and fossa that anchor the geniohyoid muscle). They terminate in the substance of the tongue itself. The fan-shape of fiber directions means that the most posterior fibers pull the back of the tongue forward (sticking the tongue out) and that the most anterior fibers depress and tuck in the tip of the tongue. You can bend the tongue to one side or the other by firing the genioglossus muscle on that side only. Symmetric tongue protrusion and deviation are essential clinical tests of the function of cranial nerve XII (the **hypoglossal nerve**).

The **hyoglossus** runs from the hyoid bone to the sides of the back of the tongue, and it helps the other tongue muscles to depress and position the back of the tongue during swallowing (Fig. 7.54). It is innervated by cranial nerve XII (the **hypoglossal nerve**). The **styloglossus** mimics the hyoglossus, but the styloglossus approaches the tongue from above rather than from below. It is anchored to the busy styloid process behind the jaw joint, and it elevates the sides of the tongue, which is a natural movement when swallowing liquid. It is innervated by cranial nerve XII (the **hypoglossal nerve**).

TABLE 7.8   EXTRINSIC MUSCLES OF THE TONGUE

MUSCLE	ORIGIN	INSERTION	INNERVATION	ACTION
Genioglossus	Genial tubercles of mandible	Bed of tongue	Hypoglossal nerve (cranial nerve XII)	Protrudes and depresses the tongue
Hyoglossus	Hyoid bone	Side and bottom of tongue	Hypoglossal nerve (cranial nerve XII)	Depresses and retracts the tongue
Styloglossus	Styloid process and stylohyoid ligament	Side and bottom of tongue	Hypoglossal nerve (cranial nerve XII)	Retracts the tongue, and draws its sides upward into a trough
Palatoglossus	Palatine aspect of soft palate	Side of tongue	Vagus nerve (cranial nerve X)	Elevates back of tongue

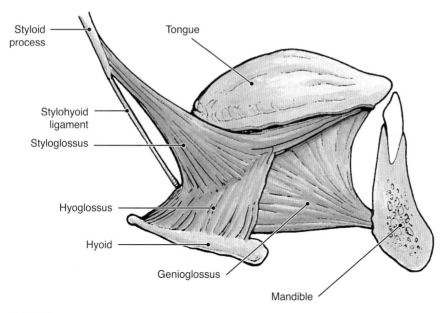

Styloid process

Tongue

Stylohyoid ligament

Styloglossus

Hyoglossus

Hyoid

Genioglossus

Mandible

FIGURE 7.54   **Muscles of the tongue—II.**

The other extrinsic muscles of the tongue reach it from nearby connective tissue moorings. The hyoglossus ascends from the hyoid bone. The styloglossus swoops down from the busy styloid process. The palatoglossus taps into the back of the tongue from underneath the palatoglossal fold of the oral mucosa. (From Moore KL, Agur AMR. Essential Clinical Anatomy, 2nd Edition. Baltimore: Lippincott Williams & Wilkins, 2002. Figure 8.10, p. 563.)

The **palatoglossus** is a thin slip of muscle that arcs down from the back of the soft palate to the back-corner fold of the tongue. You recognize where it is instantly when you ask the patient to say "Ahhh" and you examine the palatoglossal arch of mucous membrane that defines the gateway from the mouth to the pharynx. The palatoglossus muscle is simply the mobile mesodermal tissue deep to the ectodermal arch. When it contracts, it more tightly defines the chute from mouth to pharynx and helps to elevate the back of the tongue. It is the one muscle attached to the tongue that is not innervated by cranial nerve XII (the **hypoglossal nerve**). Instead, it is innervated by cranial nerve X (the **vagus nerve**) as part of the pharyngeal plexus composed of cranial nerve IX (the **glossopharyngeal nerve**) and cranial nerve X (the **vagus nerve**).

Prime mover of the head

The **sternocleidomastoid** is angled from above, behind, and lateral to below, in front, and medial, so it can move the head in many ways, either acting alone or in concert with its partner on the other side. In fact, the sternocleidomastoid is the prime mover of the head. (See Table 7.9.) Acting alone, it swivels the head toward the opposite side of the body; acting together with its partner on the other side, the muscles can powerfully flex the head forward (Fig. 7.55).

The sternocleidomastoid is innervated by cranial nerve XI (the **accessory nerve**) and by contributing fibers from the second and third cervical spinal nerves. It bulges prominently against the skin of the neck when stretched. This makes it easy to find when you physically examine a patient, and it helps you to orient yourself to the display

TABLE 7.9   PRIME MOVER OF THE HEAD

MUSCLE	ORIGIN	INSERTION	INNERVATION	ACTION
Sternocleido-mastoid	Sternum and clavicle	Mastoid process of temporal	Accessory nerve (cranial nerve XI), some fibers from C2-C3	Rotates head to the opposite side; when both contract, they flex the head

of sensory nerves that radiate from approximately the midpoint on its lateral edge. Isolated lesions of cranial nerve XI (the **accessory nerve**) and, thus, paralysis of the sternocleidomastoid are uncommon, but such lesions can result accidentally during a surgical approach to lymph nodes that cluster around the external jugular vein.

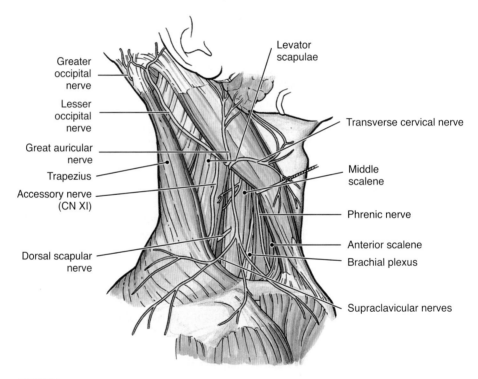

FIGURE 7.55   **Prime movers of the head.**

The trapezius and the sternocleidomastoid derive from the same embryonic tissue, are innervated by the same cranial nerve (cranial nerve XI, the accessory nerve), and arise essentially from the same arc along the base of the skull. They insert broadly along the scapular and clavicular bony arc below the head. The trapezius also is a powerful stabilizer, retractor, elevator, depressor, and rotator of the scapula. CN = cranial nerve. (Adapted from Moore KL, Agur AMR. Essential Clinical Anatomy, 2nd Edition. Baltimore: Lippincott Williams & Wilkins, 2002. Figure 9.4A, p. 603.)

Keep in mind the value of a functional approach to head and neck anatomy. A spatial approach is more academic than clinical, and you can spend valuable time trying to master spatial relationships that you can only "see" in a dissected head. Remember the "clinical head"—the head the patient brings to you—and master the functions of cranial nerves.

Muscles of the Appendicular Skeleton

Regions of the trunk bud outward during embryonic development and become the limbs, which are struts of the body that enable posture and movement, the loss of which is highly distressing to most patients. The muscles of the limbs are most active when you move the body. These muscles reach back to anchor on the trunk both for leverage and to ensure that the trunk moves with the limbs. Learning the **actions** of limb muscles is a straightforward exercise in memorization. Knowing what muscles are **active** during typical movements of the arm and leg, however, is a more clinical, but more ambiguous, objective. Because no limb movement uses just one muscle, clinical evaluation of muscle and nerve damage in the limb can be complicated. In this section, you will learn the basic attributes of the limb muscles.

Muscles of the upper limb

The upper limb is all about the hand, because the hand is what sets humans apart from other animals—and, in many ways, even from other primates. The muscles of the upper limb are designed to secure the arm against the body and to provide both power and precision to finger and thumb movements. We depend so much on our hands that even minor disabling conditions deeply affect our sense of well-being.

The proximal upper limb muscles provide stability and strength to the position of the shoulder and upper arm. They are bulky muscles that pull, lift, and spin, but they are not designed in precision. As you move across the next joint, the elbow joint, you will find simple pull muscles and little or no rotation. Somewhere in the highly mobile upper limb, a joint has to be concerned with the need to move just forward and backward, and the elbow is that joint.

Across the wrist joint, mesoderm differentiates into dedicated, small, and targeted muscles of precision. Power is sacrificed somewhat for the benefits of mobility and flexibility. Even though each finger is capable mostly of just flexing, extending, abducting, and adducting, they cooperate with one another and, especially, with the more mobile thumb to create an infinite number of composite grips and interfaces with the material world. The same instrument that can squeeze juice indiscriminantly from an orange can strike any of 88 piano keys with precision and perfect timing, and the tips of that instrument can pull a human body up a rock face and thread a needle. How can the muscles of the hand be anything less than fascinating?

We begin with the muscles that connect the upper limb to the trunk of the body from which it buds. Some of them simply bridge the scapula to the nearest anchors on the axial skeleton. Others, including the very powerful **latissimus dorsi** and **pectoralis major**, skip over the scapula and attach to the humerus. This distinction is important because it allows you to position your shoulder independently of moving your arm. This muscular strategy enables our movements to be fluid rather than "herky-jerky" or robotic. (See Table 7.10.)

Trapezius

The **trapezius** is a prominent "shoulder shrugging" muscle in the upper part of the back. It attaches in the midline of the body all the way from the bony protuberance on the occipital bone to the spines of the lowest thoracic vertebrae. From that long line of origin, it converges toward the point where the clavicle and scapula come together. This is the **acromion process**, or the "highest" knob atop of the shoulder. The trapezius casts an angle between the neck and shoulder, and muscular people can appear to have no neck at all. This muscle is frequently tense, because many routine activities use it.

TABLE 7.10   SCAPULAR MUSCLES OF THE UPPER LIMB

MUSCLE	ORIGIN	INSERTION	INNERVATION	ACTION
Trapezius	Spines of C7-T12 vertebrae, the nuchal ligament of cervical vertebrae C1-C6, the external occipital protuberance and superior nuchal line of the back of your skull	**Superior** fibers on lateral 1/3 of the clavicle, **middle** fibers on acromion and spine of the scapula, and **inferior** fibers insert on scapular spine	Cranial nerve XI (accessory nerve) and ventral rami of C3-C4	Superior fibers **elevate, rotate,** and **stabilize** scapula; middle fibers **adduct,** or retract, and stabilize scapula; and inferior fibers **depress** and stabilize scapula
Rhomboid major	Spinous processes of T2-T5	Medial border of scapula below rhomboid minor	**Dorsal scapular nerve (C5)**	Elevates, retracts, and fixes scapula
Rhomboid minor	Nuchal ligament and spinous processes of C7 and T1	Medial border of the scapula below scapular spine	**Dorsal scapular nerve (C5)**	Elevates, retracts, and fixes scapula
Levator scapulae	Transverse processes of C1-C4	Superior angle of the vertebral border of the scapula	**Dorsal scapular nerve (C5)** and ventral rami of C3-C4	Elevates, **downwardly rotates,** and **fixes** the scapula
Serratus anterior	Ribs 1 through 8 or 9, lateral to pectoralis minor	Medial border of the ventral surface of scapula	**Long thoracic nerve** (ventral rami of C5-C7)	Protracts and abducts scapula, holds scapula along posterior thoracic wall, rotates scapula, and elevates arm from horizontal to vertical
Pectoralis major	Clavicle and sternum	Intertubercular groove of proximal humerus	**Medial** and **lateral pectoral nerves** (C5-T1)	Adducts and medially rotates humerus, draws shoulder anteriorly and medially
Pectoralis minor	Outer surfaces of ribs 2-5	Coracoid process of scapula	**Medial pectoral nerve** (ventral rami of C8 and T1) and, sometimes, lateral pectoral nerve (C5-C7)	Stabilizes scapula by drawing it forward, medially, and downward; if scapula is fixed, it elevates the ribs.
Latissimus dorsi	Spinous processes of T7-T12, the thoracolumbar fascia, iliac crest, ribs 9-12, and the inferior angle of the scapula	Intertubercular groove of proximal humerus	**Thoracodorsal nerve** (middle subscapular nerve of brachial plexus, C6-C8)	Extends, adducts, and **medially rotates** the humerus
Deltoid	**Anterior** fibers on the lateral part of the clavicle, **middle** fibers on the acromion process, and **posterior** fibers on the scapular spine	Deltoid tuberosity of the humeral shaft	**Axillary nerve** (C5-C6)	**Anterior** fibers **flex** and **medially rotate** the humerus, **middle** fibers **abduct** of the humerus, and **posterior** fibers **extend** and **laterally rotate** the humerus

(continued)

TABLE 7.10   SCAPULAR MUSCLES OF THE UPPER LIMB (continued)

MUSCLE	ORIGIN	INSERTION	INNERVATION	ACTION
Teres major	Lateral side of scapula, near the bottom	Lesser tubercle of the humerus	Lower subscapular nerve (C5-C6)	Adduct, extend, and medially rotate the humerus
Teres minor	Lateral border of the scapula	Shoulder joint capsule and greater tubercle of the humerus	Axillary nerve (C5-C6)	Laterally rotates, adducts, and stabilizes the humerus
Supraspinatus	Above the spine of the scapula	Capsule of the shoulder joint and on the greater tubercle of the humerus	Suprascapular nerve (C4-C6)	Initiate the abduction of the humerus
Infraspinatus	Below the scapular spine	Greater tubercle of the humerus	Suprascapular nerve (C4-C6)	Laterally rotates and stabilizes the humerus
Subscapularis	Ventral surface of the scapula	Shoulder joint capsule and lesser tubercle of humerus	Upper and lower subscapular nerves (C5-C7)	Medially rotates and stabilizes the humerus

The trapezius steers the scapula. It can raise it, lower it, and pull it inward—all the while enabling the arm to deal with other forces. Paralysis results in drooping of the shoulder and inability to raise the arm above the head.

Five other muscles anchor the scapula to the body, mostly under cover of more prominent superficial muscles. Three of them span the vertebral border of the scapula and tie it to different parts of the backbone. One runs a strange course from the vertebral border around the ribs and onto the front part of the rib cage. The final one ties a projecting knob of the scapula (the **coracoid process**) to the front of the ribs under cover of pectoralis major.

Three muscles make up a kind of "battery" of scapula retractors (Fig. 7.56). These three muscles are:

- Rhomboid major
- Rhomboid minor (lies superior to rhomboid major)
- Levator scapulae

These muscles primarily tug the shoulder blade back toward the vertebral column, but the direction of their fibers also allows some raising of the scapula. The levator muscle is angled so much that when it contracts, it "tips" the angle of the scapula toward the arm, which, for example, rotates the right scapula clockwise (as seen from behind) if other forces also are trying to depress the shoulder joint.

Serratus Anterior   The scapula "lays" against the rib cage and can slide back and forth as well as up and down as different muscles pull on it. The **serratus anterior** is a large muscle that owns most of the action along the "armpit" border of the scapula (Fig. 7.57). Like the arc of a fishing line about to be cast, the muscle ranges from the far inside border of the scapula in the back, around to the front surface of the rib cage. When its fibers shorten, it does the complete opposite of retraction—it pulls the

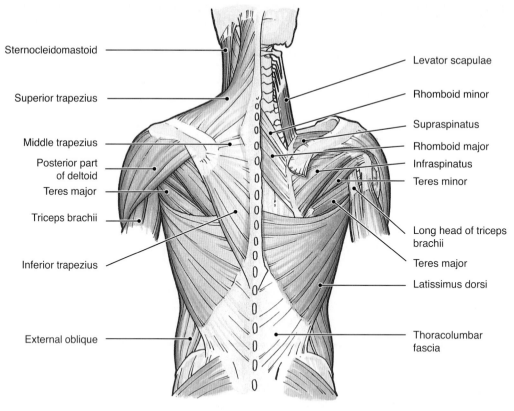

Sternocleidomastoid

Superior trapezius

Middle trapezius

Posterior part
of deltoid

Teres major

Triceps brachii

Inferior trapezius

External oblique

Levator scapulae

Rhomboid minor

Supraspinatus

Rhomboid major

Infraspinatus

Teres minor

Long head of triceps
brachii

Teres major

Latissimus dorsi

Thoracolumbar
fascia

FIGURE 7.56   **Upper extremity muscles anchored to the vertebral column.**

(From Moore KL, Agur AMR. Essential Clinical Anatomy, 2nd Edition. Baltimore: Lippincott Williams & Wilkins, 2002. Figure 7.11, p. 426.)

vertebral border of the scapula around toward the breast. Of course, the muscle never acts alone. It mostly exists to resist the powerful capacity of the trapezius and the rhomboids to pull the scapula backwards.

The serratus anterior would drift into anatomic obscurity were it not for the fact that its nerve supply runs along the outer surface of the muscle instead of the deep, or inner, surface. The **long thoracic nerve** reaches down from its origin in the armpit to lay across the surface of the muscle in the "ticklish" portion of the ribs, just below the armpit. Because surgery in this area sometimes is necessary to address tumors and breast cancers, the nerve can be cut accidentally. Damage to the long thoracic nerve will paralyze the serratus anterior, which makes it unable to resist the muscle tone in the trapezius and the rhomboids. This condition is known as a **winged scapula**, in which the vertebral border of the scapula is lifted off of the rib cage and appears to protrude against the skin (Fig. 7.58).

Pectoralis Minor   The **pectoralis minor** (see Fig. 7.57) lies deep to pectoralis major, and it does not connect to the humerus. It anchors the scapula to the front of the rib cage, which means that when you fix the scapula, this muscle can move the rib cage. People who are exhausted from physical exertion tend to rest their upper body weight by putting their hand on their knees. This fixes the scapula and enables the pectoralis minor to be an accessory muscle of respiration.

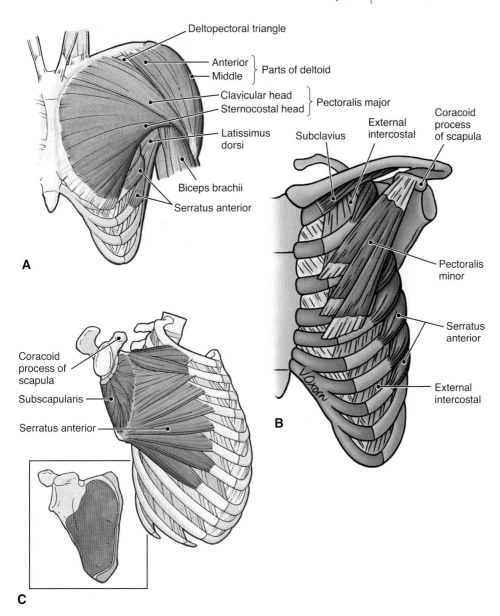

FIGURE 7.57   **Upper extremity muscles anchored to the chest wall.**

(**A**) Pectoralis major. (**B**) Pectoralis minor, smaller and deeper. (**C**) Serratus anterior, blue attachment, and subscapularis, red attachment. (From Moore KL, Agur AMR. Essential Clinical Anatomy, 2nd Edition. Baltimore: Lippincott Williams & Wilkins, 2002. Figure 7.10, p. 423.)

An insignificant muscle (the **subclavius**) binds the clavicle to the first rib in between its joint with the scapula and its joint with the sternum. The innervation of subclavius appears to be from the ventral rami of C5 and C6, and its apparent action is to stabilize the clavicle against unusual movements at either of its ends.

Two of the strongest muscles in the body originate on the trunk and bypass the scapula to insert directly on the humerus. They "override" the short muscles that connect the scapula to the humerus, and they do not depend on the position of the scapula

FIGURE 7.58   **Winging of the scapula.**

Because the long thoracic nerve approaches serratus anterior superficially, the nerve is at risk in relatively minor chest wall lacerations. With the serratus anterior paralyzed, there is no resistance to the powerful scapular retractors. (From Bickley LS and Szilagyi P. Bates' Guide to Physical Examination and History Taking, 8th Edition. Philadelphia: Lippincott Williams & Wilkins, 2003.)

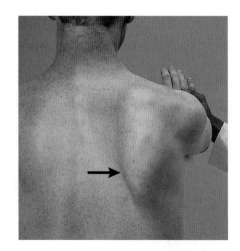

to do their job. These muscles are the complementary **latissimus dorsi** in the back and **pectoralis major** in the front. They powerfully return the arm toward the body from an outstretched and resisted position. They are associated so much with the concept of "upper body strength," in fact, that they are landmark "profile" muscles for bodybuilders.

Latissimus Dorsi   When the arm hangs down at rest, the **latissimus dorsi** (see Fig. 7.56) is not very powerful. With the arm raised upward and outward, however, and especially with palms up, the latissimus dorsi powerfully restores the arm to a resting position. Because of its broad origin and narrow insertion, arching across the back of the armpit, this muscle forms part of the fold of skin and muscle felt there (the **posterior axillary fold**).

Pectoralis Major   The **pectoralis major** (see Fig. 7.57) acts like the latissimus dorsi, but relative to the front half of the body. Both muscles insert in a groove on the anterior side of the top of the humerus, so an incredible amount of muscle force acts on a small portion of the front of the arm bone. The muscles powerfully swing the arm around, and the pectoralis major in particular is an active muscle of pushing and throwing.

Now it is time to consider the muscles that connect the scapula to the humerus. When the scapula is "fixed" in a stable position by the muscles discussed above, the scapulohumeral muscles enable twisting and tweaking of the upper arm in its socket. They also powerfully flex or extend the elbow joint. Think of throwing a baseball, hitting a tennis ball, wrestling with the dog, or tinkering with the car engine. These familiar activities need the scapulohumeral muscles and, frequently, lead to the strain or tearing of them. You may recognize the muscle names or groups already: the **rotator cuff**, **biceps**, and **triceps**.

The Rotator Cuff   Four muscles cooperate to twist the humerus in a semispherical range against the scapula. In one sense, they are the functional ligaments of the shoulder joint—even if they are as elastic as all muscle tissue. The **rotator cuff muscles** are unusual in that they insert directly into a joint capsule. This confirms their collective function as elastic ligaments of this extremely mobile synovial joint. You can remember them as the "S-I-T-S" muscles, according to the first letters of their names (**supraspinatus, infraspinatus, teres minor,** and **subscapularis**) (Fig. 7.59).

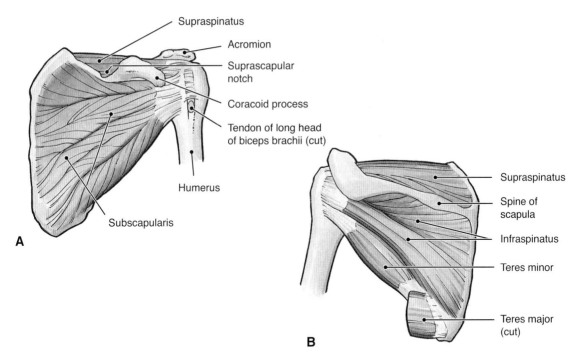

FIGURE 7.59   **Rotator cuff muscles. A, anterior; B, posterior.**

The supraspinatus (**A** and **B**), infraspinatus (**B**), teres minor (**B**), subscapularis (**A**) canvas the perimeter of the glenohumeral joint capsule. (From Moore KL, Agur AMR. Essential Clinical Anatomy, 2nd Edition. Baltimore: Lippincott Williams & Wilkins, 2002. Figure 7.12, p. 425.)

Supraspinatus   The **supraspinatus** "unlocks" the arm from resting at the side. When it pulls, it lifts the arm out the first 15° to 30° degrees of motion, which is just enough angle in the shoulder joint for the deltoid to be effective when it contracts. Paralysis of this muscle is noticeable, because patients must lean their bodies to the affected side to allow their arm to drop far enough away for the deltoid to take over. Selective paralysis is possible because the nerve to supraspinatus, the **suprascapular nerve** (C4-**C5**-C6), leaves the brachial plexus early and runs vulnerably across the root of the neck.

Infraspinatus and Teres Minor   The **teres minor** is more closely related to the **infraspinatus** than it is to teres major, which is why the teres minor is part of the rotator cuff but teres major is not. The supraspinatus, infraspinatus, and teres minor take origin from almost the entire posterior surface of the scapula and form the back side of the rotator cuff of the head of the humerus. The infraspinatus and teres minor laterally rotate the arm. The infraspinatus shares the **suprascapular nerve** with the supraspinatus, whereas the teres minor is motored by the **axillary nerve**.

Subscapularis   The **subscapularis** is hidden between the scapula bone and the rib cage against which it glides. It attaches to the whole front face of the scapula and then converges through the armpit to become the rotator cuff muscle on the front side of the joint. In this position, it medially rotates the arm in the shoulder joint. It is served by the **upper subscapular nerve** and **lower subscapular nerve** (C5-C6-C7).

Flexing and extending the arm and forearm are important and powerful movements. Some of the muscles discussed above can flex or extend the arm, but forearm movement is another matter. Three powerful muscles dedicated to this and one helper muscle (the **coracobrachialis**) complete the scapulohumeral group. (See Table 7.11.)

Deltoid   The **deltoid** (Fig. 7.60) grabs onto the "roof" of bone on top of the shoulder joint. This roof is made up of the scapular spine in back and the clavicle in front. The muscle awning then converges to a point insertion on the shaft of the humerus below the insertions of **pectoralis major** and **latissimus dorsi**. Because the deltoid starts above the humerus and both in front of and behind it, it raises the humerus in all directions. Because the deltoid fibers "drop off" their awning so steeply, however, they are not very good at initiating abduction (raising the arm forward, backward, or to the side); a separate muscle (the supraspinatus; see above) starts that process. The deltoid is innervated by the **axillary nerve (C5-6)**, principally by its C5 component.

Teres Major   The **teres major** (Fig. 7.61) is a compact muscle that mirrors the latissimus dorsi muscle and helps it to form the posterior fold of the underarm. It acts like latissimus dorsi, except its anchor is the scapula (a mobile bone) instead of the vertebral column. The teres major is innervated by the **lower subscapular nerve**, a C5-C6 branch off of the posterior cord of the brachial plexus.

Biceps Brachii   The **biceps brachii** (see Fig. 7.60) may be the most familiar muscle in the body. As the name implies, it draws from two heads of origin: a long head, and a short head. The long head originates from a bump at the top of the shoulder joint capsule (the **glenoid tubercle**). It runs through the shoulder joint, and it emerges through the bottom by traveling in the groove between the two tubercles of the humerus. The short head originates from the coracoid process of the scapula. The powerful attachment to the radius means that when biceps brachii contracts, it helps to supinate the forearm. Another way to think of this is that the most powerful action of this muscle is when the hand is "palm up." To flex the forearm with the "palm down" requires a muscle that attaches to the ulna, not to the radius. That muscle is the **brachialis**. The entire family of biceps brachii, coracobrachialis, and brachialis is served by the **musculocutaneous nerve** (C5-C7).

TABLE 7.11   MAJOR FLEXORS AND EXTENSORS OF THE FOREARM

MUSCLE	ORIGIN	INSERTION	INNERVATION	ACTION
Coracobrachialis	Coracoid process of scapula	Front shaft of humerus	Musculocutaneous nerve (C5-C6)	Flexes the arm
Brachialis	Shaft of humerus	Ulna	Musculocutaneous nerve (C5-C6)	Flexes the forearm
Biceps brachii	Long head from glenoid tubercle; short head from coracoid process of scapula	Radius	Musculocutaneous nerve (C5-C6)	Flexes and supinates the forearm, assists flexion of the arm
Triceps brachii	Infraglenoid tubercle of scapula and the posterior shaft of the humerus	Olecranon process of the ulna	Radial nerve (C6-C8)	Powerfully extends the forearm

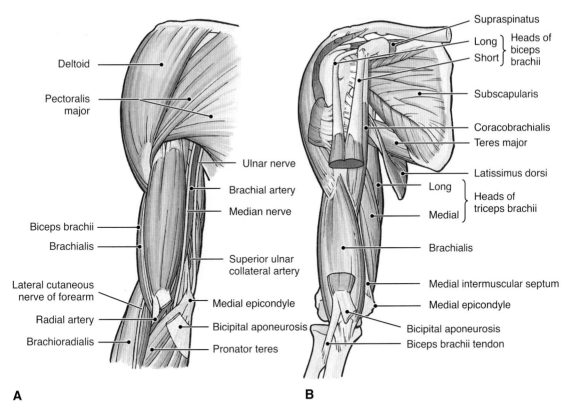

FIGURE 7.60   **Muscles that abduct and flex the arm and forearm.**

(**A**) Anterior view, superficial layer, featuring the deltoid and biceps brachii. (**B**) Anterior view, deep layer, featuring the coracobrachialis and brachialis. (From Moore KL, Agur AMR. Essential Clinical Anatomy, 2nd Edition. Baltimore: Lippincott Williams & Wilkins, 2002. Figure 7.17, p. 444.)

Coracobrachialis and Brachialis   To the extent that the biceps muscle crosses two joints (the shoulder and the elbow), it can be described as a flexor of both the arm and the forearm. Deep to biceps are two muscles that mimic the biceps but cross only one of the two joints each. The **coracobrachialis** is the arm flexor deep to biceps (see Fig. 7.60), and the **brachialis** is the forearm flexor deep to biceps. The brachialis is dedicated to the elbow joint, and it can flex the elbow regardless of the position of the forearm and hand. Thus, it accompanies biceps, and it takes over for the biceps when the arm is pronated.

Triceps Brachii   The **triceps brachii** (see Fig. 7.61) is the dominant muscle in the extensor compartment of the arm. A very small muscle, the **anconeus**, is devoted to the back of the elbow joint, but otherwise, the triceps is the whole show. As with all other muscles of extension in the arm and forearm, the triceps is served by the **radial nerve** (C5-T1), which is the large-caliber outcome of the posterior cord of the brachial plexus.

The muscles that we have discussed so far control movement at the shoulder and elbow joints. The wrist joint is next, and it is crossed by numerous muscles invested in control of the wrist and movement of the fingers. The simplest way to think about these

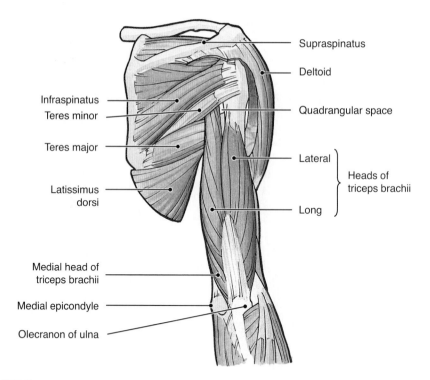

Supraspinatus

Deltoid

Infraspinatus

Teres minor

Quadrangular space

Teres major

Lateral ⎱
          ⎰ Heads of
            triceps brachii

Latissimus
dorsi

Long

Medial head of
triceps brachii

Medial epicondyle

Olecranon of ulna

FIGURE 7.61   **Muscles that extend and rotate the arm and forearm.**

Note that the latissimus dorsi and teres major insert anteriorly on the humerus, deeply out of view in this illustration. The triceps brachii extends the arm further against the shoulder with a limited range of motion and strength but powerfully and exclusively extends the forearm at the elbow. (From Moore KL, Agur AMR. Essential Clinical Anatomy, 2nd Edition Baltimore: Lippincott Williams & Wilkins, 2002. Figure 7.18A, p. 445.)

muscles is to divide them into a group that flexes and a group that extends. Some of them will impact the elbow joint because of their origin, and some of them will drive the finger joints because of their insertion. Innervation patterns track the brachial plexus, in the sense that all muscles of extension are served by the **radial nerve** outcome of the posterior cord, whereas all flexion muscles are served by the **median nerve** and **ulnar nerve** outcomes of the lateral cord and the medial cord, respectively.

Flexion Compartment
The flexion compartment muscles fan out from a more or less common anchor point along the medial epicondyle of the humerus to reach all of the possible links in the joint system of the arm. (See Table 7.12.) Of course, each muscle has a primary action, but you should appreciate that by virtue of their design, the muscles can act as synergists or stabilizers in support of each other.

Palmaris Longus   Not everybody has a **palmaris longus muscle** (Fig. 7.62). It rests just under the skin, and it inserts into the "webbing," or **palmar aponeurosis**, of the hand. The tendon pushes up against the skin when you pinch the thumb and little finger together and flex at the wrist. The name "palmaris longus" implies the presence of a **palmaris brevis muscle**. This slip of muscle tissue will be found at the base of the palm in the padding along the pinky-finger side. It is a subcutaneous muscle that is innervated by the ulnar nerve; when it shortens, it tightens the skin of the palm, just like its long partner.

TABLE 7.12   MAJOR FLEXORS OF THE WRIST AND FINGERS

MUSCLE	ORIGIN	INSERTION	INNERVATION	ACTION
Palmaris longus	Common flexor tendon on the medial epicondyle of the humerus	Palmar fascia	Median nerve (C7–C8)	Tightens the skin of the palm
Flexor carpi ulnaris	Common flexor tendon	Carpal bones and base of fifth metacarpal	Ulnar nerve (C7–C8)	Flexes wrist
Flexor carpi radialis	Common flexor tendon	First and second metacarpal	Median nerve (C6–C7)	Flexes wrist
Flexor digitorum superficialis	Common flexor tendon	Middle phalanx of each finger	Median nerve (C7–T1)	Flexes proximal and middle phalanges
Flexor digitorum profundus	Shaft of ulna and interosseous membrane	Distal phalanx of each finger	Fibers to first and second digits by median nerve (C8–T1), fibers to third and fourth digits by ulnar nerve (C8–T1)	Flexes distal phalanges (fingertips)
Flexor pollicis longus	Radius and interosseous membrane	Distal phalanx of thumb	Median nerve (C8–T1)	Flexes distal phalanx of thumb
Pronator teres	Common flexor tendon	Shaft of radius	Median nerve (C6–C7)	Pronates radius
Pronator quadratus	Lower shaft of ulna	Lower shaft of radius	Median nerve (C7–C8)	Pronates radius

Flexor Carpi Ulnaris and Flexor Carpi Radialis   The **flexor carpi ulnaris** and **flexor carpi radialis** are muscles dedicated to position control and flexion of the wrist. The flexor carpi ulnaris is served by the ulnar nerve, whereas the flexor carpi radialis is served by the median nerve. The tendon of flexor carpi radialis lies immediately medial to the position of the radial artery, so it can be used as a guide for obtaining a radial pulse at the wrist.

Flexor Digitorum Superficialis and Flexor Digitorum Profundus   The **flexor digitorum superficialis** and **flexor digitorum profundus** are muscles that work together to flex all the finger joints. The superficialis tendons do not reach across the distal interphalangeal joint. The neurovascular bundles destined for the hand travel in the "plane" between the superficialis and profundus muscle bellies. The **median nerve** provides motor supply to almost all the tendons. The medial two tendons of the flexor digitorum profundus are motored by the **ulnar nerve**. This difference can accentuate the appearance of a lower brachial plexus injury, in which the ulnar nerve is disabled. In such cases, the patient will be unable to curl the fourth and fifth finger joints with the same amount of power.

Flexor Pollicis Longus   The thumb is so important in daily life that it receives its own dedicated muscle groups, both long and short. The flexor pollicis brevis is described below with the other hand muscles. The **flexor pollicis longus** is the only flexor muscle that reaches all the way to the tip of the thumb. Its deeply embedded origin draws on both bones of the forearm and on the interosseous membrane between them. It is powered by the **median nerve**.

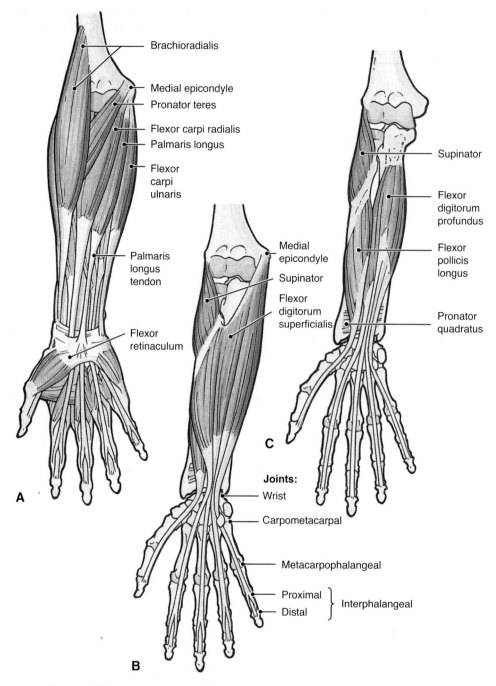

FIGURE 7.62   **Wrist and finger flexors and pronators.**

(**A**) Anterior view of the forearm showing the most superficial muscles. Note that the brachioradialis, which is visible here, derives from the extension side of the forearm, where it functions and is innervated accordingly. (**B**) Deep to the wrist flexors and pronator teres is the flexor digitorum superficialis, the tendons of which insert on the middle phalanges. (**C**) The deepest layer of flexors includes a dedicated flexor of the thumb, the flexor pollicis longus, and the flexor digitorum profundus, the tendons of which insert on the distal phalanges. (From Moore KL, Agur AMR. Essential Clinical Anatomy, 2nd Edition. Baltimore: Lippincott Williams & Wilkins, 2002. Figure 7.21, p. 452.)

Pronator Teres and Pronator Quadratus   Together, the **pronator teres** and **pronator quadratus** roll the forearm inward with control and some power. For most people, the opposite movement (**supination**) is the more powerful movement. When standing at rest, the arms are more likely to be in a slightly pronated position than in the standard anatomic position (palms forward, supinated), so in some respects, the pronator muscles can be seen as "restorative" muscles for use when the arms are in a supinated position. They are powered by the median nerve.

Extension Compartment

The muscles of the extension compartment (Fig. 7.63) fan out from the lateral side of the humerus and forearm to reach all the possible links in the joint system of the wrist and hand. (See Table 7.13.) All these muscles are innervated by the radial nerve, which is the large nerve derived from the posterior cords of the brachial plexus. In general, they lack the power of the flexor group, and no muscle bellies are found beyond the wrist onto the back of the hand. Of course, each muscle has a primary action, but by virtue of their design, the muscles can act as synergists or stabilizers in support of each other.

Supinator   The pronator muscles and the **supinator** antagonize one another, and they work together when the arm needs to be locked in an intermediate position. The muscles originate on opposite parts of the elbow complex and insert on virtually the same "lever point" of the convex shaft of the radius. They combine to "steer" the forearm and position the hand for precise actions. Powerful supination recruits the biceps brachii muscle and is performed with the elbow slightly flexed.

Brachioradialis   The **brachioradialis** is a prominent muscle in the superficial bulk of the extensor muscle group, and it is innervated by the nerve of the extensor compartment (the **radial nerve**). Because at rest the arm is comfortably in a mostly pronated position, this muscle transitionally governs the wrist position between frank flexion and frank extension (see Fig. 7.62). It stabilizes the hand in activities that require a "ski-pole holding," or a "bringing a cup to your mouth," vector.

Extensor Carpi Radialis Brevis and Extensor Carpi Radialis Longus   For all practical purposes, the **extensor carpi radialis brevis** and **extensor carpi radialis longus muscles** are a single muscle unit with two tendons. Together with the **extensor carpi ulnaris,** they complement the flexor group for providing stability of the wrist, particularly when the hand is clenched into a tight grip or fist. As with other compartment muscles that act at the wrist, much of the obligation is in stabilizing a joint (in this case, numerous joints) that is designed for flexible movement. This enables power and precision movements below the wrist regardless of the actual wrist posture.

Extensor Digitorum   In the extension compartment, only the **extensor digitorum** serves all the phalangeal joints, but its insertion splits across the middle and distal interphalangeal joints in a manner similar to that of the two digital flexor muscles. The **extensor hood** that results from the broad passage of the finger tendons provides attachment for the specialized lumbrical muscles (see below).

Extensor Indicis, Digiti Minimi, and Extensor Pollicis Longus   You enjoy more power and precision when you extend the thumb, index finger and little finger compared to the other digits, perhaps because of dedicated muscles such as the **extensor indicis** for the index finger and the **extensor pollicis longus** for the thumb. The

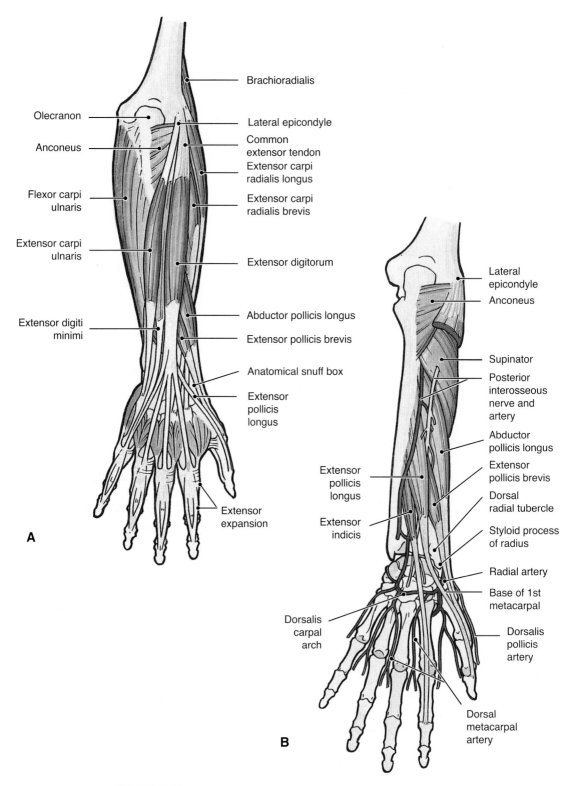

FIGURE 7.63 **Wrist and finger extensors and abductors.**

(**A**) Posterior view, featuring wrist extensors originating from the common extensor tendon on the lateral humeral epicondyle. The brachioradialis is barely visible in this view (see Fig. 7.62). (**B**) Deep view of the extensor compartment, featuring the powerful supinator and three muscle bellies dedicated to the thumb. (From Moore KL, Agur AMR. Essential Clinical Anatomy, 2nd Edition. Baltimore: Lippincott Williams & Wilkins, 2002. Figure 7.22A,C, p. 455.)

TABLE 7.13   MAJOR EXTENSORS OF THE WRIST AND FINGERS

MUSCLE	ORIGIN	INSERTION	INNERVATION	ACTION
Anconeus	Lateral epicondyle of humerus	Posterior shaft of ulna	Radial nerve (C5-C7)	Unlocks a tightly flexed elbow joint
Supinator	Lateral epicondyle of humerus and posterior ulna	Shaft of radius	Radial nerve (C5-C6)	Supinates the radius
Brachioradialis	Shaft of humerus	Radius, just superior to styloid process	Radial nerve (C5-C7)	Holds forearm between pronation and supination ("ski-pole holding" position), assists in elbow flexion
Extensor carpi radialis brevis	Common extensor tendon on lateral epicondyle of humerus	Base of third metacarpal	Radial nerve (C7-C8)	Extends wrist
Extensor carpi radialis longus	Common extensor tendon	Base of second metacarpal	Radial nerve (C6-C7)	Extends wrist
Extensor carpi ulnaris	Common extensor tendon	Base of fifth metacarpal	Radial nerve (C7-C8)	Extends wrist
Extensor digitorum	Common extensor tendon	Middle and distal phalanx of each finger	Radial nerve (C7-C8)	Extends all finger joints
Extensor indicis	Distal shaft of ulna	Extensor expansion of second digit	Radial nerve (C7-C8)	Extends index (first) finger
Extensor digiti minimi	Common extensor tendon	Extensor expansion of fifth digit	Radial nerve (C7-C8)	Extends fifth finger
Extensor pollicis longus	Ulna and interosseous membrane	Distal phalanx of thumb	Radial nerve (C7-C8)	Extends all joints of the thumb
Extensor pollicis brevis	Radius and interosseous membrane	Proximal phalanx of thumb	Radial nerve (C7-C8)	Extends proximal joint of thumb
Abductor pollicis longus	Ulna, radius, and interosseous membrane	Base of first metacarpal	Radial nerve (C7-C8)	Abducts thumb

extensor pollicis longus forms a prominent tendon in the wrist when the thumb is abducted and extended. It acts in close concert with the brevis muscle and with the nearby abductor pollicis longus muscle. Remember that the base of the thumb can swivel more freely than the other fingers can, making the distinctions between flexion, extension, abduction, and adduction more of a spherical blur.

Extensor Pollicis Brevis and Abductor Pollicis Longus   The tendons of the **extensor pollicis brevis** and **abductor pollicis longus** form the other border of the "anatomic snuffbox" at the base of the thumb (see Fig. 7.63B). Their origins are halfway up the forearm, and they travel obliquely to the rest of the extensor group. This is why you can clearly see their tendon lines under the skin when you fully stretch them by pronating and adducting your wrist. These muscles provide gross power movements to the base of the thumb, "staging" it for more precise movements at the interphalangeal joint.

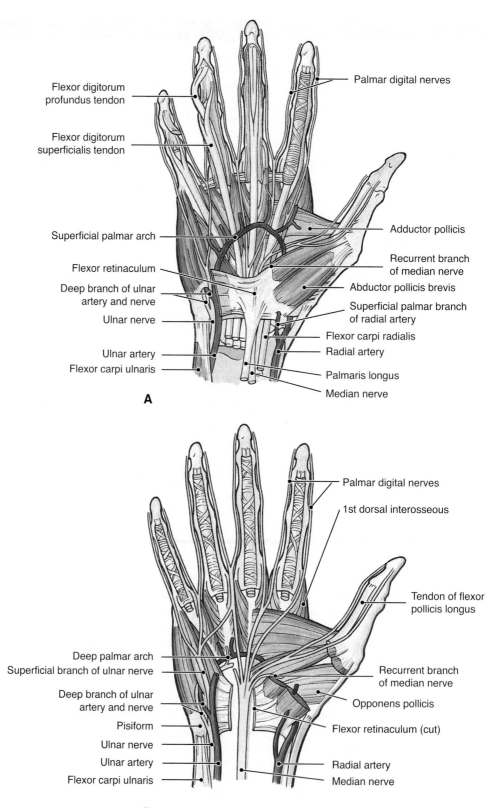

Flexor digitorum profundus tendon

Flexor digitorum superficialis tendon

Palmar digital nerves

Superficial palmar arch

Flexor retinaculum

Deep branch of ulnar artery and nerve

Ulnar nerve

Ulnar artery

Flexor carpi ulnaris

Adductor pollicis

Recurrent branch of median nerve

Abductor pollicis brevis

Superficial palmar branch of radial artery

Flexor carpi radialis

Radial artery

Palmaris longus

Median nerve

A

Palmar digital nerves

1st dorsal interosseous

Tendon of flexor pollicis longus

Deep palmar arch
Superficial branch of ulnar nerve

Deep branch of ulnar artery and nerve

Pisiform

Ulnar nerve

Ulnar artery

Flexor carpi ulnaris

Recurrent branch of median nerve

Opponens pollicis

Flexor retinaculum (cut)

Radial artery

Median nerve

B

Muscles of the hand

The culmination of a grasping hand is the muscular palm, which is outfitted with two big pads of muscles for the thumb and the little finger (Fig. 7.64). These are the **thenar eminence** and the **hypothenar eminence**, respectively. The hypothenar eminence more or less provides symmetry to the palm, but its muscles are not nearly as powerful or precise as the muscles of the thenar eminence. The thenar eminence is the star of the show, with three muscles that govern the dexterity of the thumb. All the muscles in the hand are in the palmar half. On the "back," or dorsum, of the hand are several tendons and loose-fitting skin but no dedicated muscles. (See Table 7.14.)

Ray Muscles

The middle finger acts as a kind of axis for the hand—two fingers on one side, and a finger and a thumb on the other side. Each finger can move from side to side, which is called **abduction** if the finger moves away from the axis and **adduction** if the finger moves toward the axis. Because the middle finger rests on the axis, any movement to the side it makes is abduction. The muscles that abduct and adduct the finger bones are called the **interossei muscles**, and these muscles are divided into a dorsal group and a palmar group:

- **Dorsal Interossei:** The **dorsal interossei** abduct the digits around the axis of the third digit. Thus, the middle finger receives two of the four dorsal interossei muscles because it abducts itself on both sides. The pinky and thumb do not receive this muscle because they have dedicated abductor muscles in the thenar and hypothenar eminences.
- **Palmar Interossei:** The **palmer interossei** adduct the digits around the axis of the third digit. Thus, the middle finger has no palmar interossei because it rests in the central axis. The human body has few examples of asymmetry, but this is one of them. Tissue is conserved, but capacity is retained.

Some joints in the body can flex very tightly, creating angles across the joints of much less than 90°. In a tightly closed fist, for example, the fingers curl into two sharp turns. Tendons that run over the tops of the fingers cannot easily extend one of the finger joints without extending all of them. Part of the problem is that the tendon must overcome not just one but three acute angles. Enter the lumbricals, which are muscles designed to help the fingers unbend gracefully and fluidly.

Lumbricals

The **lumbricals** (Fig. 7.65) move the finger joints when the hand is in a tight fist. These muscles arise from the tendons of flexor digitorum profundus and share the same unusual innervation pattern: The ulnar nerve serves the medial two, and median nerve serves the lateral two. They insert onto the extensor hood, effectively helping the hood to extend the fingers when the rest of the extensor digitorum tendon is fixed. Likewise, they assist their tendon of origin, the flexor digitorum profundus, to flex the metacarpophalangeal joint when the larger tendon is compromised.

FIGURE 7.64   **Intrinsic muscles of the hand.**

(A) Both the base of the thumb and the base of the fifth finger contain a short flexor, abductor, and "opposer" muscle. **(B)** The thumb is further empowered with a large adductor muscle, which is the only thumb muscle innervated by the ulnar nerve. (From Moore KL, Agur AMR. Essential Clinical Anatomy, 2nd Edition. Baltimore: Lippincott Williams & Wilkins, 2002. Figure 7.28, p. 474.)

TABLE 7.14   MUSCLES OF THE HAND

MUSCLE	ORIGIN	INSERTION	INNERVATION	ACTION
Dorsal interossei	Metacarpals of each digit	Radial side of first and second digit proximal phalanx; ulnar side of second and third proximal phalanx	Ulnar nerve (C8-T1)	Abducts second, third and fourth digits
Palmar interossei	Metacarpals of second, fourth, and fifth digits	Radial side of fourth and fifth digit proximal phalanx; ulnar side of second digit proximal phalanx	Ulnar nerve (C8-T1)	Adducts second, fourth, and fifth digits
Lumbricals	Tendons of flexor digitorum profundus	Extensor complex and tendon of the corresponding finger	Median nerve (C8-T1) for lumbricals 1–2, ulnar nerve (C8-T1) for lumbricals 3–4	Flexes metacarpophalangeal joints, extends the interphalangeal joints
Abductor digiti minimi	Pisiform bone and adjacent ligaments	Proximal phalanx of fifth digit	Ulnar nerve (C8-T1)	Abducts the fifth digit
Flexor digiti minimi	Hamate bone and flexor retinaculum	Proximal phalanx of fifth digit	Ulnar nerve (C8-T1)	Flexes the fifth digit
Opponens digiti minimi	Hamate bone and flexor retinaculum	Fifth digit metacarpal	Ulnar nerve (C8-T1)	Draws base of fifth digit toward the palm, enabling phalanges to oppose the thumb
Abductor pollicis brevis	Scaphoid, trapezium, and flexor retinaculum	Proximal phalanx of thumb	Median nerve (C8-T1)	Abducts thumb
Flexor pollicis brevis	Various carpal bones and flexor retinaculum	Proximal phalanx of thumb	Median nerve (C8-T1)	Assists flexor pollicis longus in flexing the thumb
Opponens pollicis	Trapezium and flexor retinaculum	Metacarpal of the thumb	Median nerve (C8-T1)	Turns base of thumb inward toward palm, enabling phalanges to oppose the fifth digit
Adductor pollicis	Oblique head from trapezoid, capitate, and second, third, and fourth metacarpals; transverse head from shaft of third metacarpal	Proximal phalanx of thumb	Ulnar nerve (C8-T1)	Adducts thumb across surface of the palm

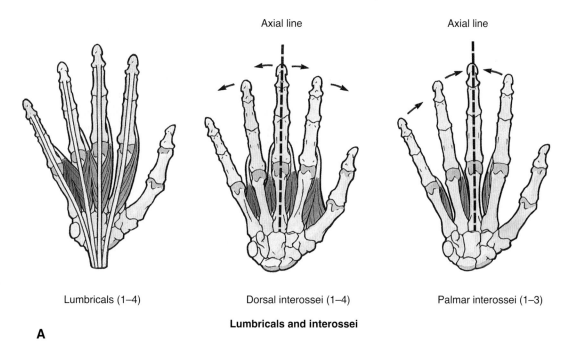

Lumbricals (1–4)   Dorsal interossei (1–4)   Palmar interossei (1–3)

Lumbricals and interossei

A

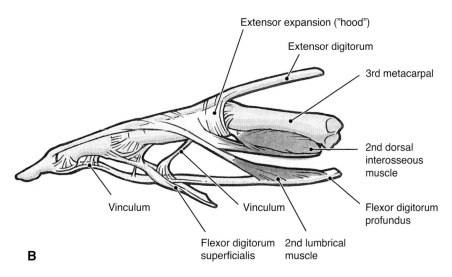

B

FIGURE 7.65   **Finger movers.**

(**A**) Palmar and dorsal interossei. The third, or middle, digit is the axis against which the other fingers abduct and adduct. (**B**) The unique need of the digit to be able to extend one joint while flexing another is addressed by the pathway of the lumbrical muscles, which originate on the powerful flexor digitorum profundus tendons but insert into the extensor tendon hood. (From Moore KL, Agur AMR. Essential Clinical Anatomy, 2nd Edition. Baltimore: Lippincott Williams & Wilkins, 2002. Figure 7.10, p. 472; Figure 7.23C, p. 457.)

The grasping muscles can be divided into two groups:

- **Hypothenar Muscles:** The **hypothenar muscles** are innervated by the **ulnar nerve.** The fifth digit is outfitted with dedicated muscles for abduction (**abductor digiti minimi**), flexion (**flexor digiti minimi**), and opposition (**opponens digiti minimi**) but, in fact, is hardly more mobile than the other fingers (see Fig. 7.64). These muscles of the hypothenar eminence provide some symmetry to the bordering of the palm of the hand, and they may assist in "cupping" the palm, or deepening the center of the palm in certain grip postures. The majority of ulnar nerve fibers that serve these muscles come from the T1 ventral ramus.

- **Thenar Muscles:** The **thenar muscles** are innervated by **median nerve.** The muscles of the thenar eminence (**abductor pollicis brevis**, **flexor pollicis brevis**, and **opponens pollicis**) are very important for proper function of the thumb, which in turn is critical to a sense of well-being. These muscles are well developed (compared to the muscles of the hypothenar eminence), and they act in concert to give your thumb as much range of motion as possible (see Fig. 7.64). The majority of median nerve fibers that serve these muscles come from the C8 ventral ramus. The nerve itself, the **recurrent branch of the median nerve,** is at risk, because it passes for a short distance just under the skin of the palm, at approximately the exact place where the hand would hit the ground when you brace for a fall. The recurrent branch of the median nerve also can be compromised in carpal tunnel syndrome. Loss of function in the thenar eminence can be very distressing to the patient, because these muscles are used for so many routine activities.

The hand includes one more important muscle that is neither a ray muscle nor an eminence muscle. Recall that the thumb does not receive an interosseous muscle for abduction or adduction. Abduction is accomplished by the dedicated abductor pollicis longus and brevis, but what about adduction? Indeed, a dedicated **adductor pollicis,** deeply embedded in the palm, pulls the thumb inward across the skin of the palm (see Fig. 7.64). This motion is not powerful in and of itself (try squeezing your thumb against the side of your hand), but it is a powerful resistor of unwanted thumb abduction, such as when you are trying to maintain a squeeze around a large object. The adductor pollicis is innervated by the ulnar nerve and is the only muscle attached to the thumb to be so innervated.

Muscles of the lower limb

The lower extremity supports the body weight in a standing posture and mobilizes the weight in motion. In many ways, the anatomic arrangement of the lower extremity parallels that of the upper extremity, but in key functional areas, the compromises that the lower extremity must make to bear weight are obvious.

The joints of the lower extremity are analogous to the joints of the upper extremity. The hip joint is analogous to the shoulder joint, except that the hip joint does not suspend freely from the trunk of the body. The bones of the hip are jointed quite securely to the trunk and to each other. Just as the shoulder joint has rotator cuff muscles that support its joint cavity, so does the hip joint. The knee joint is analogous to the elbow joint, except that it bends in the "opposite" direction. Its extension muscles, the **quadriceps femoris muscles,** also are more powerful than its flexion muscles, in part because they function to restore bipedal, or resting, posture.

Distally, the next joint is where the differences really magnify. The wrist joint and hand bones are all about mobility and flexibility; the ankle joint and foot bones are all about compromise. They must keep the body in balance as it moves, so they are much more "packed" together. The ankle joint is not intended to abduct or adduct but, rather, to keep the leg from wobbling as it powerfully flexes and extends the foot. You should think of the musculoskeletal anatomy of the lower limb in terms of how joints achieve mobility and stability.

Several upper limb muscles connect the scapula, or "girdle bone" of the limb, to the trunk skeleton. These include the rhomboids, levator scapulae, and serratus anterior muscles. The lower extremity has no such need, because the hip, or "girdle bone" of the lower limb, has joined to the sacrum of the trunk skeleton and replaced elastic muscle tissue with more rigid ligament connective tissue protecting the joint. Only one muscle, the **quadratus lumborum**, bridges the trunk skeleton to the hip bone, and its function seems to be more to close off a gap in the back of the abdomen than to maneuver the hip against the trunk.

Gluteal Muscles

The **gluteal muscles** loosely parallel the shoulder group: powerful movers of the hip joint (gluteal muscles), and a "rotator cuff" of stabilizers buried deeply beneath them. Most of them are innervated by nerves of the sacral plexus: combinations of ventral rami from adjacent spinal nerves in the sacral region of the cord.

Gluteus Maximus   You should not mistake the **gluteus maximus** (Fig. 7.66) for the bulge of the gluteal region. The "buttock" is composed of this muscle in the upper and lateral part and a fat pad in the lower and medial part. This muscle is recruited primarily when you need to extend the limb from a very flexed position, such as climbing a hill or a flight of stairs. The gluteus maximus is innervated by the **inferior gluteal nerve,** principally by its first and second sacral nerve components. It has an interesting attachment, in the sense that in addition to an expected insertion on bone (the **femur**), it also inserts on the deep fascia of the side of the thigh (**fascia lata**). When it contracts, it tightens this deep fascia strap all the way down to the tibia, providing a virtual plank of stability parallel to the femur during motion. (See Table 7.15.)

Gluteus Medius and Gluteus Minimus   The **gluteus medius** and **gluteus minimus** maintain balance when you stride. Striding is "second nature" to most people because of the efficiency with which these muscles keep your body "in line" as you move. You must balance the body on one limb only during striding, and this inclines (literally) the body to fall toward the unsupported side. The gluteus medius and gluteus minimus wrench the upper body over the hip joint on the side of the foot making contact or, at the least, resist the tendency of the body to follow gravity. **Failure of the gluteus minimus, gluteus medius, or both to maintain an erect trunk posture during unipedal stance results in a positive Trendelenburg sign, or Trendelenburg gait, when bipedal. This suggests a lesion in the superior gluteal nerve, particularly of the L5 spinal nerve** (see Fig. 7.66B). The gluteus medius is a preferred site of intramuscular injection to avoid hitting the large sciatic nerve, which travels just deep to the middle of the gluteus maximus muscle.

The next set of muscles constitutes an unofficial "rotator cuff" of the hip. They insert side by side along the greater trochanter of the femur, and they mostly resist overrotation of the femur. Each of them is capable, technically, of an independent action, but they probably act in concert as elastic ligaments as much as they act in voluntary control of movement.

Piriformis   The **piriformis** must pass through the greater sciatic notch to reach the femur. The surface anatomy of the piriformis is important to recognize, because several nerves and vessels lie in relation to it. The piriformis runs a course approximately

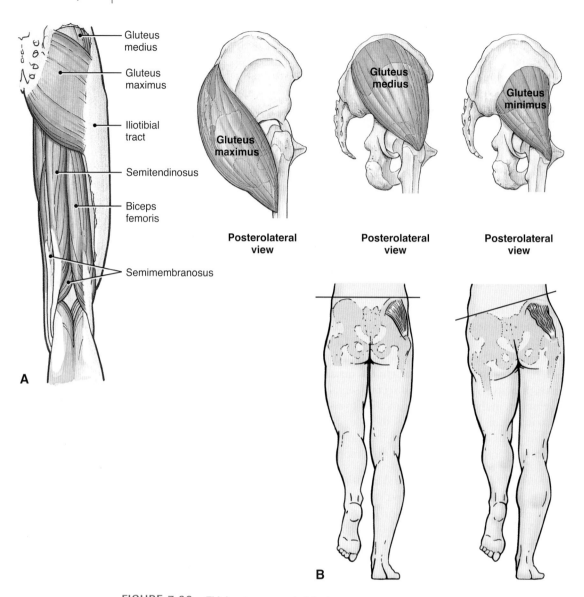

Gluteus medius

Gluteus maximus

Iliotibial tract

Semitendinosus

Biceps femoris

Semimembranosus

A

Gluteus maximus

Posterolateral view

Gluteus medius

Posterolateral view

Gluteus minimus

Posterolateral view

B

FIGURE 7.66   **Thigh extensors and abductors.**

The gluteal muscles, from superficial to deep, are shown (**A**). The large gluteus maximus muscle is most effective when the lower limb is already flexed and needs to be extended, such as when climbing a flight of stairs. The gluteus medius is a powerful hip abductor. It balances the trunk during striding against the pull of gravity toward the side that is not stepping on the ground. Damage to the superior gluteal nerve (particularly the L5 component) causes the trunk to "collapse" toward the unsupported side of the body. This is a positive Trendelenburg sign, or gait (**B**). The hamstring muscles (**A**) flex the leg and include the biceps femoris laterally and the semitendinosus and semimembranosus medially. (From Agur A, Dalley AF. Grant's Atlas of Anatomy, 11th Edition. Baltimore: Lippincott Williams & Wilkins, 2005. Figures 5.5 and 5.4, pp. 368–369; from Moore KL, Agur AMR. Essential Clinical Anatomy, 2nd Edition. Baltimore: Lippincott Williams & Wilkins, 2002.)

TABLE 7.15 MUSCLES OF THE GLUTEAL REGION

MUSCLE	ORIGIN	INSERTION	INNERVATION	ACTION
Gluteus maximus	Ilium, sacrum, and sacrotuberous ligament	Shaft of the femur and fascia of the iliotibial band	Inferior gluteal nerve (L5-S2)	Extends hip joint by pulling femur backward, tightens iliotibial band to stabilize hip and knee joints
Gluteus medius	Ilium	Greater trochanter of femur	Superior gluteal nerve (L5-S1)	Abducts femur and aids in external rotation of the hip; with gluteus minimus, it supports the trunk in unipedal posture
Gluteus minimus	Ilium, below gluteus medius	Greater trochanter of femur and hip joint capsule	Superior gluteal nerve (L5-S1)	Abducts femur and (somewhat) medially rotates hip; with gluteus medius, it supports the trunk in unipedal posture
Piriformis	Ventral surface of sacrum	Greater trochanter of femur	Nerve to piriformis (L5-S2)	Externally rotates femur
Obturator internus	Inside margin of obturator foramen	Greater trochanter of femur	Nerve to obturator internus (L5-S2)	Externally rotates femur, abducts femur when it is flexed
Gemellus superior	Ischial spine	Greater trochanter of femur	Nerve to obturator internus (L5-S2)	Externally rotates femur, and abducts femur when it is flexed
Gemellus inferior	Ischial tuberosity	Greater trochanter of femur	Nerve to quadratus femoris and inferior gemellus (L4-S1)	Externally rotates femur, abducts femur when it is flexed
Quadratus femoris	Ischial tuberosity	Crest between greater and lesser trochanter of femur	Nerve to quadratus femoris and inferior gemellus (L4-S1)	Externally rotates femur, adducts femur
Obturator externus	External margins of obturator foramen	Trochanteric fossa of femur	Obturator nerve (L2-4)	Externally rotates femur, adducts femur
Tensor fascia lata	Iliac crest	Iliotibial band of fascia	Superior gluteal nerve (L4-S1)	Tenses iliotibial band to stabilize hip and knee joint

between three palpable points: the posterior superior iliac spine, the tip of the coccyx, and the top of the greater trochanter of the femur (Fig. 7.67). **Piriformis syndrome** is a troublesome condition in which spasm of the muscle appears to irritate the neighboring sciatic nerve, with the result of radiating pain and tingling down the leg. Given the deeply embedded position of the piriformis, surgical release of the muscle is quite invasive.

Obturator Internus   The **obturator internus** (*obturator* is from the Latin for "to occlude") originates around the inner ring of the obturator foramen. As its name implies, this muscle, rather than traveling through this gargantuan foramen, instead occludes it and passes around the lesser sciatic notch to reach the femur. It must make a 90° turn at this point, so its leverage is limited. Shorter, twinned muscles on either side of its tendon (the **gemellus superior** and the **gemellus inferior**) develop to assist its leverage as a lateral rotator (see Fig. 7.67).

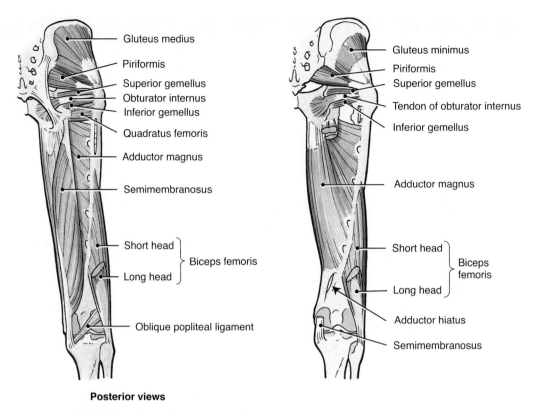

Posterior views

FIGURE 7.67   **Hip rotators.**

The posterior buttock houses a battery of external, or lateral, hip rotators. (**A**) Posterior view, superficial. The obturator internus muscle is assisted by parallel gemellus muscles. (**B**) The gluteus minimus, which is deep to the gluteus maximus, completes the arc of rotators superiorly. Its anteriormost fibers may enable it to medially rotate the hip. (From Agur A, Dalley AF. Grant's Atlas of Anatomy, 11th Edition. Baltimore: Lippincott Williams & Wilkins, 2005. Figure 5.5, p. 369.)

Quadratus Femoris   The "rotator cuff" muscles of the hip joint form an arc and exist more or less in one functional plane. The next muscle in this arc, inferiorly speaking, is **quadratus femoris**. Just like the lower rotator muscles of the shoulder joint, this muscle also can adduct the long bone to which it attaches.

Obturator Externus   The **obturator externus** lies deep to the gemelli layer, between the inferior gemellus and the quadratus femoris. It is the only muscle of the gluteal region that is innervated by a lumbar plexus nerve. It is the most deeply embedded muscle of the hip joint region.

Tensor Fascia Lata   The very existence of the **tensor fascia lata** (see Fig. 7.69) testifies to the specialized nature of the human lower limb. As its name implies, this muscle grows inside a fascial sleeve and inserts onto a specialized thickening of the deep fascia on the lateral side of the thigh. By tensing this fascia, the soft tissue of the limb cylinder "hardens" as much as possible to stiffen the side wall of the strut as you stride. The tensor fascia lata is assisted by the gluteus maximus (see above), which also inserts on the fascia lata.

Hip Flexors and Knee Extensors
The anterior region of the thigh includes some deep muscles that originate up in the trunk, as well as more superficial muscles such as the powerful quadriceps femoris. (See Table 7.16.)

Iliacus and Psoas Major   The **iliacus** and **psoas major** (Fig. 7.68) share a joint insertion on the lesser trochanter of the femur; other than that, they are an unlikely partnership. The bulky psoas major attaches in a step-like fashion to the sides of the lumbar vertebrae and strikes a visible angle of repose in the background of a standard abdominal radiograph. The iliacus is a flat muscle that occupies the iliac fossa before its fibers converge with the psoas major to cross over the pubic ramus and under the inguinal ligament. These muscles are internal "sit-up" muscles: powerful flexors of the hip when the leg is stationary, or powerful elevators of the thigh when the trunk is stationary. A small **psoas minor** muscle may be present (50–60% of individuals). This weak muscle originates from the sides of the T12 and L1 vertebrae, becoming tendinous almost immediately. The tendon travels along the ventral surface of the psoas major to insert on the **iliopubic eminence** of the pelvic brim.

TABLE 7.16   MUSCLES OF THE ANTERIOR THIGH

MUSCLE	ORIGIN	INSERTION	INNERVATION	ACTION
Iliacus	Iliac fossa	With psoas major on lesser trochanter of femur	Lumbar plexus and femoral nerve (L2-4)	Flexes the femur when the trunk is fixed, or flexes the trunk when the limb is fixed
Psoas major	Transverse processes and discs of T12-L5	With iliacus on lesser trochanter of femur	Lumbar plexus and femoral nerve (L2-L4)	Flexes the femur when the trunk is fixed, or flexes the trunk when the limb is fixed
Sartorius	Anterior superior iliac spine ("A-S-I-S")	Medial shaft of proximal tibia	Femoral nerve (L2-L4)	"Spins" your shin up toward the opposite knee, as when you sit with your ankle crossed on your knee—the hip is rotated, and the hip and leg are weakly flexed
Rectus femoris	One head on anterior inferior iliac spine, 1 head on ilium and hip joint capsule	Tibial tuberosity through the patellar ligament	Femoral nerve (L2-L4)	Flexes hip joint and extends leg
Vastus lateralis	Shaft of femur and lateral intermuscular septum	Tibial tuberosity through the patellar ligament	Femoral nerve (L2-L4)	Extends leg
Vastus medialis	Shaft of femur and lateral intermuscular septum	Tibial tuberosity through the patellar ligament	Femoral nerve (L2-L4)	Extends leg
Vastus intermedius	Shaft of femur and lateral intermuscular septum	Tibial tuberosity through the patellar ligament	Femoral nerve (L2-L4)	Extends leg
Articularis genu	Lower part of shaft of femur	Suprapatellar bursa of knee joint	Femoral nerve (L2-L4)	Retracts synovial membrane so that it stays between the patella and femur

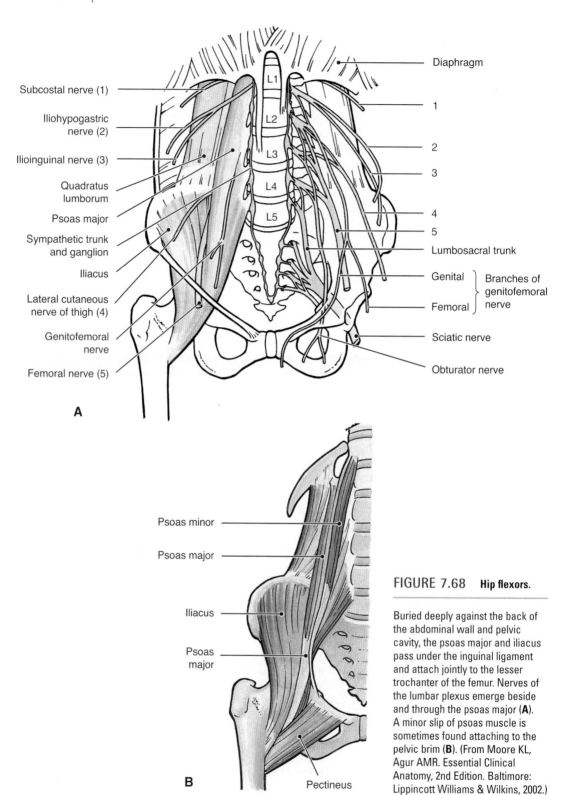

Subcostal nerve (1)

Iliohypogastric
nerve (2)

Ilioinguinal nerve (3)

Quadratus
lumborum

Psoas major

Sympathetic trunk
and ganglion

Iliacus

Lateral cutaneous
nerve of thigh (4)

Genitofemoral
nerve

Femoral nerve (5)

Diaphragm

1

2

3

4

5

Lumbosacral trunk

Genital ⎱ Branches of
         ⎰ genitofemoral
Femoral   nerve

Sciatic nerve

Obturator nerve

L1
L2
L3
L4
L5

A

Psoas minor

Psoas major

Iliacus

Psoas
major

B   Pectineus

FIGURE 7.68   Hip flexors.

Buried deeply against the back of
the abdominal wall and pelvic
cavity, the psoas major and iliacus
pass under the inguinal ligament
and attach jointly to the lesser
trochanter of the femur. Nerves of
the lumbar plexus emerge beside
and through the psoas major (**A**).
A minor slip of psoas muscle is
sometimes found attaching to the
pelvic brim (**B**). (From Moore KL,
Agur AMR. Essential Clinical
Anatomy, 2nd Edition. Baltimore:
Lippincott Williams & Wilkins, 2002.)

Sartorius   The **sartorius** (Fig. 7.69) crosses both the hip joint and the knee joint, but its slim caliber and sinuous path suggest that it is a tether as much as a contractor. This elegant muscle inserts with a muscle from the medial compartment (the **gracilis**) and a muscle from the posterior compartment (the **semitendinosus**) to form a fan-like attachment to the tibia that looks like a goosefoot. The combined insertion is called, therefore, the **pes anserinus.** Together, these muscles probably help to keep the knee and trunk from deviating too far in any one direction.

Rectus Femoris   The **rectus femoris** is one of the four quadriceps femoris muscles, which join together through the patella to powerfully extend the tibia. The quadriceps muscles are innervated by the **femoral nerve**; of the four, the rectus femoris is the only one that also crosses the hip joint. The other three arise from the femur itself and are called the **vasti muscles,** or **vastus group muscles.**

Vastus Lateralis, Vastus Medialis, and Vastus Intermedius   The robust vastus lateralis, vastus medialis, and vastus intermedius have a single mission—to extend the knee. As with most movements of the lower limb, however, the distal attachment typically is the fixed attachment—that is, the movement is actually of the body above the

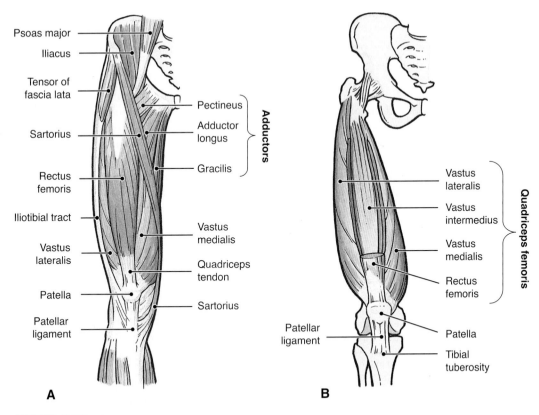

FIGURE 7.69   Leg extensors.

The powerful quadriceps muscle group blankets the anterior thigh (**A**). The rectus femoris crosses both the hip joint and the knee joint, whereas the vasti muscles (**B**) cross only the knee joint. (From Moore KL, Agur AMR. Essential Clinical Anatomy, 2nd Edition. Baltimore: Lippincott Williams & Wilkins, 2002. Figure 6.9B,C, p. 334.)

joint as the foot stays fixed on the ground. In this sense, then, these muscles actually extend the body over the knee. Therefore, although they are fully capable of extending the knee joint and kicking the foot forward, their real power is that of elevating the rest of the body above the knee joint, such as during sprinting or stair-climbing.

Articularis Genu   Because the knee joint withstands so much stress and muscle force, it is more elaborate than any other synovial joint in the body (see above). One of the most unusual anatomies of the knee joint is the **articularis genu**. This muscle attaches to a synovial membrane, which is one of the softest tissues in the body, and its job is to keep the membrane of the knee joint from getting pinched under the pressure of the patella when the knee is tightly flexed.

Hip Adductors

The **hip adductors** (Fig. 7.70) maintain balance and alignment but are not worked powerfully or repetitively to the same degree as other muscles are; therefore, they seem less defined on the surface of the thigh. This reflects the efficiency of the bony strut for maintaining posture with a minimum of muscle exertion. The hip adductors originate from the loop of pelvis bone that rims the obturator foramen, and they insert in broader fans along the shaft of the femur (and, in one case, the tibia). They are innervated by the **obturator nerve**, which, like the femoral nerve, is composed of spinal nerve segments L2-L4. (See Table 7.17.)

Pectineus   The **pectineus** forms the floor of the femoral triangle, at the front of the thigh, where the femoral neurovascular bundle is vulnerable.

Adductor Longus, Adductor Brevis, and Adductor Magnus   The adductor group—the **adductor longus**, the **adductor brevis**, and the **adductor magnus**—forms a more or less continuous sheet that tethers the femur toward the midline. Fibers of the adductor magnus that reach the lowest attachment are called the **hamstring fibers**. These fibers actually pull away from the bulk of the muscle belly to form a tight cord of tendon that inserts on a bump on the epicondyle of the femur. The separation forms a natural archway through the muscle (the **adductor hiatus**), and the femoral artery takes advantage of it to reach around the knee joint posteriorly.

FIGURE 7.70   Thigh adductors.

The medial compartment musculature attaches the pubis and ischium to the femur along virtually its entire shaft. The gracilis crosses the knee joint to join semitendinosus of the posterior compartment and sartorius of the anterior compartment along the medial tibia. (From Agur A, Dalley AF. Grant's Atlas of Anatomy, 11th Edition. Baltimore: Lippincott Williams & Wilkins, 2005. Fig. 5.15B, p. 355.)

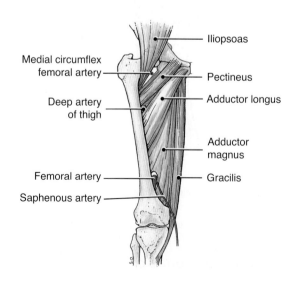

- Iliopsoas
- Medial circumflex femoral artery
- Pectineus
- Deep artery of thigh
- Adductor longus
- Adductor magnus
- Femoral artery
- Gracilis
- Saphenous artery

TABLE 7.17   MUSCLES OF THE MEDIAL THIGH

MUSCLE	ORIGIN	INSERTION	INNERVATION	ACTION
Pectineus	Superior pubic ramus	Pectineal line of the femur	Femoral nerve (L2-L3), sometimes obturator (L2-L4)	Adducts and flexes femur
Adductor longus	Body of pubis bone	Linea aspera of femur	Obturator nerve (L2-L4)	Adducts and flexes femur
Adductor brevis	Body of pubis and inferior pubic ramus	Pectineal line of femur	Obturator nerve (L2-L4)	Adducts and flexes femur
Adductor magnus	Inferior pubic ramus and ischial tuberosity	Long attachment to back of shaft of femur, from gluteal tuberosity to adductor tubercle	Obturator nerve (L2-L4), fibers to adductor tubercle by tibial part of sciatic nerve (L4-S3)	Adducts femur
Gracilis	Pubis and ischiopubic ramus	Medial shaft of proximal tibia	Obturator nerve (L2-L4)	Adducts femur and medially rotates the knee joint

Gracilis   The **gracilis** is the medial compartment muscle that joins the sartorius to form the pes anserinus insertion on the tibia. As its name implies, it is a long and delicate muscle—a true strap muscle.

Hip Extensors and Knee Flexors

The **hip extensors** and **knee flexors** are the familiar **hamstring muscles**. (See Table 7.18.) They commence the long list of muscles in the posterior compartment of the lower extremity that are served by the sciatic nerve bundle, which takes fibers from L4-S3 of the spinal cord all the way to the tips of the toes (as the **tibial nerve** and **fibular nerve**). The hamstring muscles are much less powerful than the quadriceps muscles, a ratio of "front-to-back" power that reverses below the knee. The lower extremity joints alternate in flexion–extension range of motion relative to standing posture, so the girth of muscle mass across the joint corresponds.

TABLE 7.18   MUSCLES OF THE POSTERIOR THIGH

MUSCLE	ORIGIN	INSERTION	INNERVATION	ACTION
Biceps femoris	Long head from ischial tuberosity; short head from shaft of femur	Head of fibula nerve (L4-S3), short head by common fibular nerve (L4-S3)	Long head by tibial knee, assists in extending the hip joint	Flexes leg at the knee, assists in extending the hip joint
Semitendinosus	Ischial tuberosity	Medial shaft of proximal tibia	Tibial nerve (L4-S3)	Flexes leg at the knee, assists in extending the hip joint
Semimembranosus	Ischial tuberosity	Medial condyle of tibia	Tibial nerve (L4-S3)	Flexes leg at the knee, assists in extending the hip joint

Biceps Femoris, Semitendinosus, and Semimembranosus   The **biceps femoris** is the lateral hamstring muscle (see Figs. 7.66A and 7.67). One head attaches to the ischial part of the hip bone, and one head derives entirely from the femur. After merging, the muscle crosses the knee joint and attaches to the head of the fibula. The long head, or the ischial attachment, is motored by the tibial part of the sciatic nerve bundle. The short head, or the femoral attachment, is motored by the fibular part.

The **semitendinosus** is the posterior compartment muscle that completes the pes anserinus (see Fig. 7.66A). Together with the gracilis and the sartorius, the semitendinosus tethers the hip to the inner part of the knee, much like an upside-down telephone pole. The three muscles anchor the hip joint to the center of gravity. None of them is powerful individually, but acting as a team, they can register unstable tipping in any direction to the brain and offer some resistance in response.

The fascia of the **semimembranosus** expands near its attachment to the tibia. It is so close to the knee joint that it contributes thickened fibers to it in the form of an **oblique popliteal ligament**. Together, the semimembranosus and semitendinosus form the medial half of the hamstring group. The hamstring muscles have a tendency to "pull," or strain, or even outright rupture, from their moorings on the ischium, because they are somewhat hyperextended in a fully erect posture. When sprinters, for example, thrust their coiled limb into a burst of forward motion, the rapid and full extension of the thigh can be too much strain too fast for the hamstrings.

Muscles of the leg

Just as the thigh has three muscle compartments, so, too, does the leg. In this case, however, the muscle mass is biased toward the posterior compartment because of the force that is needed to lift the heel off the ground (**plantarflexion**). The other two compartments are the anterior compartment, for flexing the ankle the other way (**dorsiflexion**), and the minor lateral compartment.

Plantarflexors and Invertors of the Foot (Posterior Compartment)
The **gastrocnemius** and **soleus** in the posterior compartment drive the ankle but not the foot (Fig. 7.71). These muscles become the powerful **Achilles tendon** leading to the heel. Deep to them are three powerful muscles that use the ankle as a fulcrum and drive plantarflexion of the foot and toes. Because the heel is like the elbow, in the sense that tendons cannot cross the very back of it, these deep tendons reach the sole of the foot by passing along the medial side of the ankle joint underneath a tough flexor retinaculum. A small muscle dedicated to the knee joint completes the array. All muscles of the this compartment are innervated by the **tibial nerve**. (See Table 7.19.)

Popliteus   The **popliteus** actually penetrates the knee joint capsule to unlock a tight bone-to-bone alignment of the femur and tibia when the knee is fully extended. Its base attachment within the knee joint capsule is on the lateral femoral condyle and lateral meniscus of the knee joint. Its base attachment on the tibia is below and outside of the joint capsule. When this muscle contracts, it flexes and medially rotates the knee joint by spinning the femur and the tibia in opposite directions. With the femur and tibia "unlocked" from their fit, the large hamstring muscles can exert leverage to continue flexing the knee.

Gastrocnemius and Soleus   The **gastrocnemius** and **soleus** are similar to the biceps brachii and brachialis, respectively. Gastrocnemius crosses two joints; soleus crosses only one. The real joint of movement, however, is the distal one, the ankle

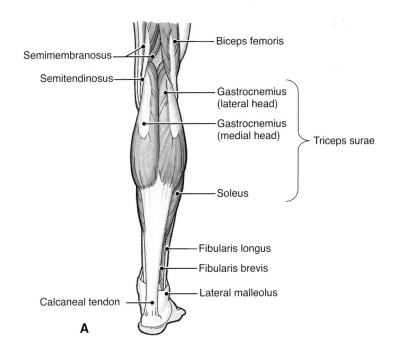

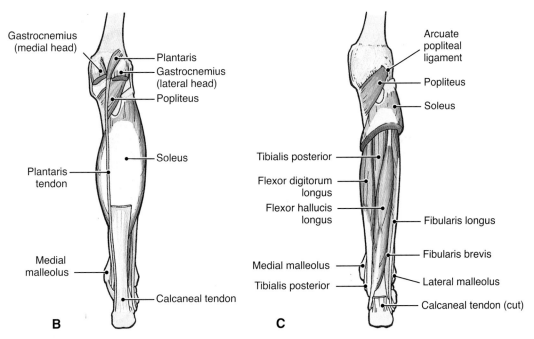

FIGURE 7.71   **Ankle, foot, and toe flexors.**

(**A**) Superficial calf muscles. (**B**) Intermediate calf. The soleus joins the gastrocnemius to form the powerful calcaneal tendon (Achilles tendon). (**C**) Deep layer of the posterior compartment. Because of a weight-bearing heel, each of these muscles must cross the side of the ankle rather than the center of the limb. (From Moore KL, Agur AMR. Essential Clinical Anatomy, 2nd Edition. Baltimore: Lippincott Williams & Wilkins, 2002. Figure 6.23B–D, p. 366.)

TABLE 7.19　MUSCLES OF THE LEG

MUSCLE	ORIGIN	INSERTION	INNERVATION	ACTION
Popliteus	Shaft of tibia above the soleal line	Lateral femoral condyle and lateral meniscus of knee joint	Tibial nerve (L4-S3)	Flexes and rotates the femur against the tibia as you "unlock" the knee joint
Gastrocnemius	One head from each femoral condyle	As the calcaneal tendon (with soleus) onto the calcaneus	Tibial nerve (L4-S3)	Plantarflexes the ankle joint, assists in flexing the knee joint
Soleus	Shaft of tibia and fibula deep to gastrocnemius	As the calcaneal tendon (with gastrocnemius) onto calcaneus	Tibial nerve (L4-S3)	Plantarflexes the ankle joint
Posterior compartment				
Tibialis posterior	Tibia, fibula, and interosseous membrane	Several foot bones - navicular; medial and intermediate cuneiform; bases of second, third, fourth metatarsal	Tibial nerve (L4-S3)	Inverts and plantarflexes the foot
Flexor digitorum longus	Tibia	Distal phalanges of the 4 lesser toes	Tibial nerve (L4-S3)	Plantarflexes the ankle joint, flexes all joints of the toes
Flexor hallucis longus	Interosseous membrane and fibula	Distal phalanx of the first toe	Tibial nerve (L4-S3)	Plantarflexes the ankle joint, flexes the first toe
Lateral compartment				
Fibularis longus	Fibula	Medial cuneiform and first metatarsal	Superficial fibular nerve (L4-S3)	Plantarflexes ankle joint, everts the foot
Fibularis brevis	Fibula and intermuscular septum	Tuberosity of fifth metatarsal	Superficial fibular nerve (L4-S3)	Plantarflexes ankle joint, everts the foot
Anterior compartment				
Tibialis anterior	Tibia	Medial cuneiform and first metatarsal	Deep fibular nerve (L4-S3)	Dorsiflexes ankle joint, inverts the foot
Extensor hallucis longus	Interosseous membrane and fibula	Distal phalanx of first toe	Deep fibular nerve (L4-S3)	Dorsiflexes ankle joint, extends the first toe
Extensor digitorum longus	Tibia, fibula, interosseous membrane and intermuscular septum	Intermediate and distal phalanges of the 4 lesser toes	Deep fibular nerve (L4-S3)	Dorsiflexes ankle joint, extends the lesser toes
Fibularis tertius	Fibula	Base of fifth metatarsal	Deep fibular nerve (L4-S3)	Assists dorsiflexion and eversion of the foot

joint. These two powerful muscles elevate the calcaneus, or plantarflex the foot. Because in resting posture the foot is more dorsiflexed than it is plantarflexed, the range of motion called plantarflexion is considerable.

Plantaris   The **plantaris** has a very small belly and an extremely long, stringy tendon, not unlike the palmaris longus in the upper limb. Variations include both absence and duplication of the muscle. It originates on the lateral femoral condyle, and it inserts beside the calcaneal tendon on the calcaneus. Given its weak proportion compared to neighboring muscles, its action probably is moot. At one time, it might have had a role in maintaining fascial tension in the skin of the sole of the foot (again analogous to palmaris longus), but given the fully bipedal human foot, that effort is moot.

Tibialis Posterior, Flexor Digitorum Longus, and Flexor Hallucis Longus
A trio of deeper muscles in the posterior leg—**tibialis posterior, flexor digitorum longus,** and **flexor hallucis longus**—assists with plantarflexion; they primarily invert the foot (tibialis posterior) or drive the toes (flexor digitorum longus and flexor hallucis longus). As with the ray muscles of the hand, two sets of digital flexors are available. In the foot, the flexor digitorum longus tendons are the ones that reach across all toe joints to insert on the distal phalanges. Also as in the hand, one digit enjoys a separate, dedicated muscle assemblage—the big toe, or **hallux**.

The flexor hallucis longus is very important for a sense of well-being, because this muscle is used to "toe-off" at the end of the stride. A disproportionate amount of power during the final phase of striding resides in the big toe, so without good joint alignment and full use of flexor hallucis longus, it is difficult—if not impossible—to stride comfortably. The flexor hallucis longus is the dominant muscle of our sense of foot position and leverage.

Foot Dorsiflexors
The muscles that dorsiflex the foot are found in the anterior compartment of the leg, just lateral to the sharp medial border of the tibial shaft. (See Table 7.19.) Some of these muscles also invert the foot and extend the toes. Dorsiflexion and toe extension are not powerful movements, but they are essential for maintaining a smooth gait. Excessive dorsiflexion, such as when running in ill-fitting shoes, results in painful "shin-splints." The nerve of this compartment is the other branch of the common fibular nerve, the deep fibular. Injury to this nerve debilitates the only muscles that are capable of dorsiflexion, which means that a patient's foot will "drop" as he or she raises the leg with each stride.

The **tibialis anterior** (Fig. 7.72) complements the **tibilias posterior** as a primary actor on the ankle joint. They share inversion capability, but they oppose each other in flexion. The **extensor hallucis longus** likewise complements a muscle of the posterior compartment, the **flexor hallucis longus**. Its tendon projects prominently against the skin when the big toe is extended. The **extensor digitorum longus** manages the lesser toes from one base muscle belly in the leg. Its tendons extend across the final interphalangeal joint to insert just behind the nail beds. As its name implies, there is a distinct **extensor digitorum brevis**, unlike the configuration in the back of the hand. The extensor digitorum brevis is the only muscle arising in the dorsum of the foot. The **fibularis tertius** is a muscle slip, sometimes absent, that looks like a mutant extra belly of extensor digitorum longus and inserts at the base of the fifth metatarsal (Fig. 7.73).

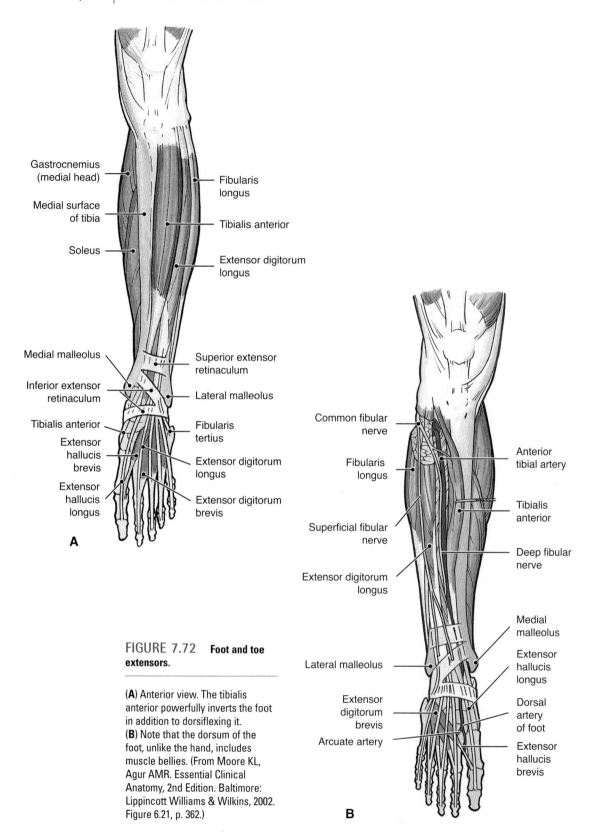

Gastrocnemius (medial head)

Medial surface of tibia

Soleus

Fibularis longus

Tibialis anterior

Extensor digitorum longus

Medial malleolus

Inferior extensor retinaculum

Tibialis anterior

Extensor hallucis brevis

Extensor hallucis longus

Superior extensor retinaculum

Lateral malleolus

Fibularis tertius

Extensor digitorum longus

Extensor digitorum brevis

A

Common fibular nerve

Fibularis longus

Superficial fibular nerve

Extensor digitorum longus

Lateral malleolus

Extensor digitorum brevis

Arcuate artery

Anterior tibial artery

Tibialis anterior

Deep fibular nerve

Medial malleolus

Extensor hallucis longus

Dorsal artery of foot

Extensor hallucis brevis

B

FIGURE 7.72   Foot and toe extensors.

(**A**) Anterior view. The tibialis anterior powerfully inverts the foot in addition to dorsiflexing it. (**B**) Note that the dorsum of the foot, unlike the hand, includes muscle bellies. (From Moore KL, Agur AMR. Essential Clinical Anatomy, 2nd Edition. Baltimore: Lippincott Williams & Wilkins, 2002. Figure 6.21, p. 362.)

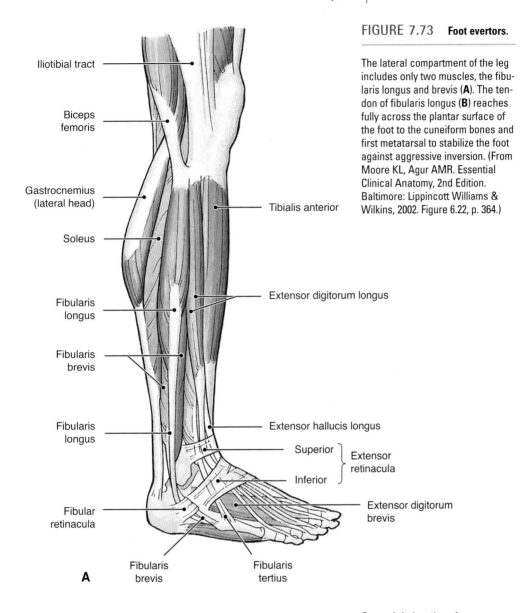

Iliotibial tract

Biceps femoris

Gastrocnemius (lateral head)

Soleus

Fibularis longus

Fibularis brevis

Fibularis longus

Fibular retinacula

Tibialis anterior

Extensor digitorum longus

Extensor hallucis longus

Superior ⎫
⎬ Extensor retinacula
Inferior ⎭

Extensor digitorum brevis

A

Fibularis brevis

Fibularis tertius

FIGURE 7.73   Foot evertors.

The lateral compartment of the leg includes only two muscles, the fibularis longus and brevis (**A**). The tendon of fibularis longus (**B**) reaches fully across the plantar surface of the foot to the cuneiform bones and first metatarsal to stabilize the foot against aggressive inversion. (From Moore KL, Agur AMR. Essential Clinical Anatomy, 2nd Edition. Baltimore: Lippincott Williams & Wilkins, 2002. Figure 6.22, p. 364.)

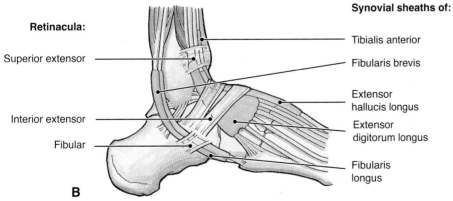

Retinacula:

Superior extensor

Interior extensor

Fibular

Synovial sheaths of:

Tibialis anterior

Fibularis brevis

Extensor hallucis longus

Extensor digitorum longus

Fibularis longus

B

Foot Evertors

The size difference between the tibia and the fibula speaks volumes. The two muscles dedicated to the fibular side of the leg help with balance, but all the power belongs to the tibia. The **fibularis longus** (see Fig. 7.73) is the primary evertor of the foot. This motion is a composite of plantarflexion and pronation and a natural culmination of taking a full stride. The fibularis longus reaches under the lateral aspect of the foot skeleton, and it attaches to the most medial bones of the plantar surface of the foot for its leverage. The **fibularis brevis** also plantarflexes and assists with eversion, but it anchors into place on the dorsal side of the foot skeleton along the prominent lateral tuberosity of the fifth metatarsal. The nerve of this compartment is the superficial branch of the common fibular nerve.

Muscles of the plantar foot

Tucked under the bony arch between the heel and the toes, the sole of the foot supports several muscles. As in the hand, there are companion pads of muscles for the little toe and big toe. Powerful short flexors, a big toe adductor, and those curious interossei muscles for spreading the toes side to side complete the similarities. All these muscles are innervated by terminal branches of the tibial nerve, called the **medial plantar nerve** and **lateral plantar nerve**. In many ways, they act to keep the toes in position by resisting counterforces rather than by acting in direct contraction. (See Table 7.20.)

The **abductor hallucis** (Fig. 7.74) is the most medial muscle in the sole of the foot. It spans the length of the medial longitudinal arch. As it crosses the metatarsophalangeal joint, it merges with the medial tendon of the **flexor hallucis brevis**. The two tendons of the flexor hallucis brevis join with the abductor hallucis medially and the adductor hallucis laterally and, in this way, pass to either side of the channel necessary for the flexor hallucis longus tendon. At this point, the joint tendons include a **sesamoid bone** that is analogous to the position of the sesamoid bones at the metacarpophalangeal joint of the thumb. The tendon of the flexor hallucis longus passes between the sesamoid bones in a kind of protective, bony house so that the crushing weight of the body travels through the sesamoids and not onto the tendon itself. Pity the patient with bunions, a condition in which this sesamoid support arch breaks down and every step can be painful. (See Clinical Anatomy Box 7.4.)

The **flexor digitorum brevis** exists only in the plantar foot, not across the ankle joint. In the upper limb, the digital flexors drive from the forearm, but in the foot, the demands of posture and locomotion mean that the flexors cannot approach the toes from straight across the calcaneus. In the muscle layer immediately deep to the flexor digitorum brevis, the tendons of the calf muscles pass forward to reach their bony attachments. The two large tendons here are the **flexor digitorum longus** and the **flexor hallucis longus**. Because these muscles pass beside the ankle joint instead of directly over the calcaneus, they enter the sole of the foot at an angle to the lesser toes. This is a problem for the tendons of the flexor digitorum longus, so an unusual **quadratus plantae muscle** develops to "align" them in the sole of the foot, parallel to the toes that they flex.

The **abductor digiti minimi** and **flexor digiti minimi brevis** constitute the pad of muscles dedicated to the fifth toe. There is no apparent analog to the opponens muscle in the hypothenar eminence of the hand. **Lumbrical muscles** analogous to those of the hand are found along the tendons of the flexor digitorum longus, just beyond

TABLE 7.20   MUSCLES OF THE FOOT

MUSCLE	ORIGIN	INSERTION	INNERVATION	ACTION
Extensor digitorum brevis	Calcaneus	Medial 3 tendons of extensor digitorum longus and on the tendon of extensor hallucis longus	Deep fibular nerve (L4–S3)	Assists dorsiflexion of metatarsopha-langeal joints
Plantar surface				
Abductor hallucis	Calcaneus	Proximal phalanx of first toe	Medial plantar nerve (L4–S3)	Abducts first toe
Flexor digitorum brevis	Calcaneus and intermuscular septum	Via 4 tendons onto middle phalanges of the 4 lesser toes	Medial plantar nerve (L4–S3)	Flexes proximal interphalangeal joint of the 4 lesser toes
Abductor digiti minimi	Calcaneus and intermuscular septum	Proximal phalanx of fifth toe	Lateral plantar nerve (L4–S3)	Abducts fifth toe
Quadratus plantae	Calcaneus	The joint tendon of flexor digitorum longus	Lateral plantar nerve (L4–S3)	Assists the tendons of flexor digitorum longus to plantarflex the lesser toes
Lumbricals	Tendons of flexor digitorum longus	Dorsal tendon hood of extensor digitorum longus	First lumbrical by medial plantar nerve; lumbricals 2–4 by lateral plantar nerve	Initiates extension of plantarflexed toes
Flexor hallucis brevis	Cuboid and lateral cuneiform	Via 2 tendons onto proximal phalanx of the first toe	Medial plantar nerve (L4–S3)	Plantarflexes the proximal joint of the first toe
Adductor hallucis	Transverse head from metatarsopha-langeal ligament and metatarsal heads of toes 2–5; oblique head from bases of metatarsals 2–4 and long plantar ligament	Proximal phalanx of first toe	Lateral plantar nerve (L4–S3)	Adducts the first toe
Flexor digiti minimi brevis	Fifth metatarsal and long plantar ligament	Proximal phalanx of fifth toe	Lateral plantar nerve (L4–S3)	Plantarflexes the fifth metatarsopha langeal joint
Plantar interossei	Medial side of metatarsals 3–5	Base of proximal phalanx of the same toe	Lateral plantar nerve (L4–S3)	Adducts the lateral 3 toes
Dorsal interossei	Base of each metatarsal	Proximal phalanx of toes 2–4	Lateral plantar nerve (L4–S3)	Abducts toes 2–4

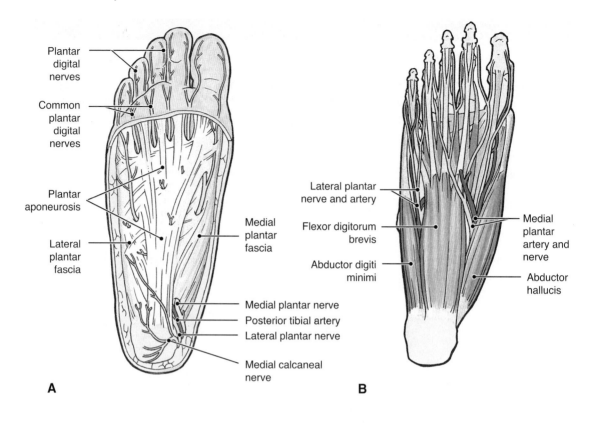

A

Plantar digital nerves

Common plantar digital nerves

Plantar aponeurosis

Lateral plantar fascia

Medial plantar fascia

Medial plantar nerve
Posterior tibial artery
Lateral plantar nerve

Medial calcaneal nerve

B

Lateral plantar nerve and artery

Flexor digitorum brevis

Abductor digiti minimi

Medial plantar artery and nerve

Abductor hallucis

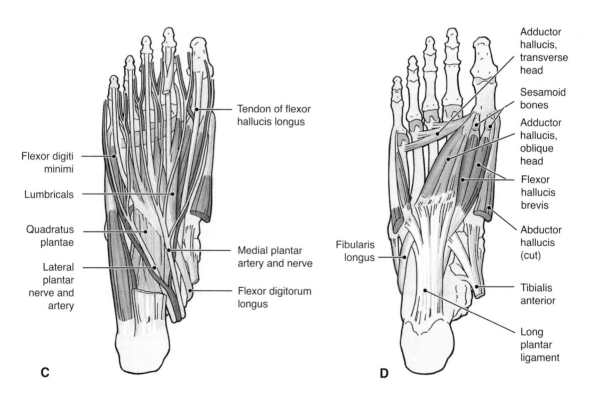

C

Flexor digiti minimi

Lumbricals

Quadratus plantae

Lateral plantar nerve and artery

Tendon of flexor hallucis longus

Medial plantar artery and nerve

Flexor digitorum longus

D

Adductor hallucis, transverse head

Sesamoid bones

Adductor hallucis, oblique head

Flexor hallucis brevis

Abductor hallucis (cut)

Fibularis longus

Tibialis anterior

Long plantar ligament

CLINICAL ANATOMY

Box 7.4
HALLUX VALGUS (BUNIONS)

The pressure exerted on the "ball" of the foot, where the heads of the metatarsals press against the skin, is tremendous. The sesamoid bones that grow in the tendons of the flexor hallucis brevis "pedestal" the first metatarsal above contact with the ground, but these can become displaced. The skew of the first metatarsophalangeal joint that results from misdirected force through these displaced sesamoids results in hallux valgus, or a **bunion**. The body's ability to adapt to stressful conditions is its own downfall here, because a bunion only aggravates over time. Because the course of the important "toe-off" muscle, the flexor hallucis longus, depends on proper alignment of the sesamoids, hallux valgus prevents normal stride and weight-bearing. The pain associated with stressful degeneration of the metatarsophalangeal joint only compounds the misery.

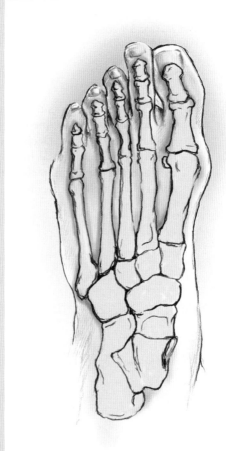

Bunions.

FIGURE 7.74   **The sole of the foot.**

(**A**) Plantar fascia. To prevent the skin of the foot from sliding, a tough plantar fascia blankets the underlying muscle bed from the calcaneus to the metatarsals. (**B**) The lesser toes receive tendons from a short flexor muscle, and both the big toe and little toe receive their own abductors. (**C**) The long flexor tendons enter the plantar muscle compartment deep to the short flexors. The angle of the flexor digitorum longus tendon is anchored to the calcaneus by the quadratus plantae muscle to effect a more direct pull on the toes. These tendons include lumbricals, as in the hand. (**D**) The powerful flexor hallucis longus tendon passes between the heads of flexor hallucis brevis and between the sesamoid bones that pedestal the ball of the foot. An adductor hallucis in this deep layer opposes the abductor hallucis, and together, these muscles help to keep the weight-bearing big toe from undue excursion. (From Moore KL, Agur AMR. Essential Clinical Anatomy, 2nd Edition. Baltimore: Lippincott Williams & Wilkins, 2002. Figure 6.27, p. 373.)

FIGURE 7.75   **Toe abductors and adductors.**

The plantar and dorsal interossei muscles adduct the toes and abduct the toes, respectively, against an axis represented by the second toe. (Adapted from Moore KL, Dalley AF. Clinically Oriented Anatomy, 5th Edition. Baltimore: Lippincott Williams & Wilkins, 2006. Figure 5.14-III, p. 661.)

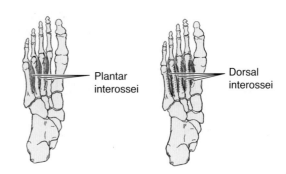

Plantar interossei

Dorsal interossei

the attachment of the tendons to the quadratus plantae. A substantial **adductor hallucis** keeps the big toe in line with the other toes; it resists the temptation of the big toe to splay out to the side. Deepest in the sole of the foot are the interossei, three **plantar interossei** and four **dorsal interossei**. As in the hand, the plantar group adducts the toes, and the dorsal group abducts the toes. In the case of the foot, however, the central axis is actually the second toe, not the third, as would be strictly analogous to the hand (Fig. 7.75).

8

Integument

INTRODUCTION

Beginning an anatomy book with the integument, or "skin," seems logical because the integument constitutes almost all of what you see when you look at the body. In truth, however, the integument is barely studied in gross anatomy courses. The vast majority of it constitutes the same structure (skin), which has fascinating tissue layers but which is taught more thoroughly in the histology curriculum. The relationship between epidermis and dermis, with the attendant specializations of hair follicles, sweat glands, and nails (Fig. 8.1), represents the interface of the embryologic dermomyotome with the overlying ectoderm layer.

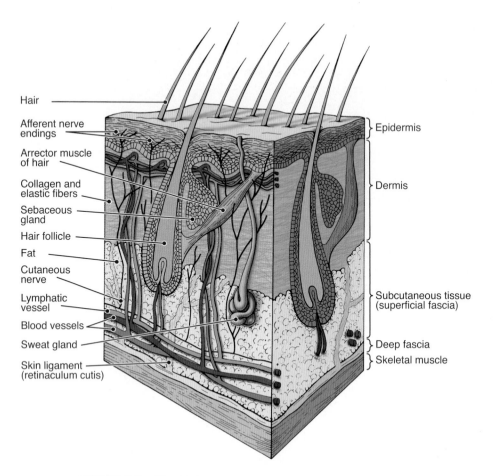

Hair

Afferent nerve
endings

Arrector muscle
of hair

Collagen and
elastic fibers

Sebaceous
gland

Hair follicle

Fat

Cutaneous
nerve

Lymphatic
vessel

Blood vessels

Sweat gland

Skin ligament
(retinaculum cutis)

Epidermis

Dermis

Subcutaneous tissue
(superficial fascia)

Deep fascia

Skeletal muscle

FIGURE 8.1   **The skin in cross-section.**

Sympathetic innervation drives erection of hair follicles, expression of sweat, and vasoconstriction. The superficial fascia varies in thickness and texture, and in parts of the body, the deep fascia layer thickens into an effective compartment border and/or attachment site for muscles. (From Moore KL, Agur AMR. Essential Clinical Anatomy, 2nd Edition. Baltimore: Lippincott Williams & Wilkins, 2002. Figure 1.3. p. 9.)

ECTODERM

Other aspects of the integument are so fascinating that they eclipse a gross anatomy course and become their own medical specialty. Tooth enamel, for example, derives from ectoderm (skin) rather than from mesoderm. In a gross anatomy course, you may be expected to learn the names and position of the teeth, but the real study belongs to dentistry, not to general medicine. Likewise, the lens of the eye, which derives from the same surface ectoderm that produces skin elsewhere, is more a focus (pardon the pun!) of ophthalmology and optometry than of medical gross anatomy.

MAMMARY GLAND

One major clinical structure is embedded in the superficial fascia of the skin—the **mammary gland**. This gland is a modified sweat gland derived from ectoderm (Fig. 8.2). Because of the prevalence of cancerous tissue growth in this gland, its blood supply and lymphatic drainage must be well understood (Fig. 8.3). The breast is richly supplied from four arterial sources:

- **Internal thoracic artery** (also known as the internal mammary artery)
- **Lateral thoracic artery**
- **Thoracoacromial trunk** (via the pectoral branches)
- **Anterior intercostal artery** and **posterior intercostal artery**

The prevalence of breast cancer mandates that you learn the lymphatic drainage of the breast, which is mapped opportunistically away from four "quadrant areas" (Fig. 8.4). The axillary pathway is primary, at least in the sense that lymph nodes at this location are called sentinel nodes, because the spread of cancer away from the gland tissue via the lymphatic channels can be detected here either clinically or through self-examination.

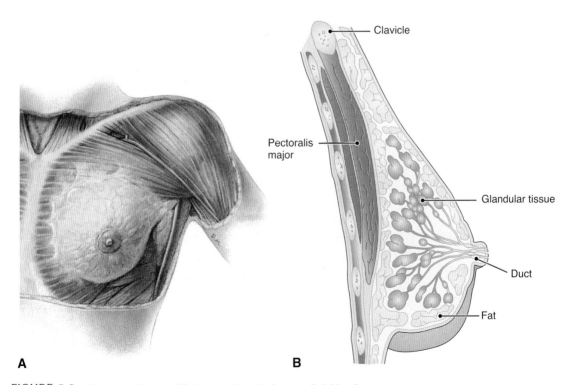

A   **B**

FIGURE 8.2   **The breast is a modified sweat gland in the superficial fascia.**

(**A**) Anterior view. (**B**) Lateral view sagittal section showing mammary gland tissue suspended in the proliferation of superficial fascia. (From Agur A, Dalley AF. Grant's Atlas of Anatomy, 11th Edition. Baltimore: Lippincott Williams & Wilkins, 2005; from Bickley LS, Szilagyi P. Bates' Guide to Physical Examination and History Taking, 8th Edition. Philadelphia: Lippincott Williams & Wilkins, 2003.)

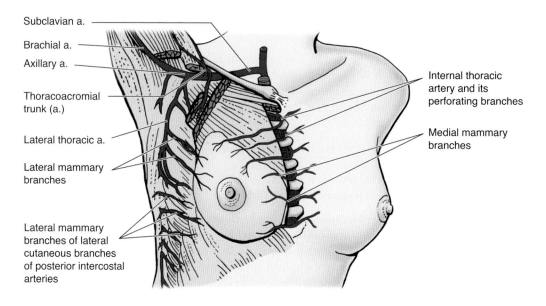

Subclavian a.

Brachial a.

Axillary a.

Thoracoacromial trunk (a.)

Lateral thoracic a.

Lateral mammary branches

Lateral mammary branches of lateral cutaneous branches of posterior intercostal arteries

Internal thoracic artery and its perforating branches

Medial mammary branches

FIGURE 8.3   **Arterial supply to the breast.**

a. = artery. (From Moore KL, Dalley AF. Clinically Oriented Anatomy, 5th Edition. Baltimore: Lippincott Williams & Wilkins, 2006. Figure 1.21A, p. 107.)

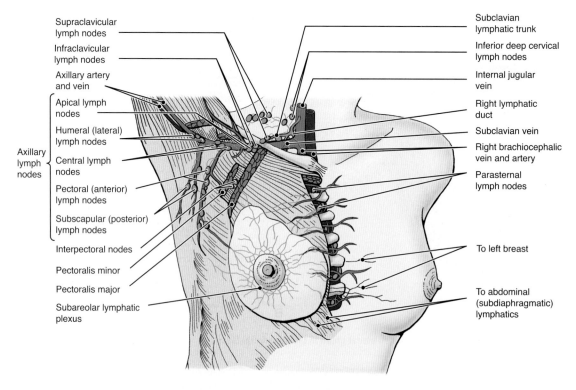

Supraclavicular lymph nodes

Infraclavicular lymph nodes

Axillary artery and vein

Apical lymph nodes

Humeral (lateral) lymph nodes

Central lymph nodes

Pectoral (anterior) lymph nodes

Subscapular (posterior) lymph nodes

Interpectoral nodes

Pectoralis minor

Pectoralis major

Subareolar lymphatic plexus

Axillary lymph nodes

Subclavian lymphatic trunk

Inferior deep cervical lymph nodes

Internal jugular vein

Right lymphatic duct

Subclavian vein

Right brachiocephalic vein and artery

Parasternal lymph nodes

To left breast

To abdominal (subdiaphragmatic) lymphatics

FIGURE 8.4   **Lymphatic drainage of the breast.**

Cancerous tissue that metastasizes from the breast follows lymphatic routes. (From Moore KL, Dalley AF. Clinically Oriented Anatomy, 5th Edition. Baltimore: Lippincott Williams & Wilkins, 2006. Figure 1.22A, p. 108.)

Index